W9-ACF-552

Student Learning Guide to accompany

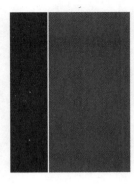

Basic Pharmacology for Nurses

Thirteenth Edition

Bruce D. Clayton, BS, RPh, Pharm D

Professor of Pharmacy Practice
College of Pharmacy & Health Sciences
Butler University
Indianapolis, Indiana

Yvonne N. Stock, MS, BSN, RN

Professor of Nursing
Health Occupations Department
Iowa Western Community College
Council Bluffs, Iowa

Mosby
An Affiliate of Elsevier

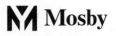
Mosby

An Affiliate of Elsevier
11830 Westline Industrial Drive
St. Louis, Missouri 63146

© 2004, 2001, 1997 Mosby, Inc. All rights reserved.

No part of this publication may be reproduced or transmitted in any form or by any means, electronic or mechanical, including photocopy, recording, or any information storage and retrieval system, without permission in writing from the publisher, except for the printing of complete pages, with the copyright notice, for instructional use and not for resale.

Permissions may be sought directly from Elsevier Inc. Rights Department in Philadelphia, Pennsylvania USA: telephone: (+1)215-238-7869, fax: (+1)215-238-2239, e-mail: healthpermissions@elsevier.com. You may also complete your request on-line via the Elsevier Science homepage http://www.elsevier.com, by selecting "Customer Support" and then "Obtaining Permissions."

Notice

Pharmacology is an ever-changing field. Standard safety precautions must be followed but as new research and clinical experience broaden our knowledge, changes in treatment and drug therapy may become necessary or appropriate. Readers are advised to check the most current product information provided by the manufacturer of each drug to be administered to verify the recommended dose, the method and duration of administration, and contraindications. It is the responsibility of the treating physician, relying on experience and knowledge of the patient, to determine dosages and the best treatment for each individual patient. Neither the Publisher nor the author assumes any liability for any injury and/or damage to persons or property arising from this publication.

The Publisher

Vice President, Publishing Director: Sally Schrefer
Managing Editor: Lee Henderson
Developmental Editor: Celia Cruz
Project Manager: Gayle May

Printed in USA.
International Standard Book Number 0-323-02360-6

04 05 06 07 08   6 5 4 3 2

To the Student

This study guide was created to assist you in achieving the objectives of each chapter in *Basic Pharmacology for Nurses, Thirteenth Edition*, and establishing a solid base of knowledge in nursing pharmacology. Completing the exercises in each chapter in this guide will help to reinforce the material studied in the textbook and learned in class. Such reinforcement also helps students to be successful on the NCLEX-PN.

STUDY HINTS FOR ALL STUDENTS

Ask Questions!

There are no stupid questions. If you do not know something or are not sure, you need to find out. Other people may be wondering the same thing but may be too shy to ask. The answer could mean life or death to your patient. That is certainly more important than feeling embarrassed about asking a question.

Chapter Objectives

At the beginning of each chapter in the textbook are objectives that you should have mastered when you finish studying that chapter. Write these objectives in your notebook, leaving a blank space after each. Fill in the answers as you find them while reading the chapter. Review to make sure your answers are correct and complete. Use these answers when you study for tests. This should also be done for separate course objectives that your instructor has listed in your class syllabus.

Key Terms

At the beginning of each chapter in the textbook are key terms that you will encounter as you read the chapter. The key terms are in color the first time they appear in the chapter. Phonetic pronunciations are provided for terms that students might find difficult to pronounce. The terms that were assigned simple phonetic pronunciations were selected because they are either (1) difficult medical, nursing, or scientific terms or (2) other words that may be difficult for students to pronounce. The goal is to help the student reader with limited proficiency in English to develop a greater command of the pronunciation of scientific and nonscientific English

terminology. It is hoped that a more general competency in the understanding and use of medical and scientific language may result.

Key Points

Use the Key Points at the end of each chapter in the textbook to help with review for exams.

Reading Hints

When reading each chapter in the textbook, look at the subject headings to learn what each section is about. Read first for the general meaning. Then reread parts you did not understand. It may help to read those parts aloud. Carefully read the information given in each table and study each figure and its caption.

Concepts

While studying, put difficult concepts into your own words to see if you understand them. Check this understanding with another student or the instructor. Write these in your notebook.

Class Notes

When taking lecture notes in class, leave a large margin on the left side of each notebook page and write only on right-hand pages, leaving all left-hand pages blank. Look over your lecture notes soon after each class, while your memory is fresh. Fill in missing words, complete sentences and ideas, and underline key phrases, definitions, and concepts. At the top of each page, write the topic of that page. In the left margin, write the key word for that part of your notes. On the opposite left-hand page, write a summary or outline that combines material from both the textbook and the lecture. These can be your study notes for review.

Study Groups

Form a study group with some other students so you can help one another. Practice speaking and reading aloud. Ask questions about material you are not sure about. Work together to find answers.

References for Improving Study Skills

Good study skills are essential for achieving your goals in nursing. Time management, efficient use of study time, and a consistent approach to studying are all beneficial. There are various study methods for reading a textbook and for taking class notes. Some methods that have proven helpful can be found in *Saunders Student Nurse Planner: A Guide to Success in Nursing School*. This book contains helpful information on test taking and preparing for clinical experiences. It includes an example of a "time map" for planning study time and a blank form that the student can use to formulate a personal time map.

ADDITIONAL STUDY HINTS FOR ENGLISH AS SECOND-LANGUAGE (ESL) STUDENTS

Vocabulary

If you find a nontechnical word you do not know (e.g., *drowsy*), try to guess its meaning from the sentence (e.g., *With electrolyte imbalance, the patient may feel fatigued and drowsy*). If you are not sure of the meaning, or if it seems particularly important, look it up in the dictionary.

Vocabulary Notebook

Keep a small alphabetized notebook or address book in your pocket or purse. Write down new non-technical words you read or hear along with their meanings and pronunciations. Write each word under its initial letter so you can find it easily, as in a dictionary. For words you do not know or for words that have a different meaning in nursing, write down how they are used and sound. Look up their meanings in a dictionary or ask your instructor or first-language buddy. Then write the different meanings or usages that you have found in your book, including the nursing meaning. Continue to add new words as you discover them. For example:

primary
- of most importance; main: *the primary problem or disease*
- the first one; elementary: *primary school*

secondary
- of less importance; resulting from another problem or disease: *a secondary symptom*
- the second one: *secondary school (in the United States, high school)*

First Language Buddy

ESL students should find a first-language buddy – another student who is a native speaker of English and who is willing to answer questions about word meanings, pronunciations, and culture. Maybe your buddy would like to learn about your language and culture as well. This could help in his or her nursing experience as well.

Quick Review of Drug Classifications

ACE inhibitors Prevent the synthesis of angiotensin II, a potent vasoconstrictor; used to treat hypertension and heart failure

Acetylcholinesterase inhibitors Promote the accumulation of acetylcholine, resulting in prolonged cholinergic effects

Adrenergic Produce effects similar to the neurotransmitter norepinephrine; see Chapter 13

Adrenergic blocking agents Inhibit the adrenergic system, preventing stimulation of the adrenergic receptors

Aldosterone receptor antagonists Block stimulation of mineralocorticoid receptors by aldosterone, thus reducing high blood pressure by reducing sodium reabsorption

Aminoglycosides Gentamicin, tobramycin, and related antibiotics; particularly effective against gram-negative microorganisms; noted for potentially dangerous toxicity

Analgesics Narcotic and nonnarcotic; relieve pain without producing loss of consciousness or reflex activity

Androgens These steroid hormones produce masculinizing effects

Angiotensin II receptor antagonists Also known as ARBs (angiotensin receptor blockers); act by binding to angiotensin II receptor sites, preventing angiotensin II (a very potent vasoconstrictor) from binding to receptor sites in vascular smooth muscle, brain, heart, kidneys, and adrenal gland, thus blocking the blood pressure–elevating and sodium-retaining effects of angiotensin II

Anesthetics For example, local anesthesia, general anesthesia; cause a loss of sensation with or without a loss of consciousness

Antacids Reduce the acidity of the gastric contents

Antianginals Used to prevent or treat attacks of angina pectoris

Antianxiety Used to treat anxiety symptoms or disorders; also known as minor tranquilizers or anxiolytics, although the term *tranquilizer* is avoided today to prevent the misperception that the patient is being tranquilized

Antiarrhythmics Used to correct cardiac arrhythmias (any heart rate or rhythm other than normal sinus rhythm.)

Antibiotics Used to treat infections caused by pathogenic microbes; the term is often used interchangeably with antimicrobial agents

Anticholinergic Block the action of acetylcholine in the parasympathetic nervous system; also known as cholinergic blocking agents, antispasmodics, and parasympatholytic agents

Anticoagulants Do NOT dissolve existing blood clots, but do prevent enlargement or extension of blood clots

Anticonvulsants Suppress abnormal neuronal activity in the CNS, preventing seizures

Antidepressants Relieve depression

Antidiabetics Also known as hypoglycemics; include insulin (used to treat type 1 diabetes mellitus) and oral hypoglycemic agents (used in the treatment of type 2 diabetes mellitus)

Antidiarrheals Relieve or control the symptoms of acute or chronic diarrhea

Antiemetics Used to prevent or treat nausea and vomiting

Antifungals Used to treat fungal infections

Antiglaucoma Used to reduce intraocular pressure

Antigout Used in the treatment of active gout attacks or to prevent future attacks

Antihistamines Used to treat allergy symptoms; may also be used to treat motion sickness, insomnia, and other nonallergic reactions

Antihypertensives Used to treat elevated blood pressure (hypertension)

Antilipemics Used to reduce serum cholesterol and/or triglycerides

Antimicrobials Chemicals that eliminate living microorganisms pathogenic to the patient; also called antibiotics or antiinfectives

Antineoplastics Also called chemotherapy agents; used alone or in combination with other treatment modalities such as radiation, surgery, or biologic response modifiers for the treatment of cancer

Antiparkinson's Used in the treatment of Parkinson's syndrome and other dyskinesias

Antiplatelets Prevent platelet clumping (aggregation), thereby preventing an essential step in formation of a blood clot

Antipsychotics Used in the treatment of severe mental illnesses; also known as major tranquilizers or neuroleptics, although the term *tranquilizer* is avoided today to prevent the misperception that the patient is being tranquilized

Antipyretics Used to reduce fevers associated with a variety of conditions

Antispasmodics Actually anticholinergic agents

Antithyroid Used to treat the symptoms of hyperthyroidism; also known as thyroid hormone antagonists

Antituberculins Used to prevent or treat an infection caused by *Mycobacterium tuberculosis*

Antitussive Used to suppress a cough by acting on the cough center of the brain

Antiulcer agents These drugs, such as histamine-2 antagonists, decrease the volume and increase the pH of gastric secretions

Antivirals Used to treat infections caused by pathogenic viruses

Bronchodilators Stimulate receptors within the tracheobronchial tree to relax and dilate the airway passages, allowing a greater volume of air to be exchanged and improving oxygenation

Beta blockers Inhibit the activity of sympathetic transmitters, norepinephrine, and epinephrine; used to treat angina, arrhythmias, hypertension, and glaucoma

Calcium channel blockers Also called calcium ion antagonists, slow channel blockers or calcium ion influx inhibitors; inhibit the movement of calcium ions across the cell membrane; used to decrease arrhythmias, slow rate of contraction of the heart, and cause dilation of blood vessels

Carbapenems Antibiotics (imipenem, ertapenem, meropenem) that have a broad spectrum of activity against gram-positive and gram-negative bacteria; they act by inhibiting cell wall synthesis

Carbonic anhydrase inhibitors Interfere with the production of aqueous humor, thereby reducing intraocular pressure associated with glaucoma

Cell-stimulating agents Improve immune function by stimulating the activity of various immune cells

Cholinergic Also known as parasympathomimetics; produce effects similar to those of acetylcholine

Cholinesterase inhibitors These enzymes destroy acetylcholine, the cholinergic neurotransmitter

Coating agent This drug, sucralfate, forms a complex that adheres to the crater of an ulcer, protecting it from aggravation from gastric secretions

Colony-stimulating factors Stimulate progenitor cells in bone marrow to increase numbers of leukocytes, thereby improving immune function

v

Corticosteroids These hormones are secreted by the adrenal cortex of the adrenal gland

Cycloplegics Anticholinergic agents that paralyze accommodation of the iris of the eye

Cytotoxics Agents that cause direct cell death; often used for cancer chemotherapy

Decongestants Reduce swelling in the nasal passages caused by a common cold or allergic rhinitis

Digestants Combination products containing digestive enzymes used to treat various digestive disorders and to supplement deficiencies of natural digestive enzymes

Digitalis glycosides A class of drugs, also known as cardiac glycosides, that increase the force of contraction and slow the heart rate, thereby improving cardiac output

Diuretics Act to increase the flow of urine

Emetics Used to induce vomiting

Estrogens Steroids that cause feminizing effects

Expectorants Liquefy mucus by stimulating the natural lubricant fluids from the bronchial glands

Fluoroquinolones Ciprofloxacin and related agents; widely used broad-spectrum antibiotics

Gastric stimulants Used to increase stomach contractions, relax the pyloric valve, and increase peristalsis in the gastrointestinal tract; result in a decrease in gastric transit time and more rapid emptying of the intestinal tract

Glucocorticoids Also known as adrenocorticosteroids; are used to regulate carbohydrate, fat, and protein metabolism

Gonadal hormones Hormones produced by the testes in the male and ovaries in the female

Herbals Plant products usually sold as food supplements; may have pharmacologic effects that are not evaluated or regulated by the FDA

Histamine (H$_2$) antagonists Decrease the volume and increase the pH of gastric secretions both during the day and the night

HMG-CoA reductase enzyme inhibitors Also known as the statins; antilipemic agents that inhibit hydroxymethyl-glutaryl coenzyme A (HMG-CoA) reductase enzyme, the enzyme that stimulates the conversion of HMG-CoA to mevalonic acid, a precursor in the biosynthesis of cholesterol, thus reducing the potential for atherosclerosis

Hyperuricemics Used to decrease the production of and increase the excretion of uric acid

Hypnotics Used to produce sleep

Insulins Hormone required for glucose transport to the cells

Lactation suppressants Used to prevent physiologic lactation

Laxatives Act by a variety of mechanisms to treat constipation

Low molecular weight heparins Derivatives of heparin; anticoagulants for the prophylactic treatment of pulmonary thromboembolism and deep vein thrombosis

Macrolides Erythromycin, azithromycin, and related antibiotics

MAO inhibitors: Agents that block monoamine oxidase, thereby preventing the degradation and prolonging the action of norepinephrine and serotonin

Mineralocorticoids Steroids that cause the kidneys to retain sodium and water

Miotics Cause constriction of the iris

Mucolytics Reduce the thickness and stickiness of pulmonary secretions by acting directly on the mucous plugs to dissolve them

Muscle relaxants Relieve muscle spasms

Mydriatics Cause dilation of the iris

Neuromuscular blockers Skeletal muscle relaxants used to produce muscle relaxation during anesthesia; reduce the use and side effects of general anesthetics; used to ease endotracheal intubation and prevent laryngospasm

Nitrates Metabolize to nitric oxide, a potent vasodilator used to treat angina

Nonsteroidal antiinflammatory drugs (NSAIDs) These "aspirin-like" drugs are chemically unrelated to the salicylates but are prostaglandin inhibitors

Opioids Centrally acting analgesic agents related to morphine

Oral contraceptives Used for birth control; administered orally

Oral hypoglycemics Used in type 2 diabetes mellitus to improve glucose metabolism and lower blood glucose levels

Progestins Steroids regulating endometrial and myometrial function; used alone or in combination with estrogen for oral contraception

Protease inhibitors Saquinavir, ritonavir, indinavir, and related drugs; block the maturation of human immunodeficiency virus; used to treat HIV infections

Salicylates Effective as analgesics, antipyretics, and antiinflammatory agents

Sedatives Given to an individual to produce relaxation and rest; do not necessarily produce sleep

Selective serotonin reuptake inhibitors (SSRIs) Antidepressants that act by specifically blocking the reuptake of serotonin, thus prolonging its action

Serotonin antagonists Used to block serotonin; prevent emesis induced by chemotherapy, radiation therapy, and surgery

Statins (HMG-CoA reductase inhibitors) Agents that block the synthesis of cholesterol

Stool softeners or fecal softeners Draw water into the stool, thereby softening it

Sympatholytics Interfere with the storage and release of norepinephrine

Sympothomimetics Mimic the action of dopamine, norepinephrine, and epinephrine

Thrombolytics A specific group of drugs (alteplase, anistreplase, streptokinase or urokinase) given to dissolve existing blood clots

Thyroid hormone antagonists Used to counteract or block the action of excessive formation of thyroid hormones

Thyroid hormones Used when thyroid hormones are not being produced or are not produced in sufficient quantities to meet the body's physiologic needs

Tricyclic antidepressants Inhibit the reuptake of norepinephrine and serotonin (include doxepin, amitriptyline, and imipramine)

Uricosuric agents Act on the tubules of the kidneys to enhance the excretion of uric acid

Urinary analgesics Produce a local anesthetic effect on the mucosa of the ureters and bladder to relieve burning, pain, urgency, and frequency associated with urinary tract infections (UTIs)

Urinary antimicrobials Substances excreted and concentrated in the urine in sufficient amounts to have an antiseptic effect on the urine and the urinary tract

Uterine relaxants Used to primarily prevent preterm labor and delivery

Uterine stimulants Increase the frequency or strength of uterine contractions

Vaccines Suspensions of either live, attenuated, or killed bacteria or viruses administered to induce immunity against infection of specific bacteria or viruses

Vasodilators Relax the arteriolar smooth muscle, causing dilation of the blood vessels

Contents

CHAPTER 1

Definitions, Names, Standards, and Informational Sources

Syllabus

CHAPTER CONTENT

CHAPTER OBJECTIVES

Definitions
1. State the origin and definition of *pharmacology*.
2. Explain the meaning of therapeutic methods.

Drug Names (USA)
1. Describe the process used to name drugs.
2. Differentiate among the chemical, generic, official, and brand names of medicines.

Drug Names (Canada)
1. Differentiate between the *official* drug and the *proper* names of a medicine.

Sources of Drug Standards (USA)
1. List official sources of American drug standards.

Sources of Drug Standards (Canada)
1. List official sources of Canadian drug standards.

Sources of Drug Information (USA)
1. List and describe literature resources for researching prescription and nonprescription medications.

2. List and describe literature resources for researching drug interactions and drug compatibilities.

Sources of Drug Information (Canada)
1. Describe the organization of the *Compendium of Pharmaceuticals and Specialties* and the information contained in each colored section.
2. Describe the organization of the *Canadian Self-Medication*.

Sources of Patient Information
1. Cite literature resources for reviewing information to be given to the patient concerning prescribed medications.

Drug Legislation (USA)
1. List legislative acts controlling drug use and abuse.
2. Differentiate among Schedule I, II, III, IV, and V medications, and describe nursing responsibilities associated with the administration of each type of drug.

Drug Legislation (Canada)
1. List legislative acts controlling drug use and abuse.
2. Differentiate between Schedule F and Controlled Drugs and describe nursing responsibilities with each.

New Drug Development
1. Describe the procedure outlined by the FDA to develop and market new medicines.

KEY TERMS

pharmacology
therapeutic methods
medicine

Copyright © 2004 Mosby Inc. All rights reserved.

drug
chemical name
generic name
official name
trademark
brand name
proprietary name
over-the-counter (OTC) drugs
illegal drugs
*The United States Pharmacopeia (USP)/National
Formulary (NF)*
*US Dictionary of USAN and International Drug
Names*
European Pharmacopoeia
American Drug Index
American Hospital Formulary Service
Drug Interaction Facts
Drug Facts and Comparisons
Handbook on Injectable Drugs
Handbook of Nonprescription Drugs
Martindale—The Complete Drug Reference
Medical Letter
Mosby's Drug Consult
Natural Medicines Comprehensive Database
Physicians' Desk Reference (PDR)
Electronic databases
*Compendium of Pharmaceuticals and Specialties
(CPS)*
*Patient Self-Care: Helping Patients Make Therapeutic
Choices*
Compendium of Self-Care Products
USP DI
Therapeutic Choices
Tyler's Honest Herbal
Federal Food, Drug, and Cosmetic Act, 1938
Controlled Substances Act, 1970
Scheduled Drugs
Food and Drugs Act, 1927
Food and Drug Regulations 1953, 1954, 1979
Controlled Drugs and Substance Act, 1997
Nonprescription Drugs
Preclinical research
Clinical research
New drug application review
Postmarketing surveillance
Orphan Drugs

ASSIGNMENTS

Read textbook, pp. 1-13.
Study the Key Terms associated with the chapter
content.
Study Review Sheets for Chapter 1.
Complete Chapter 1 Practice Quiz.
Complete Chapter 1 Exam.

WEB RESEARCH ACTIVITIES

1. Go to the library in your school and have the
   librarian demonstrate the electronic database
   services available for the study of pharmacology.
2. Use a computer to access the Internet site
   http://www.medlineplus.gov and open the National Library of Medicine's Medline Plus site.
   At the site, identify the information contained in
   the following sections:

Health Topics

Drug Information

Medical Encyclopedia

Dictionary

News

Directories

Other Resources

3. Using http://www.centerwatch.com/patient/
   drugs/druglist.html, identify two new drugs
   approved by the FDA in 2003 and two drugs approved in 2002.

COLLABORATIVE ACTIVITIES

*Complete the following activities and questions to pre-
pare for in-class discussion and group work that may
be assigned by the instructor.*

A. Controlled Substances

Turn to p. 92 and examine the names of the medicines listed on the controlled substance inventory
form. Compare the drugs listed with those found
on the controlled substance inventory form at your

Copyright © 2004 Mosby Inc. All rights reserved.

clinical practice setting assignment. What additional drugs are listed in the clinical practice setting? Discuss possible reasons for such differences.

B. New Drugs/Research

Discuss the nurse's role in clinical research involving new drug products being administered in a clinical site.

C. Activity Designed to Acquaint the Student with the *PDR*

Section 2 of the *PDR*: Identify the generic and brand names of the following drugs using this section of the *PDR*:

Generic name: *Brand name:*

1. Theophylline ethylenediamine extended-release tablets
2. Indomethacin suppositories
3. Rifampin tablets

Section 3 of the *PDR*: Give an example of a drug in the following therapeutic classes:

1. Hypolipidemic agent—

2. Proton pump inhibitor—

3. Calcium channel blocker—

Section 4 of *PDR*: A patient describes a medicine she is taking at home as about 3/4" long, capsule-shaped, with oval ends, orange with MSD697 printed on one side. Using this information, can you identify the medication using Section 4? If you were unable to identify it, what would you do?

Section 5 of *PDR*: Examine and list the major categories of information found in a package insert that accompanies a drug. Discuss the value of information found in a package insert to the nurse in the clinical setting.

Copyright © 2004 Mosby Inc. All rights reserved.

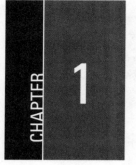

CHAPTER 1

Definitions, Names, Standards, and Informational Sources

Practice Quiz

COMPLETION

Complete the following statements or answer questions using Key Terms from Chapter 1.

1. The study of drugs and the actions they have in the human body is _____.
2. The actual substance that causes the response in a living organism is a(n) _____.
3. How do chemical names differ from brand names and generic names?

Use the textbook and other drug resources (e.g., PDR) to identify the brand name or generic name and additional brand names for each drug listed.

Generic name:	Brand name:	Other Brand names:
4. Aspirin		
5.	Tylenol®	
6.	Pepto-Bismol®	
7.	Maalox®	
8. Ibuprofen		
9.	Tums®	

Summarize the content found in each of the following pharmacy resource books:

10. *American Drug Index*

11. *American Hospital Formulary Service, Drug Information*

12. *Facts and Comparisons*

13. *Martindale—The Complete Drug Reference*

14. *Handbook of Nonprescription Drugs*

15. *Medical Letter*

16. *Physicians' Desk Reference* (PDR)

CONTROLLED SUBSTANCES

For each medicine listed, identify the DEA schedule. Use the textbook and other resources.

Medicine	DEA Schedule
17. Darvocet N®	C-
18. Diazepam	C-
19. Flurazepam	C-
20. LevoDromoran	C-
21. Meperidine	C-
22. Morphine Sulfate	C-
23. Tylenol® with codeine no. 2	C-
24. Tylenol® with codeine no. 3	C-
25. Tylenol® with codeine no. 4	C-
26. Percodan®	C-
27. Tylox® Capsules	C-

DRUG LEGISLATION

Critical Thinking

28. What is the purpose of the Controlled Substances Act of 1970?
29. When can a nurse be in possession of controlled substances without it being considered a crime?
30. What information is found in *Tyler's Honest Herbal* reference and of what significance is it to the nurse during patient education?
31. What drug information resources are immediately available on the clinical unit where you are assigned? Is there an electronic database available in addition to hardcopy materials?
32. Outline the procedures used for the development of new drugs.
33. Explain why manufacturers do not aggressively develop new medicines for rare diseases.

Copyright © 2004 Mosby Inc. All rights reserved.

Student Name _____

REVIEW QUESTIONS

_____ 1. Medicines are most commonly classified by:
  a. brand or generic name.
  b. chemical name.
  c. proprietary name.
  d. body systems, clinical use, or physiology.

_____ 2. The *Physicians' Desk Reference* is available:
  a. electronically and in book form.
  b. on every nursing unit.
  c. biannually.
  d. as a package insert with each drug.

Copyright © 2004 Mosby Inc. All rights reserved.

CHAPTER 2

Principles of Drug Action and Drug Interactions

Syllabus

CHAPTER CONTENT

Basic Principles (p. 14)
Drug Action (p. 17)
Variable Factors Influencing Drug Action (p. 18)
Drug Interactions (p. 19)

CHAPTER OBJECTIVES

Basic Principles

1. Identify five basic principles of drug action.
2. Explain nursing assessments necessary to evaluate potential problems associated with the absorption of medications.
3. Describe nursing interventions that can enhance drug absorption.
4. List three categories of drug administration and state the routes of administration for each category.
5. Differentiate between general and selective drug distribution mechanisms.
6. Name the process that inactivates drugs.
7. Identify the meaning and significance to the nurse of the term *half-life* when used in relation to drug therapy.

Drug Action

1. Compare and contrast the following terms used with regard to medications: *desired action, side effects, adverse effects, allergic reactions*, and *idiosyncratic reactions*.

Variable Factors Influencing Drug Action

1. List factors that cause variations in the absorption, metabolism, distribution, and excretion of drugs.

Drug Interactions

1. State the mechanism by which drug interactions may occur.
2. Differentiate among the following terms used with regard to medications: *additive effect,*

synergistic effect, antagonistic effect, displacement, interference, and *incompatibility*.

KEY TERMS

receptors
pharmacodynamics
agonists
antagonists
partial agonists
ADME
pharmacokinetics
absorption
enteral
parenteral
percutaneous
distribution
drug blood level
metabolism
biotransformation
excretion
half-life
desired action
side effects
adverse effects
toxicity

parameters
idiosyncratic reaction
allergic reaction
urticaria
hives
carcinogenicity
teratogen
placebo effect
nocebo effect
placebo
tolerance
drug dependence
drug accumulation
drug interaction
unbound drug
additive drug
synergistic effect
antagonistic effect
displacement
interference
incompatibility

ASSIGNMENTS

Read textbook, pp. 14-21.
Study Key Terms associated with chapter content.
Study Review Sheets for Chapter 2.
Complete Chapter 2 Practice Quiz.
Complete Chapter 2 Exam.

WEB RESEARCH ACTIVITY

Access http://medlineplus.gov. Open the National Library of Medicine's Medline Plus site and research the term *antagonist*.

Copyright © 2004 Mosby Inc. All rights reserved.

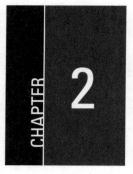

CHAPTER 2

Principles of Drug Action and Drug Interactions

Review Sheet

Note: Understanding the vocabulary associated with the study of pharmacology is fundamental to understanding the remaining information presented in the textbook. Therefore, the first step is to define and memorize the vocabulary. The second step is to apply the vocabulary learned during the pharmacology course. The third step in learning pharmacology is to apply the vocabulary during the actual clinical practice of nursing.

The QUESTION column and the ANSWER column have been offset so you can cover the answer while reading the question, allowing you to assess your knowledge. Define the following vocabulary.

Question	Answer
1. Pharmacodynamics	
2. Receptors	1. The study of drug interactions including the drug receptors and the series of events that culminates in a pharmacologic response.
3. Agonists	2. Sites on the cells where chemical bonding of drugs occurs are receptors.
4. Antagonists	3. Drugs that stimulate a response at a receptor site are agonists.
5. Partial agonists	4. Drugs that attach to receptor sites, but do NOT stimulate a response are antagonists.
6. ADME	5. Drugs that interact with a receptor to stimulate a response and concurrently inhibit other responses are partial agonists.
7. Pharmacokinetics	6. ADME is an abbreviation for the four stages of drug processing: absorption, distribution, metabolism, and excretion.
8. Absorption	7. Pharmacokinetics is the study of the mathematical relationship among the absorption, distribution, metabolism, and excretion of medicines.
9. Enteral	8. Absorption is the process by which a drug is made available to the body fluids for distribution.
10. Parenteral	9. The enteral route of drug administration is placed directly into the gastrointestinal tract by oral, rectal, or nasogastric routes.
11. Percutaneous	10. Parenteral routes of drug administration are subcutaneous (SC), intramuscular (IM), or intravenous (IV) injection.
12. Distribution	11. Percutaneous drug administration is done via inhalation, sublingual, or topical administration.

Copyright © 2004 Mosby Inc. All rights reserved.

13. Drug blood level

14. Biotransformation (metabolism)

15. Excretion

16. Half-life

17. Desired action

18. Side effects

19. Adverse effects

20. Idiosyncratic reaction

21. Allergic reactions

22. Urticaria (hives)

23. Carcinogenicity

24. Teratogen

12. The term *distribution* refers to the ways in which drugs are transported by the circulating body fluids to the sites of action (receptors) for metabolism and excretion.

13. The drug blood level measures the amount of a drug present in the blood to determine if it is within the therapeutic range, below the range (subtherapeutic), or above the range (toxic).

14. *Metabolism* and *biotransformation* are defined as the process by which a drug is inactivated (broken down). The terms are used interchangeably.

15. Excretion of a drug is the elimination of the active drug or its metabolites from the body.

16. The time required for one-half, or 50%, of the drug administered to be excreted from the body.

17. Desired action is the achievement of the expected response to the drug administered.

18. Most side effects are predictable responses seen when a specific drug is administered. (The drug monographs throughout the textbook will give suggested nursing actions that can make these anticipated reactions more tolerable to the patient.)

19. Adverse effects are side effects that are more serious and require reporting to the HCP for further orders on how to manage these reactions. These are sometimes referred to as drug toxicity reactions. Adverse effects are labeled "side effects to report" throughout this textbook. See also World Health Organization definition on p. 17.

20. Idiosyncratic reactions are reactions that are not predictable; they are unusual or abnormal responses to the drug administered.

21. An allergic reaction, also called a *hypersensitivity reaction*, occurs in an individual who has previously taken the drug and is sensitized to it. With repeat administration, antibodies formed when the drug was first given respond to the repeated exposure producing an undesirable response, such as severe itching, urticaria (hives), or in more severe cases, collapse of the respiratory and cardiovascular systems, known as *anaphylactic reaction* or *anaphylaxis*, a life-threatening situation.

22. Urticaria or hives are elevated, irregular, patchlike rashes on the skin accompanied by itching.

23. Carcinogenicity is the ability of a drug to cause living cells to be altered (mutate) and become cancerous.

Copyright © 2004 Mosby Inc. All rights reserved.

25. Placebo
26. Tolerance

27. Drug dependence

28. Drug accumulation

29. Drug interaction

30. Unbound drug

31. Additive effect

32. Synergistic effect

33. Antagonistic effect

34. Displacement

35. Interference

36. Incompatibility

24. A drug that causes birth defects is a teratogen.
25. A placebo is a drug dosage form that contains no active ingredients.
26. Tolerance occurs when higher doses of a drug are required to achieve the same effects that a lower dose once achieved.
27. Drug dependence, also called *addiction* or *habituation*, occurs when the individual is no longer able to control the ingestion of the drug.
28. Drug accumulation occurs when there is an excess amount of a drug in the body due to a number of possible physiologic variables. This can result in drug toxicity.
29. Drug interaction occurs when one drug being administered changes the action of other the drugs being used at the same time.
30. Unbound or free drug is the active amount of drug available to achieve the desired physiologic response.
31. Additive effect occurs when two drugs with similar actions have an increased effect.
32. Synergistic effect occurs when the combined effect of two drugs is greater than the effect of each drug given alone.
33. Antagonistic effect occurs when one drug interferes with the action of another.
34. Displacement occurs when one drug is moved from the protein binding sites by a second drug. This usually increases the activity of the first drug because it is now unbound.
35. Interference occurs when one drug inhibits the metabolism or excretion of a second drug, causing increased activity of the second drug.
36. Incompatibility occurs when one drug is chemically incompatible with another drug, resulting in deterioration of the drug.

Copyright © 2004 Mosby Inc. All rights reserved.

Principles of Drug Action and Drug Interactions

Practice Quiz

TRUE OR FALSE

Mark "T" for true or "F" for false for each statement.
Correct all false statements.

_____ 1. Percutaneous route is the administration of drugs by subcutaneous, intramuscular, or intravenous injection.

_____ 2. Enteral route is the administration of drugs to the gastrointestinal tract.

_____ 3. Agonists stimulate a response at a receptor site on the cells.

_____ 4. Partial agonists stimulate some responses while inhibiting others at a receptor site on the cells.

_____ 5. Parenteral route is the administration of drugs by inhalation, sublingual, or topical methods.

_____ 6. Receptors are specific sites within the body where a drug acts.

_____ 7. Antagonists cause a drug response at a receptor site.

_____ 8. Absorption refers to the ability of a drug to be integrated into the body fluids.

_____ 9. Metabolism is the activation of a drug for use by the body.

_____ 10. Distribution is the transportation of a drug within the body fluids for utilization within the body.

_____ 11. Excretion of a drug is the elimination of a drug from the body.

_____ 12. Biotransformation is another term for excretion of a drug.

_____ 13. Drug blood level is a measurement of the amount of drug present in the blood at the specific time of the blood draw.

COMPLETION

Finish each of the following statements using the correct term.

14. A drug interaction that produces an increased action is known as a(n) _____ effect.

15. Two drugs with similar actions that produce an effect substantially greater than either drug administered alone are said to be _____.

16. When one drug moves the original drug administered from a binding site to produce an increased drug effect, this is known as _____.

17. Drug _____ is defined as one drug chemically destroying a second drug if mixed together prior to administration.

18. Drug tolerance is _____.

19. Drug dependence is _____.

20. An adverse drug reaction is also known as _____.

MULTIPLE CHOICE

Choose the BEST answer from those provided.

_____ 21. The primary routes for drug excretion are
   a. skin and lungs.
   b. gastrointestinal tract and the skin.
   c. renal tubules and GI tract.
   d. lungs and renal tubules.

_____ 22. Drug distribution occurs by
   a. decreasing body protein levels.
   b. transport in blood and lymphatic systems.
   c. keeping the drug at toxic levels.
   d. increasing the amount of adipose tissue.

Copyright © 2004 Mosby Inc. All rights reserved.

_____ 23. A partial agonist is a drug that stimulates
    a. action at receptor sites within the circulating blood.
    b. one response and inhibits another response.
    c. no response when attached to a receptor site.
    d. a response at a receptor site.

_____ 24. Another name for an idiosyncratic reaction is a(n)
    a. allergic reaction.
    b. unexpected reaction.
    c. teratogenic reaction.
    d. drug overresponse.

_____ 25. The literature states that the half-life of a particular drug is 8 hours. This means _____% of the drug will have been excreted in this time period.
    a. 25
    b. 30
    c. 50
    d. 75

_____ 26. A *desired* drug action is
    a. the predictable/usual response to the drug.
    b. an unusual or idiosyncratic response to a drug.
    c. capable of inducing cell mutations.
    d. the development of symptoms that should be reported to the prescribing physician.

REVIEW QUESTIONS

_____ 1. A patient takes 50 mg of a drug that has a half-life of 12 hours. What percentage of the dose remains in the body 36 hours after the drug is administered?
    a. 50 mg (100%)
    b. 25 mg (50%)
    c. 12.5 mg (25%)
    d. 6.25 mg (12.5%)

_____ 2. The portion of a drug that is pharmacologically active is known as the:
    a. protein-bound drug.
    b. unbound drug.
    c. drug tolerance level.
    d. incompatibility factor.

_____ 3. A person who has an increased metabolic rate (e.g., hyperthyroidism) would generally require a dosage that is:
    a. normal.
    b. lower than normal.
    c. higher than normal.
    d. based on thyroid function levels.

Copyright © 2004 Mosby Inc. All rights reserved.

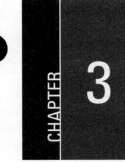

Drug Action Across the Life Span

Syllabus

CHAPTER CONTENT

Changing Drug Action Across the Life Span (p. 22)
    Drug Absorption (p. 22)
    Drug Distribution (p. 23)
    Drug Metabolism (p. 24)
    Drug Elimination (p. 24)
    Therapeutic Drug Monitoring (p. 25)
Nursing Implications when Monitoring Drug
    Therapy (p. 26)
    Use of Monitoring Parameters (p. 26)

CHAPTER OBJECTIVES

1. Discuss the effects of patient age on drug action.
2. Cite major factors associated with drug absorption, distribution, metabolism, and excretion in the pediatric and the geriatric populations.
3. Cite major factors associated with drug absorption, distribution, metabolism, and excretion in men and women.

KEY TERMS

gender-specific
    medicine
passive diffusion
hydrolysis
intestinal transit
protein binding

drug metabolism
metabolites
therapeutic drug
    monitoring
polypharmacy

ASSIGNMENTS

Read textbook, pp. 22-30.
Study Key Terms associated with chapter content.
Study Review Sheet for Chapter 3.
Complete Chapter 3 Practice Quiz.
Complete Chapter 3 Exam.

WEB RESEARCH ACTIVITY

Access http://www.medlineplus.gov and open the National Library of Medicine's Medlineplus site. Open Health Topics and in the search box, insert: pregnancy and drugs. Select and read information on one topic; e.g., Pregnancy and Drug Dilemma.

Copyright © 2004 Mosby Inc. All rights reserved.

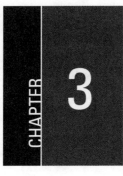

Drug Action Across the Life Span

CHAPTER 3

Review Sheet

The QUESTION column and the ANSWER column have been offset so you can cover the answer while reading the question, allowing you to assess your knowledge. Define the following vocabulary.

Question

1. What are common terms used to refer to individuals of different ages up to 5 years old?

2. What is the meaning of *gender-specific medicine*?

3. What are the underlying rationales for the erratic absorption of intramuscular (IM) drugs in both the neonate and the geriatric population?

4. Define *passive diffusion*. (Research other sources.)

5. Define *carrier-mediated diffusion*. (Research other sources.)

6. Define *active transport*. (Research other sources.)

7. State two factors that influence drug absorption from the gastrointestinal tract.

Answer

1. Fewer than 38 weeks = premature, 0–1 months = newborn or neonate, 1–24 months = infant or baby, 1–5 years = young child.

2. Gender-specific medicine is a new area of pharmacology that studies the differences in the response of females and males to prescribed drugs.

3. The underlying rationales for the erratic absorption of IM drugs are differences in muscle mass and blood flow to muscles and muscular inactivity in the bedridden patient.

4. Passive diffusion is the most common mechanism associated with drug absorption. It requires no cellular energy and involves the movement of a drug from an area of high concentration to an area of low concentration.

5. Carrier-mediated diffusion, or facilitated transport or diffusion, occurs when the drug molecules combine with a carrier substance such as an enzyme or other protein. An example is glucose combining with insulin to be carried from the bloodstream into the cell, moving from an area of high concentration (the bloodstream) to an area of low concentration (the cell). In other words, the drug needs help to pass across the cell membrane and the insulin passively provides the transport. This passive process requires no cellular energy.

6. Active transport involves the movement of drug molecules from an area of low concentration to an area of high concentration. This process requires cellular energy to accomplish the movement.

Copyright © 2004 Mosby Inc. All rights reserved.

8. Summarize the gastric pH in a premature infant, newborn, infant, adult, and elder.

9. Compare gastric emptying time in a premature infant, adult, and elder.

10. Look up the term *hydrolysis* in a dictionary.

11. In the newborn, what factor affects the absorption of drugs during the process of hydrolysis?

12. If gastric emptying time increases, what happens to the speed of absorption of a drug?

13. What is the purpose of performing therapeutic drug monitoring?

14. What effect does the route of drug administration have on drug absorption?

15. List accurate methods of measuring oral liquid medications.

16. What nursing actions are appropriate when "off-label use" of medications is prescribed?

17. Why is transdermal absorption of a drug in an elder difficult to predict?

7. Passive diffusion and gastric emptying time influence the absorption of drugs in the intestinal tract. Both passive diffusion and gastric emptying time are dependent on pH.

8. The gastric pH values are:
   premature   6–8
   newborn   6–8; decreases to 2–4 in 24 hours
   infant   1–3
   adult   1–3
   elder   pH is increased due to decreasing number of acid-secreting cells

9. Premature infants and geriatric patients have slower gastric emptying time; therefore, the drug is in contact with the absorptive tissue longer. This may result in more absorption and a higher serum concentration of the drug in the blood.

10. Hydrolysis is the chemical alteration or decomposition of a compound with water.

11. In an infant, the absence of enzymes needed for hydrolysis of certain drugs influences the ability of the drug to be absorbed.

12. The faster the gastric emptying time, the less time the drug has to be absorbed; therefore, drug absorption is decreased.

13. Assays measure blood levels of specific drugs, providing a means to identify needed dosage adjustments.

14. In general, drug absorption is affected by: dosage form (e.g., liquid versus enteric-coated tablets); route of drug administration (e.g., oral, intramuscular, inhalation); solubility of the drug; gastrointestinal function; the condition of the absorptive surface (e.g., inflamed, open skin area versus intact skin); and blood flow to and from the site.

15. Use medicine cups, droppers provided with a specific medication, or oral syringes to measure liquid forms of oral medications accurately.

16. "Off-label use" of medications is legal; however, nurses should check reliable references or with the pharmacist for further information. In all cases, monitor the patient carefully for side effects or adverse effects whenever the medicine is administered.

Copyright © 2004 Mosby Inc. All rights reserved.

18. What factors affect drug distribution?

19. Examine Table 3-1 on p. 24 of the text. Compare the total percentage of body water in a premature infant, a full-term infant, a 1-year-old infant, and a male adult. What conclusion(s) did you reach?
20. What effect will a higher percentage of total body water have on drug absorption?
21. Research the meaning of *lipid-soluble* and *water-soluble*.

22. Define *protein binding*.

23. What happens to the concentration of albumin in the body after the age 40?

24. What happens to the rate of drug metabolism in the elderly?

25. How functional is the renal filtration system of preterm infants and of full-term newborns when compared to that of an adult?

26. What effect do age and renal function have on drug dosages?

27. What test is used as the best predictor to estimate renal function in the elderly?

28. Define *polypharmacy*.

17. In an elder, there is decreased dermal thickness that may increase drug absorption; however, there may be drying, wrinkling, and decreased hair follicles that decrease absorption. There is often decreased cardiac output, which results in decreased blood flow to the tissues (decreased tissue perfusion), which results in decreased drug absorption.
18. Distribution is dependent on pH, body water concentration (intracellular, extracellular, and total body water), presence and quantity of fat tissue, protein binding, cardiac output, and regional blood flow.
19. The younger the individual, the higher the percent of the total body water.
20. A higher percent of total body water means drugs that are water-soluble will be more rapidly distributed and the individual may require a higher dose of these drugs. Conversely, fat-soluble drugs would be poorly absorbed.
21. Water-soluble drugs have an affinity for body fluids and are quickly absorbed and excreted through the kidneys; therefore, water-soluble drugs often have a shorter half-life. Lipid-soluble drugs have an affinity for fat tissue in the body and will often have a longer half-life.
22. Protein binding occurs when a drug binds to proteins in the body, such as albumin. When "bound," the drug is not "free" or actively available for use at the receptor sites for action.
23. Total albumin concentration decreases after age 40, while other proteins increase. This results in an increase in unbound drug making more free drug available for action and metabolism.
24. The number of functioning hepatic cells and the blood flow decreases with aging, resulting in slower drug metabolism. As drug metabolism decreases, drug doses must be reduced to prevent accumulation of the drug, producing toxicity.
25. At birth, preterm infants have approximately 15% of the renal capacity of an adult and full-term infants have approximately 35%.
26. Drug doses must be adjusted so an adequate, therapeutic serum blood concentration is maintained. Increased age and decreased renal function often require a reduced dosage.
27. The urine creatinine test is used to estimate renal function in the elderly.

Copyright © 2004 Mosby Inc. All rights reserved.

29. Describe the safest method of initiating newly prescribed medications to a geriatric patient.

30. Identify principles of drug administration that are specifically applicable to a pregnant patient.

28. Polypharmacy is the use of multiple drugs concurrently.

29. Drug dosage should be initiated at 1/3 to 1/2 the normal adult dose and, whenever available, therapeutic drug monitoring should be completed.

30. Take a thorough drug history of all prescribed and over-the-counter medications and "street drugs" being taken. Ask specifically about any herbal remedies or nutritional supplements being taken. Ask about the use of alcohol, tobacco, and herbal products during pregnancy. Refer to Tables 3-6 and 3-7, p. 29 in the textbook.

Copyright © 2004 Mosby Inc. All rights reserved.

Student Name_____

Drug Action Across the Life Span

Practice Quiz

TRUE OR FALSE

Directions: Mark "T" for true and "F" for false for each statement. <u>*Correct all false statements.*</u>

_____ 1. The elderly population includes persons 65 years and older.

_____ 2. Absorption of drugs administered intramuscularly is consistent and predictable.

_____ 3. Transdermal drug absorption has a predictable rate.

_____ 4. Enteric-coated and sustained-release tablets are absorbed erratically if crushed.

_____ 5. Passive diffusion requires cellular energy.

_____ 6. The gastric emptying time of the elder and the premature infant are slow and result in increased drug absorption.

_____ 7. Hydrolysis involves the chemical breakdown of a compound, such as a drug, in water.

_____ 8. The elderly patient has a greater percentage of total body fluid than an infant.

_____ 9. Drug elimination is affected by the number of functional renal tubules.

_____ 10. Albumin is a protein to which drugs bind for transport.

_____ 11. "Unbound" drug is the active portion of the drug dose available for the desired drug action.

_____ 12. "Bound" drug is the portion of the drug causing the desired drug action.

_____ 13. The term *infant* is used to signify babies 0–1 month of age.

_____ 14. Gender-specific medicine studies how disease differences affect normal functions of men and women.

_____ 15. The pH environment of the gastrointestinal tract affects passive diffusion and gastric emptying time.

_____ 16. Some drugs such as erythromycin, prednisolone, diazepam, and verapamil are metabolized more rapidly in men than in women.

_____ 17. Saliva assays may be used for therapeutic drug monitoring of some types of medications.

_____ 18. "Peak" and "trough" laboratory values should be communicated promptly to the prescribing HCP.

_____ 19. Household teaspoons provide a safe, reliable measurement for drug doses.

_____ 20. Many drugs, in addition to street drugs, may be teratogenic.

REVIEW QUESTIONS

_____ 1. Protein-binding is _____ in preterm infants, therefore _____ dosage adjustments on a mg/kg basis would be required.
   a. same as in adult as; no
   b. same as in elderly as; no
   c. increased; lower
   d. reduced; higher loading

_____ 2. Enzyme systems are primarily found in the _____, therefore laboratory values to assess functioning of this organ may be a required premedication assessment.
   a. kidney
   b. liver
   c. lungs
   d. blood

_____ 3. Pediatric renal function is equivalent to that of an adult at:
   a. full-term birth.
   b. infant 4 weeks.
   c. infant 9 to 12 months.
   d. young child 2 years.

Copyright © 2004 Mosby Inc. All rights reserved.

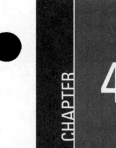

The Nursing Process and Pharmacology

Syllabus

CHAPTER CONTENT

The Nursing Process (p. 31)
Relating the Nursing Process to Pharmacology
(p. 41)

CHAPTER OBJECTIVES

The Nursing Process

1. Explain the purpose of the nursing process and methodology used to apply it to the study of pharmacology.
2. State the five steps in the nursing process and describe them in terms of a problem-solving method used in nursing practice.

Assessment

1. Describe the components of the assessment process.
2. Compare current methods used to collect, organize, and analyze information about the health care needs of patients and their significant others.

Nursing Diagnosis

1. Define the term *nursing diagnosis* and discuss the wording used in formulating nursing diagnosis statements.
2. Define the term *collaborative problem*.
3. Differentiate between a nursing diagnosis and a medical diagnosis.
4. Differentiate between problems that require formulation of nursing diagnoses and those categorized as collaborative problems, which may not require nursing diagnosis statements.

Planning

1. Identify the steps in the planning of nursing care.
2. Explain the process of prioritizing individual patient needs utilizing Maslow's hierarchy of needs.

3. Formulate measurable goal statements for assigned patients in the clinical practice setting.
4. State the behavioral responses around which goal statements revolve when planning a patient's discharge.
5. Integrate outcome/classification system(s) and critical pathways into care plans.
6. Identify the purposes of a patient care plan.
7. Differentiate between nursing interventions and therapeutic outcomes.

Nursing Intervention or Implementation

1. Compare the types of nursing functions classified as dependent, interdependent, and independent, and give examples of each.

Evaluating and Recording Therapeutic Outcomes

1. Describe the evaluation process used to establish whether patient behaviors are consistent with the identified short- or long-term goals.

Relating the Nursing Process to Pharmacology

Assessment

1. State the information that should be obtained as a part of the medication history.
2. Identify primary, secondary, and tertiary sources of information used to build a patient information base.

Nursing Diagnosis

1. Define *problem*.
2. Describe the process used to identify factors that could result in patient problems when medications are prescribed.
3. Review the content of several drug monographs to identify information that may result in patient problems from the medication therapy.

Planning

1. Identify steps used to plan nursing care in relation to a medication regimen prescribed for a patient.

Copyright © 2004 Mosby Inc. All rights reserved.

2. Describe an acceptable method of organizing, implementing, and evaluating the patient education delivered.
3. Practice developing short- and long-term patient education objectives and have them critiqued by the instructor.

Nursing Intervention or Implementation
1. Differentiate among dependent, interdependent, and independent nursing actions and give an example of each.

Evaluating Therapeutic Outcomes
1. Describe the procedure for evaluating the therapeutic outcomes obtained from prescribed medication therapy.

KEY TERMS

nursing process
nursing classification
   system
assessment
nursing diagnosis
actual nursing
   diagnosis
risk/high-risk nursing
   diagnosis
possible nursing
   diagnosis
wellness nursing
   diagnosis
syndrome nursing
   diagnosis
defining characteristics
medical diagnosis
collaborative problem
focused assessment
nursing care plan
critical care pathway
priority setting
measurable goal
   statements
patient goals
nursing actions

nursing interventions
nursing orders
anticipated therapeutic
   statements
expected outcome
   statements
nursing interventions
   or implementation
nursing actions
dependent actions
interdependent actions
independent actions
drug history
primary sources
subjective data
objective data
secondary sources
tertiary sources
drug monographs
side effects
pathophysiology
   (indications)
therapeutic intent
side effects to report
side effects to expect

ASSIGNMENTS

Read textbook, pp. 31-50.
Study Key Terms associated with chapter content.
Complete Chapter 4 Collaborative Activity.
Study Review Sheet for Chapter 4.
Complete Chapter 4 Practice Quiz.
Complete Chapter 4 Exam.

WEB RESEARCH ACTIVITY

Go to any search engine (e.g., yahoo.com) and type in "collaborative problem." Read one article on the subject.

COLLABORATIVE ACTIVITY

Complete the following activity to prepare for in-class discussion and group work that may be assigned by the instructor.

After reading the section "Nursing Process for Nausea and Vomiting," Chapter 33, pp. 470-482, identify the specific questions that could be used to gather data to develop an individualized care plan for a patient who is experiencing nausea and vomiting during pregnancy. Add questions appropriate to the person and situation.

Copyright © 2004 Mosby Inc. All rights reserved.

The Nursing Process and Pharmacology

Review Sheet

The QUESTION column and the ANSWER column have been offset so that you can cover the answer while reading the question, allowing you to assess your knowledge.

Question	Answer
1. Identify the purpose of nursing classification systems.	
2. Define *nursing diagnosis*.	1. Nursing classification systems provide a standardized language for recording and analysis of individualized nursing care delivery.
3. State the five steps of the nursing process.	2. A nursing diagnosis is a problem-solving method used in nursing.
4. Explain the purpose of the assessment phase of the nursing process.	3. The five steps of the nursing process are assessment, nursing diagnosis, planning, implementation, and evaluation.
5. What are defining characteristics?	4. Assessment is an ongoing data-gathering process used to identify existing (actual) patient problems and/or to identify patient problems that may be evolving.
6. How does a medical diagnosis differ from a nursing diagnosis?	5. Defining characteristics are existing signs and symptoms that help define the presence of a patient problem. They provide clinical evidence of an existing or developing patient problem.
7. What is a collaborative problem?	6. A medical diagnosis is a statement relating to a disease's or disorder's effect on the individual's physiological functioning. A nursing diagnosis defines a patient problem in which the nurse can intervene.
8. Why is a focused assessment beneficial to the nurse?	7. Collaborative problems require both medical or dental prescriptive orders and nursing interventions to monitor and evaluate the existing condition.
9. Differentiate among actual, risk, possible, wellness, and syndrome nursing diagnoses.	8. After establishing that a patient problem may or does exist, a focused assessment allows the nurse to concentrate the data collection process on a specific area that would help to define, validate, or negate the existence of a specific nursing diagnosis.
10. Explain the intent of using critical pathways.	9. See definitions in textbook, pp. 35-38.

Copyright © 2004 Mosby Inc. All rights reserved.

21

11. What are the four phases of the planning process used to prepare to provide patient care?

12. Use Maslow's hierarchy of needs on p. 39 of the text to label the following individual needs and prioritize them according to importance: a) need for family visitors, b) need to avoid falls while ambulating, c) need for basic care to prevent skin breakdown, d) need for praise for learning about self-care.

13. Which of the following are nursing actions?
    a. giving a bed bath
    b. forcing fluids
    c. taking vital signs
    d. developing a medical diagnosis statement

14. Label the following nursing actions as "D" for dependent, "I" for interdependent, and "ID" for independent:
    a. administering a tube feeding
    b. administering prn medications
    c. positioning patient for comfort
    d. providing oral hygiene
    e. monitoring respiratory function between treatments by respiratory therapist

15. Develop a short-term goal for a patient receiving Maalox.

16. Explain why a drug history may be beneficial.

17. Label the following statements "S" for subjective data or "O" for objective data.
    a. "My medication makes me dizzy."
    b. "Yesterday the pain medication gave me good pain relief."
    c. One hour after administration of chemotherapy the nurse charts, "Patient vomited 4 ounces greenish-tinged, watery vomitus."

18. Turn to a drug classification section in the textbook. Find the area labeled Nursing Diagnosis. Explain the difference between indications and side effects when used to designate the nursing diagnoses associated with drug therapy.

10. Critical pathways provide a sequential, detailed plan for clinical interventions within a specified time period for a particular disease or disorder.

11. Planning encompasses: a) setting priorities, b) developing measurable goal statements, c) formulating nursing interventions, and d) developing anticipated therapeutic outcomes as a basis for evaluating the patient's status.

12. During a period of ambulation, these needs would be in the following order: b, c, a, d. The priority may vary depending on variables present.

13. a, b, and c are nursing actions.

14. Items a and b are dependent, c and d are independent, and e is interdependent. Note: d could be dependent if the oral hygiene was specifically ordered by the HCP.

15. Multiple possible answers. One example is: The patient will be able to state the correct schedule for self-administration of Maalox on Tuesday, (date).

16. A drug history can be used to identify current drugs, OTC, and herbal products being taken or problems relating to drug therapy and to evaluate the need for medications.

17. Items a and b are subjective; c is objective.

Copyright © 2004 Mosby Inc. All rights reserved.

19. Develop a statement for the therapeutic intent of a sedative for a patient having surgery tomorrow morning.

20. Differentiate between side effects to expect and side effects to report.

21. List common laboratory studies used to evaluate liver (hepatic) function and those used to evaluate kidney (renal) function.

22. When are culture and sensitivity (C&S) tests taken?

23. What changes in the baseline CBC report should be reported to the HCP?

24. Why are serum drug levels monitored?

25. What patient education should be done prior to discharge for all persons with medications prescribed?

26. List a minimum of five drugs that can be monitored by a blood draw.

18. Indications are nursing diagnosis statements that exist as a result of patient problems being experienced due to disruption of normal functioning by a disease process or disorder. Side effects are patient problems that have evolved as a result of drug therapy.

19. Therapeutic intent is to "provide rest and relaxation prior to surgery."

20. Side effects to expect are those that can generally be anticipated when the drug therapy is prescribed. It is important for the nurse to teach the patient steps he/she can take to minimize the side effects to make the drug therapy more tolerable. Side effects to report, also known as adverse drug effects, are those that require notification of the physician regarding the drug's action.

21. Hepatic function tests include AST, ALT, alkaline phosphatase, LDH, and GGT. Renal function tests include serum creatinine, creatinine clearance, blood urea nitrogen (BUN), and urinalysis.

22. C&S specimens (e.g., throat culture) are usually obtained prior to initiation of antibiotic therapy for an infection.

23. Elevated WBCs, bands, "segs," and/or lymphocytes should be reported.

24. Serum drug levels are monitored to establish whether the serum blood level of the specific drug is too low or in the nontherapeutic range, within the normal range and therapeutic, or too high and toxic to the patient.

25. Patient education before discharge should include drug name, dosage, route, and specific time(s) of administration; reason for taking the drug (therapeutic outcome or intent); side effects to expect and ways these can be minimized or eliminated; side effects to report; what to do if a dose is missed; and how to have the medication prescription filled.

26. Digoxin, theophylline, gentamicin, tobramycin, lithium, lidocaine, phenytoin, procainamide, quinidine, vancomycin, cyclosporine, and chloramphenicol can be monitored by a blood draw.

Copyright © 2004 Mosby Inc. All rights reserved.

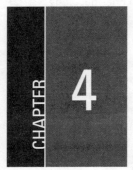

CHAPTER 4

The Nursing Process and Pharmacology

Practice Quiz

COMPLETION

Complete the following statements using Key Terms from Chapter 4.

1. Mary tells you she developed nausea and vomiting 4 hours after taking the first dose of her newly prescribed antibiotic. This would be an example of (subjective, objective) data.

2. The nursing instructor tells the student nurse to collect further data relating to this case. The collection of patient data is known as the _____ phase of the nursing process.

3. Further inquiry reveals that Mary took the antibiotic on an empty stomach. In addition to gaining further information about the nausea and vomiting, the student nurse also asks Mary to tell her of all other medications being taken, both prescription and nonprescription. This is known as taking a(n) _____. Mary indicates that she does not regularly take any other medicine.

4. After collecting the data, the student reviews the drug monograph on the antibiotic. It states that nausea and vomiting are side effects to expect if taken on an empty stomach. The student nurse compares the signs and symptoms present with the _____ listed in a nursing diagnosis resource book to establish the _____.

5. Rescheduling of the time the medication is taken is an example of a nursing _____. The student nurse suggests that Mary take the next dose of the medication with food.

6. Mary will self-administer the prescribed antibiotic with food at 6 AM, 12 noon, 6 PM, and midnight starting with the next dose. This is a _____ statement.

7. You notice on the HCP's order sheet that a lab draw is ordered for gentamicin sulfate for a patient that was assigned to you. Important information for the laboratory to know is _____.

8. When a culture and sensitivity is ordered on a patient it is important to be sure the test is performed _____ the first dose of medication is administered.

9. Nursing diagnosis statements dealing with a patient with a family history of a disease who is likely to develop the disease would be called _____ nursing diagnosis statements.

10. An example of a phrase of the nursing process called _____ is the periodic review of goals/outcomes of care.

11. A nursing minimum data set is an example of a(n) _____.

REVIEW QUESTIONS

_____ 1. A patient develops edema as a side effect to report to a prescribed medication. A gain of 5 lbs has occurred in 24 hours and 2+ edema is present in the legs. An appropriate nursing diagnosis statement would be:
   a. Fluid volume excess r/t calcium ion antagonist therapy (nifedipine) as evidenced by dependent edema (2+) and weight gain of 5 lbs in 24 hours.
   b. Fluid volume excess r/t drug therapy.
   c. Fluid volume excess r/t drug side effects evidenced by unknown etiology.
   d. Risk for fluid volume excess r/t drug side effects.

Copyright © 2004 Mosby Inc. All rights reserved.

_____ 2. The nursing diagnosis developed in question number 1 above is known as a(n):
  a. risk diagnosis.
  b. actual nursing diagnosis.
  c. collaborative nursing diagnosis.
  d. possible nursing diagnosis.

Copyright © 2004 Mosby Inc. All rights reserved.

Patient Education and Health Promotion

Syllabus

CHAPTER CONTENT

The Three Domains of Learning (p. 51)
Principles of Learning (p. 51)
Patient Education Associated with Medication
    Therapy (p. 55)

CHAPTER OBJECTIVES

The Three Domains of Learning
1. Differentiate among cognitive, affective, and psychomotor learning domain.

Principles of Learning
1. Identify the main principles of learning applied when teaching a patient, family, or group.
2. Apply the principles of learning to the content taught in pharmacology.

Patient Education Associated with Medication Therapy
1. Describe essential elements of patient education in relation to prescribed medications.
2. Describe the nurse's role in fostering patient responsibility for the maintenance of well-being and adhering to the therapeutic regimen.
3. Identify the types of information that should be discussed with the patient or significant others in order to establish reasonable expectations for prescribed therapy.
4. Discuss specific techniques used in your clinical practice setting to document patient education performed and degree of achievement attained.

KEY TERMS

cognitive domain
affective domain
psychomotor domain
objectives
ethnocentrism
scientific-biomedical
    paradigm
magicoreligious
    paradigm
holistic paradigm
health teaching

ASSIGNMENTS

Read textbook, pp. 51-58.
Study Key Terms associated with the chapter content.
Complete Chapter 5 Collaborative Activity.
Complete Chapter 5 Practice Quiz.
Complete Chapter 5 Exam.

COLLABORATIVE ACTIVITY

Complete the following activities to prepare for in-class discussion and group work that may be assigned by the instructor.

Purpose of Interview
The student will gain experience in data collection relating to medications. The data assembled will continue to be analyzed as the course progresses. For example, the techniques the individual describes for self-administration can be researched and analyzed during the study of medication administration.

Preparing for Interview
1. Read Chapter 5.
2. Go to the library and find two articles on health teaching, preferably relating to pharmacology. Read and analyze the articles for additional ideas on health teaching that might benefit you.

Copyright © 2004 Mosby Inc. All rights reserved.

3. Research recommended safe storage of medications in the home and available resources in the immediate area should an inadvertent poisoning occur.
4. Ask a friend, neighbor, or family member to participate in an interview regarding the medications currently being taken. Include both prescribed medications and over-the-counter (OTC) medicines. Stress that *NO* advice will be given regarding the medications; this is strictly a data-gathering activity.
5. In accordance with school policy, have appropriate release forms signed prior to initiating the interview.

Interview

1. Explain the purpose of the interview and stress that no medical advice will be given regarding the medications discussed.
2. Take notes, including the following information:
   a. In what type of environment was the interview conducted?
   b. List the medicines being taken by the interviewee, including those that have been prescribed by an HCP as well as those purchased over-the-counter.
   c. For each drug discussed (a minimum of three) note the following:
      1) Name of the drug
      2) Purpose for taking the drug
      3) Length of time the drug(s) have been taken (e.g., 1 week, 2 years)
      4) Instructions given regarding how or when to discontinue the medicines (e.g., "take until the entire prescription is finished")
      5) Importance of taking these drugs as prescribed
      6) Any annoying symptoms experienced since starting on the medications and what has been done to relieve them
      7) Time schedule used when taking these medicines
      8) Self-administration techniques used when taking the medications
      9) Where the drugs are stored in the household
3. If the interviewee has questions regarding the medications, suggest discussing them with the physician or pharmacist.

Note: It might be nice to send a thank-you note to the participant following the interview.

Data Analysis After the Interview

The data gathered during this interview will continue to be used as the course progresses and the student gains more knowledge of the study of pharmacology.

1. For each drug listed, state the generic and brand names.
2. Examine the drug monographs for the drugs listed. What are the anticipated therapeutic outcomes of these medicines? How does the information in the drug monograph correlate with the data provided by the interviewee?
3. Based on the length of time the drug has been taken, is it possible that drug tolerance may have occurred?
4. Read each drug monograph. Do any of the medicines being taken require gradual withdrawal upon discontinuation? What instructions should be given regarding the scheduling of the dosages? Was the time schedule the interviewee described appropriate for the medicine being taken?
5. What perception does the individual have of the importance of the medicines to the condition for which the medicines were prescribed? In the interviewee's opinion, are the medications important to the overall treatment of the condition?
6. What side effects to expect and side effects to report are listed for each drug in the monograph? Did the interviewee experience any of these? If so, were the actions used to minimize them appropriate?
7. Were the techniques of self-administration appropriate and accurate? If not, what changes should be suggested?
8. Based on the data collected, what nursing diagnosis statements are appropriate for the individual interviewed?
9. Establish goals and a health teaching plan for the person interviewed.
10. Was the person interviewed anxious to learn more about his/her medications? If so, how could you be of assistance?
11. Were drugs stored safely in the home setting? What suggestions could be made to improve the storage of or access to the medications?

Copyright © 2004 Mosby Inc. All rights reserved.

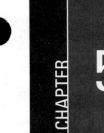

CHAPTER 5

Patient Education and Health Promotion

Practice Quiz

TRUE OR FALSE

Mark "T" for true or "F" for false for each statement.
<u>*Correct all false statements*</u>.

_____ 1. Explaining the various self-care needs to an individual and exploring his/her prior knowledge is an example of the affective domain learning.

_____ 2. Establishing an environment that is conducive to learning is essential to the overall learning process.

_____ 3. Deciding what to teach and how much to teach is essential to the learning process.

_____ 4. Utilizing an established teaching plan that all nurses can build on is important to the continuity of health teaching.

_____ 5. Health teaching is valued by all individuals equally.

_____ 6. Children may need adaptations in prepared learning materials based on their age, learning capabilities, and development.

_____ 7. It is best to explain all of the information needed for self-care so the teaching plan on the chart documents that all the health teaching was accomplished prior to discharge.

_____ 8. The magicoreligious belief system stresses that humans are under control of supernatural forces.

_____ 9. The scientific-biomedical belief system emphasizes health promotion and restoration.

_____ 10. Illness may not have the same meaning for all individuals.

REVIEW QUESTIONS

_____ 1. According to the magicoreligious belief system, health is:
   a. a supernatural agent with or without justification via sorcery.
   b. a gift as a sign of God's blessing.
   c. the fate of the world.
   d. based on mystical causes.

_____ 2. Short hospitalization stays have influenced patient education delivery by making it difficult to do all *except*:
   a. assess readiness to learn.
   b. assess learning has occurred.
   c. having time to motivate the patient.
   d. requesting referral to home health.

Copyright © 2004 Mosby Inc. All rights reserved.

A Review of Arithmetic

Syllabus

CHAPTER CONTENT

CHAPTER OBJECTIVES

Roman Numerals
1. Read and write selected numerical values using Roman numerals.

Fractions
1. Demonstrate proficiency in calculating mathematical problems using addition, subtraction, multiplication, and/or division of fractions.

Decimal Fractions
1. Demonstrate proficiency in calculating mathematical problems using the addition, subtraction, multiplication, and/or division of decimals.
2. Convert decimals to fractions and fractions to decimals.

Percents
1. Demonstrate proficiency in calculating mathematical problems using percents.
2. Convert percents to fractions, percents to decimals, decimal fractions to percents, and common fractions to percents.

Ratios
1. Demonstrate proficiency in converting ratios to percents and percents to ratios, in simplifying ratios, and in using the proportion method for solving problems.

Systems of Weights and Measures
1. Memorize the basic equivalents of the household, apothecary, and metric systems.
2. Demonstrate proficiency in performing conversion of medication problems utilizing the household, apothecary, and metric systems.

Calculation of Intravenous Fluid and Medication Rates
1. Use formulas to calculate intravenous fluid and medicine administration rates.

Fahrenheit and Centigrade (Celsius) Temperatures
1. Demonstrate proficiency in performing conversions between the centigrade and Fahrenheit systems of temperature measurement.

KEY TERMS

numerator	milligram
denominator	gram
household	kilogram
measurements	administration sets
apothecary	drip chamber
measurements	macrodrip
grain	microdrip
minim	drop factor
milliliter	rounding
centimeter	centigrade
metric system	Fahrenheit
liter	Celsius

ASSIGNMENTS

Read textbook, pp. 59-77.
Complete Chapter 6 Practice Quiz Parts 1 and 2.
Complete Chapter 6 Exam.

Copyright © 2004 Mosby Inc. All rights reserved.

Student Name_____

A Review of Arithmetic

Practice Quiz (Part 1)

EQUIVALENTS AND CONVERSION

Memorize the equivalents listed in Chapter 6, then do the following self-test. Write the answer in the blank provided.

Household Equivalents

1. 4 cups = _____ quarts
2. 1 tablespoon = _____ teaspoons
3. 8 ounces = _____ cup(s)
4. 1 pint = _____ cup(s)

Apothecary Equivalents

5. 1 fluid dram = _____ ml
6. 8 fluid drams = _____ fluid ounces
7. 8 drams = _____ grains
8. 1 dram = _____ grains

Metric Equivalents

9. 1 ml = _____ cc
10. 1 liter = _____ ml
11. 1 milligram (mg) = _____ micrograms (µg)
12. 1 gram (g) = _____ milligrams (mg)
13. 1 gram (g) = _____ grains (gr)

Conversion Rules

14. To convert grams to grains:

15. To convert grains to grams:

16. To convert milligrams to grams:

17. To convert grains to milligrams:

STOP! IF YOU HAVE NOT MEMORIZED THE EQUIVALENTS AND THE CONVERSION RULES YOU SHOULD NOT PROCEED UNTIL YOU HAVE DONE SO.

Copyright © 2004 Mosby Inc. All rights reserved.

CHAPTER 6

A Review of Arithmetic

Practice Quiz (Part 2)

ROMAN NUMERALS

Convert the following Arabic numerals to Roman numerals.

1. 5   =   _____
2. 7 1/2 =   _____
3. 4   =   _____
4. 15   =   _____
5. 20   =   _____
6. 24   =   _____

FRACTIONS

Identify the numerator or denominator for each of the following fractions as indicated.

7. 1/5   numerator is _____
8. 2/3   numerator is _____
9. 3/8   numerator is _____
10. 1 1/2   denominator is _____
11. 9/10   denominator is _____
12. 2 2/5   numerator is _____
13. 6/10   denominator is _____
14. 1 1/3   denominator is _____

Which of the following fractions is the largest? Circle your answer.

15. 1/8 or 1/16
16. 2/3 or 3/4
17. 1/100 or 1/200
18. 1/4 or 1/3
19. 3/8 or 7/8
20. 1/150 or 1/90

Reduce the following fractions.

21. 4/16   =   _____
22. 12/24   =   _____
23. 4/8   =   _____
24. 36/48   =   _____
25. 1 12/18 =   _____
26. 3 34/85 =   _____
27. 1 6/8   =   _____

28. 12 6/8   =   _____
29. 2 30/60 =   _____
30. 3/9   =   _____

Write the following fractions as decimals. When applicable, carry the decimal to thousandths and round to <u>hundredths</u>.

31. 7/8   =   _____
32. 5/6   =   _____
33. 1 3/4   =   _____
34. 2/3   =   _____
35. 15/16   =   _____
36. 1/3   =   _____
37. 5/8   =   _____
38. 7/9   =   _____
39. 1/16   =   _____
40. 1/2   =   _____

Multiply the following fractions. Reduce answers to lowest terms.

41. 1/3 × 1/4 =
42. 2/3 × 3/8 =
43. 7/8 × 1/2 =
44. 3/4 × 7/8 =
45. 1/2 × 4/7 =
46. 7/8 × 2/3 =
47. 1 1/2 × 3/4 =
48. 2 2/3 × 4/5 =

Divide the following. As appropriate, carry to hundredths and round to <u>tenths</u>.

49. 2/3 ÷ 7/8 =
50. 1/3 ÷ 1/2 =
51. 5/9 ÷ 1/4 =
52. 21.78 ÷ 1.23 =
53. 756 ÷ 12.3 =
54. 32 ÷ 1.78 =
55. 112 ÷ 0.06 =
56. 1.22 ÷ 0.32 =
57. 3.789 ÷ 0.112 =

Copyright © 2004 Mosby Inc. All rights reserved.

33

Student Name _____

Change the following percents to decimals and the fractions to percents.

58. 56%   =   _____
59. 1/150   =   _____%
60. 2/3   =   _____%
61. 75%   =   _____
62. 1/2%   =   _____
63. 3/4   =   _____%
64. 7/8   =   _____%
65. 123%   =   _____

Change the following decimals to fractions and the fractions to decimals.

66. 0.3   =   _____
67. 0.003   =   _____
68. 0.03   =   _____
69. 4/10   =   _____
70. 4/100   =   _____
71. 4/1000   =   _____

Change the following percents to ratios.

72. 75%   =   _____
73. 60%   =   _____
74. 1/2%   =   _____

Convert the following using equivalency tables.

75. 1 quart = _____ cup(s)
76. _____ ounces = 1 pint
77. 3 teaspoon = _____ tablespoon(s)
78. 2 g = _____ gr
79. 0.125 g = _____ mg
80. 6 gr = _____ mg
81. 250 mg = _____ g
82. 1 fl dram = _____ ml
83. 1 teaspoon = _____ ml
84. 6 lbs = _____ kg (round to hundredths)
85. 165 lbs = _____ kg

REVIEW QUESTIONS

Perform questions throughout the chapter.

Copyright © 2004 Mosby Inc. All rights reserved.

7

CHAPTER

Principles of Medication Administration

Syllabus

CHAPTER CONTENT

Legal and Ethical Considerations (p. 78)
Patient Charts (p. 79)
Drug Distribution Systems (p. 89)
The Drug Order (p. 93)
The Six Rights of Drug Administration (p. 95)

CHAPTER OBJECTIVES

Legal and Ethical Considerations
1. Identify the limitations relating to medication administration placed on licensed practical nurses, vocational nurses, registered nurses, and nurse clinicians in the nurse practice act in the state where you will be practicing.
2. Study the policies and procedures of the practice setting to identify specific regulations concerning medication administration by licensed practical nurses, vocational nurses, registered nurses, and nurse clinicians.

Patient Charts
1. Identify the basic categories of information available in a patient's chart.
2. Study the patient charts at different practice settings to identify the various formats used to chart patient data.
3. Cite the information contained in a Kardex and describe the purpose of this file.

Drug Distribution Systems
1. Cite the advantages and disadvantages of the ward stock system, computer-controlled ordering and dispensing system, the individual prescription order system, the unit dose system.
2. Study the narcotic control system used at your assigned clinical practice setting and compare it to the requirements of the Controlled Substance Act of 1970.

The Drug Order
1. Define the four categories of medication orders used.
2. Describe the procedure used in your assigned clinical setting for taking, recording, transcribing, and verifying verbal medication orders.

Medication Errors
1. Identify common types of drug errors and actions needed for their prevention.

The Six Rights of Drug Administration
1. Identify specific precautions needed to ensure that the *right drug* is prepared for the patient.
2. Memorize and recite standard abbreviations associated with the scheduling of medications.
3. Identify data found in the patient's chart used to determine if the patient has abnormal renal or hepatic function.
4. Describe specific safety precautions the nurse should implement to ensure that correct medication calculations are performed.
5. Review the policies and procedures of your practice setting to identify drugs for which doses must be checked by two qualified persons.
6. Describe the methods that should be used to ensure that the correct patient receives the correct medication, by the correct route, in the correct amount, at the correct time.
7. Compare each safety measure describing safe preparation and administration of medications with those procedures used at your clinical practice setting.
8. Identify appropriate nursing actions for documenting the administration and therapeutic effectiveness of each medication administered.

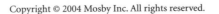

Copyright © 2004 Mosby Inc. All rights reserved.

KEY TERMS

nurse practice act
standards of care
summary sheet
consent forms
physician's order form
history and physical
    examination form
progress notes
critical pathways
nurse's notes
nursing care plan
laboratory tests record
graphic record
flow sheet
consultation reports
other diagnostic tests
medication
    administration
    record (MAR)
prn or unscheduled
    medication record
unscheduled
    medication orders
case management plan
patient education
    record

Kardex records
floor or ward stock
    system
individual prescription
    system
computer-controlled
    ordering and
    dispensing system
unit dose system
long-term care unit
    dose system
stat orders
standing orders
renewal orders
prn order
Adverse Drug Events
    (ADEs)
Computerized
    Physician Order
    Entry (CPOE)
Clinical Decision
    Making Support
    System (CDSS)
verification
transcription

ASSIGNMENTS

Read textbook, pp. 78-99.
Study Key Terms associated with chapter content.
Complete Chapter 7 Collaborative Activities.
Study Review Sheet for Chapter 7.
Complete Chapter 7 Practice Quiz.
Complete Chapter 7 Exam.

WEB RESEARCH ACTIVITY

Go to: http://www.ahrq.gov/qual/errorsix.htm and read the article on Medication Errors and Safety.

COLLABORATIVE ACTIVITIES

Complete the following activities to prepare for in-class discussion and group work that may be assigned by the instructor.

1. Research how drug orders are taken and transcribed in the clinical sites where you are assigned. Include rules for orders that are received by fax.

2. Charting Exercise
   a. What time frames are used in the clinical site where you are assigned when drugs are ordered?

Abbreviation	*Time Frame*
bid	
tid	
ac	
pc	
qid	
q 4 h	
q 6 h	
hs	

   b. Use the MAR record on the next page and other forms as appropriate from a clinical site where you are assigned to transcribe the following orders. Use military time and the customary time frames for medication scheduling.

   Chart for: Martha Washburn
                    1616 Tangerine Blvd.
                    Hometown, Pa.
                    Rm. 454—Bed 2
                    Patient No. 123456
                    Dr. Ballantyne

Physician's Order Form

Date:	Time:	Physician's Order:	Doctor:
Today	0700	acebutolol 400 mg PO, bid	
		acetaminophen 600 mg PO,	
		q 3 h, prn temperature	
		> 101.6° F	
		cefadroxil 1000 mg PO, bid	
		MOM 30 ml daily	
		prn constipation	
			Signed by Dr. Ballantyne

Copyright © 2004 Mosby Inc. All rights reserved.

MEDICATION ADMINISTRATION RECORD

NAME:	RM-BD:	Init	Signature	Title
ID NO.:	AGE:			
DIAGNOSIS:	SEX:			

| PHYSICIAN: | Ht: | Wt: |

SCHEDULED MEDICATIONS

DATE	MEDICATION-STRENGTH-FORM-ROUTE	0030-0729	0730-1529	1530-0029

** PRN MEDICATIONS**

Copyright © 2004 Mosby Inc. All rights reserved.

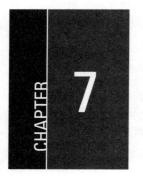

Principles of Medication Administration

Review Sheet

The Question column and the Answer column have been offset so that you can cover the answer while reading the question, allowing you to assess your knowledge.

Question	**Answer**
1. What is the Nurse Practice Act?	
2. What are the Standards of Care in relationship to nursing?	1. The Nurse Practice Act establishes the rules and regulations for the practice of nursing at the various entry levels within a practice area within each state.
3. Can an employing agency write policies that require the nurse to exceed the standards established by the state board of nursing/nursing licensing agency?	2. Guidelines for practice of nursing as defined by the Nurse Practice Act, the Joint Commission on Accreditation of Healthcare Organizations (JCAHO) and professional nursing organizations (e.g., American Nurses Association [ANA] and specialty nursing organizations).
4. What types of medications may have restrictions regarding the qualifications of an individual to administer the medicine?	3. No. Policies of the employing agency can authorize less than, but not more than, the established maximum standards.
5. What information is the nurse expected to know about a specific drug before administering it?	4. Antineoplastic medicines, Imferon, RhoGAM, allergy extracts, and heparin are administered in accordance with specific limitations of the employing agency. Most policies require doses of heparin and insulin to be checked by two qualified individuals. Additional policies are developed to identify guidelines within a particular clinical site for the administration of intravenous therapy.
6. What information should be recorded whenever a "prn" medicine is to be administered?	5. See textbook, p. 78.
7. What role do critical pathways have on the delivery of clinical care?	6. Date, time, drug name, dose, route of administration, reason for administration, and the patient's response to the medication.
8. Examine the sections on a medication administration record (MAR) to identify the categories used.	7. Critical pathways are a multidisciplinary plan used by all health care providers to track the individual's progress toward expected outcomes within a specified time period.
9. Where would information regarding a patient's possible allergies be found?	8. Medication administration records are usually divided into four sections: scheduled section, parenteral section, stat section, and prn medication section.

 Copyright © 2004 Mosby Inc. All rights reserved.

10. Explain the differences among the ward stock, computer-controlled ordering and dispensing system, individual prescription order, and unit dose drug distribution (acute and long-term care) systems.
11. Identify procedures for the electronic transmission of patient orders.
12. What are adverse drug events (ADEs)?

13. Briefly discuss newly developed computerized physician order entry (CPOE) systems that are supported by clinical decision making support systems (CDSSs).
14. Referring to the narcotic substance inventory form, Figure 7-11 in the textbook, list narcotic drugs routinely used in the acute care setting.
15. What information is recorded on the controlled substance inventory form when a controlled substance is administered?
16. Explain the differences between a stat order, standing order, prn order, verbal order, and fax order.

17. How is a drug order verified and transcribed?
18. What are the six "rights" of drug administration?
19. What tests are used to identify hepatic and renal function?

20. What methods are used to ensure correct identification of a patient prior to drug administration? (Discuss adults, children, and inpatient and outpatient settings.)

21. Review commonly used abbreviations for the scheduling of medication administration.

9. Information about a patient's allergies is recorded in the history and physical section of the chart, the Kardex, the MAR, the patient's chart holder, and on the patient's allergy bracelet.

10. See textbook, pp. 89-91.

11. Faxed orders must be signed within a specified time, often 24 hours.
12. See textbook, p. 94.

13. See textbook, pp. 89-90.

14. See Figure 7-11, p. 92.

15. The date, time, name of medicine administered, patient's name, amount wasted (if any), and the number of dosage containers (such as unit dose tablets or ampules) remaining after the drug is removed are recorded on the form. The nurse administering the medicine signs the record as well as the qualified witness if any medicine is wasted.
16. See textbook, p. 93.
17. See textbook, pp. 94-95.

18. The six "rights" of drug administration are: right drug, right time, right dose, right patient, right route, and right documentation.
19. Liver function tests include aspartate aminotransferase (AST), alanine aminotransferase (ALT), alkaline phosphatase, lactic dehydrogenase (LDH), and gamma glutamyl transferase (GGT). Renal function tests include serum creatinine, creatinine clearance, blood urea nitrogen (BUN), and urinalysis.
20. See textbook, p. 96.

21. See textbook Appendix A, Prescription Abbreviations.

Copyright © 2004 Mosby Inc. All rights reserved.

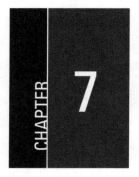

Principles of Medication Administration

Practice Quiz

MATCHING

Match the definition with the corresponding term. Definitions may be used more than once and some may not be used.

_____ 1. prn medications
_____ 2. physician's order form
_____ 3. MAR
_____ 4. "stat"
_____ 5. Kardex

a. Check this section of the patient chart when questioning details of a drug order on the MAR.
b. Give around-the-clock.
c. Give immediately.
d. Administer as required or necessary within defined limits of the drug order.
e. Record scheduled drugs administered here.
ab. Section of the patient record containing the care plan.
ac. Controlled substances are recorded here when administered.

MULTIPLE CHOICE

Select the BEST answer and write the letter selected in the space provided.

_____ 6. 6 AM in military time is
    a. 0600.
    b. 1200.
    c. 1800.
    d. 2200.

_____ 7. 2 PM in military time is
    a. 0200.
    b. 0600.
    c. 1200.
    d. 1400.

_____ 8. The inventory control record is completed when the
    a. patient asks for a controlled substance.
    b. controlled substance is removed.
    c. medication is administered.
    d. degree of pain relief is assessed.

_____ 9. The prn medication record is completed
    a. when the patient asks for a controlled substance.
    b. when the controlled substance is removed.
    c. immediately after administering the drug.
    d. when the degree of pain relief is assessed.

_____ 10. The narcotic control count is performed by
    a. the charge nurse.
    b. a nurse going off duty.
    c. a nurse coming on duty.
    d. two nurses; one from shift going off duty and one from shift coming on duty.

_____ 11. A drug on a scheduled order is given
    a. as many times as needed.
    b. at prescribed/designated intervals.
    c. one time only.
    d. immediately.

_____ 12. A student nurse may accept a verbal drug order.
    a. true
    b. false

_____ 13. When a verbal order is taken it must be co-signed and dated by the physician within
    a. 3 days.
    b. 2 days.
    c. 24 hours.
    d. 12 hours.

Copyright © 2004 Mosby Inc. All rights reserved.

_____ 14. The person responsible for the transcription of the drug order is the
   a. nurse's aide.
   b. unit secretary/ward clerk.
   c. physician.
   d. nurse.

_____ 15. When "wasting" a portion of a dose of narcotic, the nurse must have this witnessed by
   a. the prescribing physician.
   b. the charge nurse.
   c. a second qualified nurse.
   d. the medication aide.

_____ 16. When measuring a fractional dose of a medication with a volume of less than 1 ml, the most accurate method would be to use a
   a. medicine cup.
   b. tuberculin syringe.
   c. teaspoon.
   d. medicine dropper.

_____ 17. The most reliable method of calculating pediatric drug doses is using
   a. body surface area (BSA).
   b. Clark's rule.
   c. a fraction of the adult dose.
   d. Pyxis system of measurement.

_____ 18. A client has a new drug ordered bid. This means the drug will be administered
   a. once daily.
   b. two times per day.
   c. three times per day.
   d. four times per day.

_____ 19. The Pyxis system refers to a(n)
   a. narcotic inventory system.
   b. individual prescription order system.
   c. unit dose system used primarily in long-term care.
   d. electronic medication dispensing system.

_____ 20. The medication administration record (MAR) in a long-term care setting is designed to be used for
   a. 8 hours.
   b. 24 hours.
   c. 1 week.
   d. 1 month.

_____ 21. Faxed medication orders are usually signed by the health care provider within
   a. 8 hours.
   b. 12 hours.
   c. 24 hours.
   d. 48 hours.

_____ 22. Electronic database charting systems may vary but they must comply with guidelines/requirements of _____ while incorporating standards of care.
   a. American Nurses Association
   b. Joint Commission on Accreditation of Healthcare Organizations
   c. Intravenous Nurses Society
   d. National League of Nurses

_____ 23. Unit dose systems in a long-term care setting supply enough medication containers for a(n) _____ period.
   a. 8 hour
   b. 24 hour
   c. 48 hour
   d. one week

CRITICAL THINKING QUESTIONS

24. What information is included on a written prescription?
25. Explain the procedure used to check the drug name against the drug order during the preparation of medications.
26. Describe procedures used within the immediate clinical practice setting to prevent adverse drug events (ADEs).

REVIEW QUESTIONS

_____ 1. A patient refuses an essential heart medication that has been prescribed. The nurse should first:
   a. call the physician.
   b. report it to the head nurse.
   c. seek patient reasons.
   d. document refusal on MAR.

Copyright © 2004 Mosby Inc. All rights reserved.

_____ 2. General guidelines for entering nurses'
notes include completing nursing entries:
   a. whenever the patient complains.
   b. whenever the head nurse requests.
   c. on admission, after prn medications,
      and before leaving area.
   d. periodically throughout the shift as
      care needs dictate.

Copyright © 2004 Mosby Inc. All rights reserved.

Percutaneous Administration

Syllabus

CHAPTER CONTENT

CHAPTER OBJECTIVES

Administration of Creams, Lotions, and Ointments

1. Describe the topical forms of medications used on the skin.
2. Cite the equipment needed and techniques used to apply each of the topical forms of medications to the skin surface.

Patch Testing for Allergens

1. Describe the procedure used and purpose of performing patch testing.
2. Describe specific charting methods used with allergy testing.

Administration of Nitroglycerin Ointment

1. Identify the equipment needed, sites and techniques used, and patient education required when nitroglycerin ointment is prescribed.
2. Describe specific documentation methods used to record the therapeutic effectiveness of nitroglycerin ointment therapy.

Administration of Transdermal Drug Delivery Systems

1. Identify the equipment needed, sites used, techniques employed, and patient education required when transdermal medication systems are prescribed.
2. Describe specific documentation methods used to record the therapeutic effectiveness of medications administered using a transdermal delivery system.

Administration of Topical Powders

1. Describe the dosage form, sites used, and techniques employed to administer medications in topical powder form.

Administration of Medications to Mucous Membranes

1. Describe the dosage forms, sites, equipment used, and techniques for administration of medications to the mucous membranes.
2. Identify the dosage forms safe for administration to the eye.
3. Describe patient education necessary for patients requiring ophthalmic medications.
4. Compare the techniques used to administer eardrops in a patient under age 3 with those over age 3.
5. Describe the purpose, precautions necessary, and patient education required for persons requiring medications by inhalation.
6. Describe the dose forms available for vaginal administration of medications.
7. Identify the equipment needed, sites used, and specific techniques required to administer vaginal medications or douches.

Copyright © 2004 Mosby Inc. All rights reserved.

8. State the rationale and procedure used for cleansing vaginal applicators or douche tips following use.
9. Develop a plan for patient education of persons taking medications via the percutaneous routes.

KEY TERMS

creams
lotions
ointments
dressings
allergens
antigens
patch testing

transdermal patch
buccal
ophthalmic
otic
nebulae
aerosols
metered-dose inhalers

ASSIGNMENTS

Read textbook, pp. 100-117.
Study Key Terms associated with chapter content.
Study Review Sheet for Chapter 8.
Complete Chapter 8 Practice Quiz.
Complete Chapter 8 Exam.

WEB RESEARCH ACTIVITY

Go to: http://www.ahcpr.gov/clinic/cpgonline.htm.

1. Identify the areas of clinical practice guidelines available on this site.
2. Access the Pressure Ulcer Treatment Site—Clinical Guide and review Dressings AND Adjunctive Therapies.

Copyright © 2004 Mosby Inc. All rights reserved.

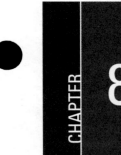
Percutaneous Administration

Review Sheet

The Question column and the Answer column have been offset so that you can cover the answer while reading the question, allowing you to assess your knowledge.

Question	**Answer**
1. What factors affect the absorption of topical medications?	
2. What is the major advantage of the percutaneous route for drug administration?	1. Factors affecting the absorption of topical medications include drug concentration, the length of time the medication is in contact with the skin, size and depth of affected area, and thickness and hydration of the skin.
3. Explain the differences among a cream, lotion, ointment, and wet dressing and cite the methods used to apply each.	2. The action of the drug is primarily limited to the site of application, thereby decreasing the systemic side effects.
4. What health teaching should be given to a patient using a topical form of medication?	3. See textbook, p. 100.
5. What is the purpose of patch testing?	4. Patients receiving topical medications should receive the following health teaching: personal hygiene measures to treat/improve underlying condition, methods of application, ways to avoid touching affected areas, and prevention of spread of infection when present.
6. Describe the method used to apply allergens and read results.	5. Patch testing is used to identify specific sensitivity to allergens.
7. List commonly used symbols for reading of reactions to allergen testing.	6. See textbook, pp. 101-103.
8. Describe the specific method used to apply nitroglycerin ointment and a nitroglycerin transdermal disk.	7. Commonly used symbols for reading allergen patch test reactions include (see also p. 102):

7. (continued)

+	1+ no wheal, 3 mm flare
++	2+ 2–3 mm wheal with flare
+++	3+ 3–5 mm wheal with flare
++++	4+ > 5 mm wheal

Question	**Answer**
9. Why is it important for the nurse to wear gloves when applying a topical ointment or transdermal patch?	8. See textbook, pp. 103-106.
10. What types of medications are available in transdermal patch form?	9. The nurse should wear gloves when administering a topical ointment or transdermal patch to avoid inadvertent absorption of the medication by the nurse through the skin.

Copyright © 2004 Mosby Inc. All rights reserved.

11. Why is it important to discard transdermal medication patches safely after removal?

12. What schedule is used for the administration of the estrogen transdermal system Ortho-Evra patch?

13. Where are sublingual and buccal forms of medication administered?

14. What is the primary advantage of the sublingual route?

15. What abbreviations are used for ophthalmic medications?

16. Describe the correct techniques for administering eye drops, eye ointments, and eye disks, including patient teaching.

17. Compare the correct technique of administering an ear (otic) drug to a child and to an adult.

18. Explain the procedure for instilling nose drops/nasal sprays into an adult and a child; include health teaching.

19. Why shouldn't oily preparations be administered by inhalation?

20. Explain how to give medications by inhalation.

21. What is a metered-dose inhaler?

22. Explain how to teach a patient to administer a medication using an inhaler.

23. Explain the correct technique for inserting a vaginal suppository and proper hygiene measures used during the course of treatment.

10. Nitroglycerin, clonidine, estrogen, nicotine, scopolamine, fentanyl, and Ortho-Evra are available in transdermal patch forms.

11. Used transdermal patches must be safely discarded because the patch may still contain some medication that could be harmful to individuals or pets for whom it is not prescribed.

12. Ortho-Evra transdermal system is worn continuously for 3 weeks, with week 4 patch-free.

13. Sublingual medications are administered under the tongue; buccal medications are administered in the back cheek area of the mouth.

14. In addition to being easy to access, the sublingual area provides rapid absorption and onset of action of the drug because the drug passes directly into the systemic circulation with no immediate pass through the liver, where extensive metabolism usually takes place.

15. All medications used in the eye should be specifically labeled FOR OPHTHALMIC USE. Abbreviations used are:
    os = left eye
    od = right eye
    ou = both eyes

16. See textbook, pp. 108-110.

17. See textbook, p. 110.

18. See textbook, pp. 111-112.

19. Oily preparations should not be administered by inhaler because oil droplets would be carried to the lungs and initiate a lipid pneumonia.

20. See textbook, pp. 113-114.

21. A metered-dose inhaler is an aerosolized, pressurized inhaler that delivers a measured amount of medication with each depression of the device.

22. See textbook, p. 114.

23. See textbook, pp. 114-115.

Copyright © 2004 Mosby Inc. All rights reserved.

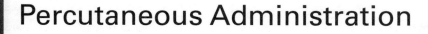

CHAPTER 8

Percutaneous Administration

Practice Quiz

CRITICAL THINKING QUESTIONS

1. When applying topical drugs, the site should be cleansed prior to application of the new dose of medication. Explain how to cleanse the site correctly.
2. Why are gloves worn when applying topical dosage forms of medication?
3. Which type of topical medication needs to be shaken well prior to administration?
4. Describe the correct techniques for application of ointments and creams.

CHARTING

Chart the essential data in the following situation. M.T. has a red, weeping, ulcerated area on the lower leg that is to be dressed using neomycin powder. Use today's date and time when doing the charting.

MEDICATION ADMINISTRATION RECORD

NAME: ID NO.: DIAGNOSIS:	RM-BD: AGE: SEX:	Init Signature Title
PHYSICIAN:	Ht:	Wt:

SCHEDULED MEDICATIONS

DATE	MEDICATION-STRENGTH-FORM-ROUTE	0030-0729	0730-1529	1530-0029

** PRN MEDICATIONS**				

Copyright © 2004 Mosby Inc. All rights reserved.

5. M.T. is to receive 1/2" of nitroglycerin topical ointment at 9 PM. Explain how to measure and apply the dose at site 8 on the figure below. Chart the medication using today's date on M.T.'s chart in the situation above.

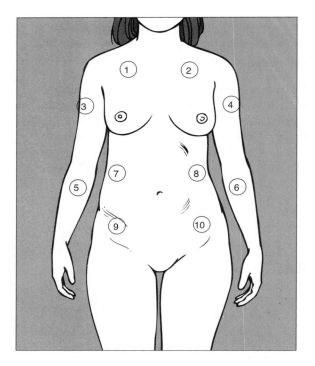

6. Explain the correct technique for applying a topical disk containing nitroglycerin and state the patient teaching that would be appropriate while performing this task.
7. A.H. is using nitroglycerin sublingually and is keeping the medication at the bedside. What data would you collect during and at the end of the shift to include in the charting?
8. Use M.T.'s chart already provided to chart the following medication:
   Timoptic one drop in both eyes at 8 AM daily
9. Describe the correct technique for instilling eye drops.
10. Explain the rationale for blocking the inner corner (canthus) of the eye for 1–2 minutes after instilling an eye medication.
11. Differentiate between the direction you pull the earlobe in a child under 3 years old and in an adult when instilling ear drops.

12. Why should you have the individual blow his/her nose gently prior to instilling nose drops or a nasal spray?
13. Describe the health teaching that should be completed when nasal spray or nose drops are being used.
14. Explain the procedure for administering a medication using a metered-dose inhaler.
15. Explain the procedure for positioning the patient, inserting the medication, and providing follow-up care to a patient having a vaginal cream inserted.

REVIEW QUESTIONS

_____ 1. How long a drug-free period is usually recommended when nitroglycerin ointment is being prescribed?
   a. 3–4 hours off q 24 hours
   b. 5–10 hours off q 24 hours
   c. 10–12 hours off q 24 hours
   d. 12–24 hours off q 24 hours

_____ 2. Fentanyl patches do not usually achieve a sufficient blood level for pain control until _____ hours after initial application.
   a. 6
   b. 8
   c. 10
   d. 12

_____ 3. The standard abbreviation used for administering a prescribed ophthalmic medication in both eyes is:
   a. os.
   b. od.
   c. ou.
   d. bil.

Copyright © 2004 Mosby Inc. All rights reserved.

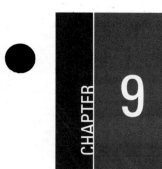

Enteral Administration

Syllabus

CHAPTER CONTENT

Administration of Oral Medications (p. 118)
Administration of Solid-Form Oral Medications
    (p. 121)
Administration of Liquid-Form Oral Medications
    (p. 123)
Administration of Medications by Nasogastric Tube
    (p. 125)
Administration of Enteral Feedings (p. 126)
Administration of Rectal Suppositories (p. 128)
Administration of a Disposable Enema (p. 130)

CHAPTER OBJECTIVES

Administration of Oral Medications
1. Correctly define and identify oral dose forms of
    medications.
2. Identify common receptacles used to administer
    oral medications.

Administration of Solid-Form Oral Medications
1. Describe general principles of administering
    solid forms of medications and the different
    techniques utilized with a medication card,
    computer-controlled distribution, and unit dose
    distribution systems.

Administration of Liquid-Form Oral Medications
1. Compare techniques used to administer liquid
    forms of oral medications using a medication
    card and unit dose systems of distribution.

Administration of Medications by Nasogastric Tube
1. Cite the equipment needed, techniques used,
    and precautions necessary when administering
    medications via a nasogastric (NG) tube.

Administration of Enteral Feedings Via Gastrostomy or Jejunostomy Tube
1. Meet the person's basic metabolic requirements
    and provide adequate nutritional intake through
    the use of enteral nutrition support.

Administration of Rectal Suppositories
1. Cite the equipment needed and techniques used
    to administer rectal suppositories.

Administration of a Disposable Enema
1. Cite the equipment needed and techniques used
    to administer a disposable enema.

KEY TERMS

capsules	unit dose packaging
lozenges	bar coded packaging
tablets	soufflé cup
elixirs	medicine cup
emulsions	medicine dropper
suspensions	oral syringe
syrups	nasogastric tube

ASSIGNMENTS

Read textbook, pp. 118-131.
Study Key Terms associated with chapter content.
Study Review Sheet for Chapter 9.
Complete Chapter 9 Practice Quiz.
Complete Chapter 9 Exam.

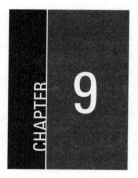

Enteral Administration

Review Sheet

The Question column and the Answer column have been offset so that you can cover the answer while reading the question, allowing you to assess your knowledge.

Question

1. When an individual is unable to swallow or has had oral surgery, an alternative route of administration is the _____ route.
2. A major advantage of using the rectal route for drug administration is _____.
3. List the composition and advantages of the following dosage forms: capsules, timed-release capsules, lozenges, tablets, elixirs, emulsions, suspensions, and syrups.
4. Why is it important to use the medicine dropper that accompanies a medication?
5. Why is an oral syringe preferred over a household teaspoon for administering a medication?

6. List the five "rights" of medication administration.
7. What is the sixth "right" of medication administration and why is it important?

8. What are the primary principles of giving a solid form and liquid form of a medication?
9. Discuss the proper method(s) of checking NG tube placement prior to the administration of a drug or an enteral formula.
10. Identify the color and pH values of gastric, intestinal, and pleural secretions, both with and without the administration of H_2 blockers (antagonists).
11. Name four general categories of enteral formulas.
12. How long can an enteral formula be left standing open with refrigeration?

Answer

1. Nasogastric

2. Bypass the digestive enzymes and avoid irritation to the esophagus and stomach.

3. See textbook, pp. 118-119.

4. The dropper has been specifically made to correspond with the viscosity of the drug to deliver the correct volume of medication.
5. An oral syringe is more accurate.

6. The five rights of drug administration are: RIGHT patient, RIGHT drug, RIGHT dosage, RIGHT time of administration, and RIGHT route of administration.
7. RIGHT documentation explains not only what was administered but also the patient's response.
8. See textbook, pp. 122, 124-125.

9. Verify NG location after initial placement using x-ray verification BEFORE administering any drug or enteral formula for the first time. (See textbook, pp. 125-126.)
10. See textbook, Method 1: pH testing of gastric contents, pp. 126-127.
11. Four general types of enteral formulas are intact (polymeric) nutrient, elemental, disease- or condition-specific, and modular nutrients.

Copyright © 2004 Mosby Inc. All rights reserved.

13. Review the procedure for NG administration of enteral formulas using bolus and continuous infusion techniques.

14. State the positioning used for a patient when he/she is receiving an NG feeding using the bolus and using a continuous delivery method.

15. How are rectal suppositories inserted?

16. What position is the patient placed in to administer a disposable enema?

12. An open enteral formula can be kept refrigerated up to 24 hours. The tubing and formula receptacle used for a continuous method of delivery such as the Kangaroo also should be changed every 24 hours.

13. See textbook, pp. 126-128.

14. Place the patient in semi-Fowler's position with head of bed (HOB) elevated 30 degrees for 30 minutes before and at least 1 hour after a bolus feeding. Most patients with a continuous feeding are maintained at a 30 to 45 degree elevation of the HOB.

15. Apply a glove or finger cot, have suppository in a solid form, use water-soluble lubricant or plain water to moisten, then insert suppository about one inch past the internal sphincter in the rectum.

16. To administer a disposable enema, place the patient on the left side.

Copyright © 2004 Mosby Inc. All rights reserved.

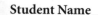

CHAPTER 9

Enteral Administration

Practice Quiz

COMPLETION

Complete the following statements.

1. Capsules are _____.
2. Timed-release tablets differ from capsules by _____.
3. Lozenges or troches are administered by _____ route and patient should be instructed to _____.
4. Elixirs are drugs dissolved in _____.
5. Syrups are drugs dissolved in _____.
6. Emulsions and suspensions are similar in that _____.
7. On the medicine cup, 1 oz (fl oz) equals _____ Tbsp.
8. On the medicine cup, 1 tsp equals _____ ml.

TRUE OR FALSE

Mark "T" for true or "F" for false for each question.
Correct all false statements.

_____ 9. The oral dropper that accompanied a specific drug is lost. The nurse should substitute a dropper from another medication for the lost one.

_____ 10. To validate the correct placement of an NG tube prior to administering a medication or enteral feeding it is acceptable to aspirate gastric contents and check the pH and color.

_____ 11. When flushing an NG tube, do not clamp the tube until all the solution has time to reach the stomach.

_____ 12. When documenting an enteral feeding, the amount administered is charted on the intake and output sheet and then is included in the intake total for each shift.

_____ 13. Intermittent tube feedings require that the unused formula mixed and dispensed by the pharmacy be discarded every 48 hours.

_____ 14. The head of the bed (HOB) is elevated 30 minutes before and 30 minutes to 1 hour after administering an intermittent tube feeding.

_____ 15. Rectal suppositories are generally inserted with the patient positioned in the Sims' position.

_____ 16. A disposable enema is administered with the patient positioned on the right side.

_____ 17. When testing gastric pH for a person NOT taking an H_2 blocker such as ranitidine, the gastric contents would have a pH of 1.0–4.0.

_____ 18. When testing gastric pH for a person who is taking an H_2 blocker such as ranitidine, the gastric contents would have a pH > 4.0.

_____ 19. Aspirated intestinal fluid should be a clear-to-straw–colored secretion.

_____ 20. Auscultation is an accurate method of checking NG tube placement.

REVIEW QUESTIONS

_____ 1. Medicines given orally are absorbed:
   a. more rapidly than via other routes.
   b. more rapidly when food is present.
   c. slower than by other routes.
   d. rapidly but erratically.

Copyright © 2004 Mosby Inc. All rights reserved.

_____ 2. When giving an intermittent enteral feeding, the residual aspirate obtained in an adult is 150 ml. The nurse should:
   a. administer the next scheduled feeding.
   b. stop feeding for 30 minutes and recheck residual.
   c. check procedural manual for guidelines.
   d. notify the health care provider if no orders are specified.

_____ 3. When giving oral medications, the nurse should *first*:
   a. give the patient water to drink.
   b. identify the patient.
   c. check all aspects of the order.
   d. sit the patient upright.

Copyright © 2004 Mosby Inc. All rights reserved.

Parenteral Administration: Safe Preparation of Parenteral Medications

Syllabus

CHAPTER CONTENT

Safe Preparation, Administration, and Disposal of Parenteral Medication and Supplies (p. 132)
Equipment Used in Parenteral Administration (p. 132)
Parenteral Dose Forms (p. 141)
Preparation of Parenteral Medication (p. 142)

CHAPTER OBJECTIVES

Equipment Used in Parenteral Administration
1. Name the three parts of a syringe.
2. Read the calibrations of the minim and cubic centimeter or milliliter scale on different types of syringes.
3. Identify the sites where the volume of medication is read on a glass syringe and a plastic syringe.
4. Give examples of volumes of medications that can be measured in a tuberculin syringe, rather than a larger volume syringe.
5. State the advantages and disadvantages of using prefilled syringes.
6. Explain the system of measurement utilized to define the inside diameter of a syringe.
7. Identify the parts of a needle.
8. Explain how the gauge of a needle is determined.
9. Compare the usual volume of medication that can be administered at one site when giving a medication by intradermal, SC, or IM routes.
10. State the criteria used for the selection of the correct needle gauge and length.
11. Identify examples of the safety-type syringes and needles.

Parenteral Dose Forms
1. Differentiate among ampules, vials, and Mix-O-Vials.

Preparation of Parenteral Medication
1. List the equipment needed for the preparation of parenteral medication.
2. Describe, practice, and perfect the preparation of medications using the various dose forms for parenteral administration.
3. Describe, practice, and perfect the technique of preparing two different drugs in one syringe, such as insulin or a preoperative medication.

KEY TERMS

barrel
plunger
tip
minim scale
milliliter scale
tuberculin syringe
insulin syringe

prefilled syringes
insulin pen
needle gauge
safety devices
ampules
vials
Mix-O-Vials

ASSIGNMENTS

Read textbook, pp. 132-148.
Study Key Terms associated with chapter content.
Study Review Sheet for Chapter 10.
Complete the Chapter 10 Practical Test.
Complete Chapter 10 Practice Quiz.
Complete Chapter 10 Exam.

WEB RESEARCH ACTIVITIES

Access: www.allergic-reactions.com
Open: 1) **Causes of Anaphylaxis** and identify common documented causes of anaphylaxis.
Open: 2) **Living with Anaphylaxis** and review questions a person with an allergy should ask about the condition.

Copyright © 2004 Mosby Inc. All rights reserved.

Open: 3) **About Epi-Pen®** and view information on prescribing information and the trainer instructions for use of the Epi-Pen®.

Access: http://www.bd.com/
Print out materials for class discussion on: Safety-Lok Syringe and Safetyguide Shielding Hypodermic Needles.

Copyright © 2004 Mosby Inc. All rights reserved.

Parenteral Administration: Safe Preparation of Parenteral Medications

Review Sheet

The Question column and the Answer column have been offset so that you can cover the answer while reading the question, allowing you to assess your knowledge.

Question	Answer
1. Define *parenteral*.	
2. What are the major advantages of parenteral medication administration?	1. Parenteral medication administration routes are intradermal, intramuscular (IM), and intravenous (IV) injections.
3. Cite specific nursing actions required during medication administration to provide for accurate, safe drug delivery to the patient.	2. See textbook, p. 132.
4. Discuss established policies and procedures used for checking and transcribing medication orders and for preparing, administering, recording, and monitoring of therapeutic responses to drug therapy in clinical sites where assigned.	3. 1) Knowledge of individual drugs ordered, prepared, and administered; 2) awareness of symptoms for which drug is prescribed as well as baseline evaluation of desired therapeutic outcomes desired; 3) understanding of nursing assessments needed to detect, prevent, or ameliorate adverse events; and 4) the nurse must exercise clinical judgment when drug orders are changed, new drugs are ordered, drug doses are missed, or when substitution of therapeutically equivalent medicines are made by the pharmacy.
5. List the parts of a syringe and the method of reading the measuring scale on the tuberculin, 3 ml, and insulin syringes.	4. Instructor needs to assist the student to identify policies developed by the school and by individual clinical sites relative to this question.
6. What volume can safely be injected at one site for intradermal, SC, IM, and IV medications?	5. Figures 10-1, 10-2, 10-6A and B, 10-7.
7. Identify the types of tips found on syringes.	6. See Table 10-1, p. 137.
8. Examine calibrations found on different types of syringes.	7. See Figure 10-4 A, B.
9. What are common manufacturers' names for prefilled syringes?	8. See Figure 10-2, 10-6A and B, 10-7.
10. Name the parts of an "insulin pen."	9. Tubex, Carpuject
11. What medication is contained in an Epi-Pen® and what is the intended use for this device?	10. See Figure 10-10.
12. The inner diameter of a needle is known as _____.	11. Epinephrine, p. 136.

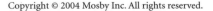

Copyright © 2004 Mosby Inc. All rights reserved.

13. Why are different length needles available for intramuscular and subcutaneous injections?

14. What do the terms *package integrity* or *package continuity* mean?

15. What are the provisions of the Needlestick Safety and Prevention Act of 2000?

16. What is the purpose of a filter needle?

17. Research safety devices developed for syringes and needles.

18. Identify the location of the OSHA-approved "sharps" containers on the clinical unit where assigned.

19. Differentiate between an ampule, a vial, and a Mix-O-Vial. Read the section on removal of medications from these containers.

20. Practice the procedures involved in the removal of a drug from an ampule, vial, and Mix-O-Vial.

12. Gauge: the larger the number, the smaller the diameter.

13. Provides a means of depositing the prescribed medication into the correct location/depth for maximum drug response in individuals of different build and age.

14. The terms *package integrity* or *package continuity* mean inspecting the container to ensure sterility of the contents has been retained.

15. The Act requires OSHA to develop and revise standards for blood-borne pathogens, monitoring and reporting of needlestick injuries, and the development of safety equipment to protect health care providers.

16. A filter needle is used to screen out glass particles that may have inadvertently fallen into the ampule during removal of its top. *Note:* After medication is removed from the ampule, remove filter needle, apply appropriate gauge and length needle for drug administration, and measure the amount of drug prescribed.

17. See Figures 10-15 through 10-19.

18. Ask your instructor.

19. See Figures 10-20, 10-21, and 10-22.

20. See Figure 10-23, pp. 142-143; Figure 10-24, p. 144; Figure 10-25, p. 145.

Copyright © 2004 Mosby Inc. All rights reserved.

Student Name_____

Parenteral Administration: Safe Preparation of Parenteral Medications

Practice Quiz

Study the chapter content, then take the practice quiz to test your knowledge.

LABEL THE SYRINGE BELOW

1.

READ THE FOLLOWING SYRINGES

2. _____

3. _____

4. _____

5. _____

6. _____

7. _____

8. _____

9. _____

10. _____

11. _____

12. _____

LABEL THE PARTS OF A NEEDLE

13.

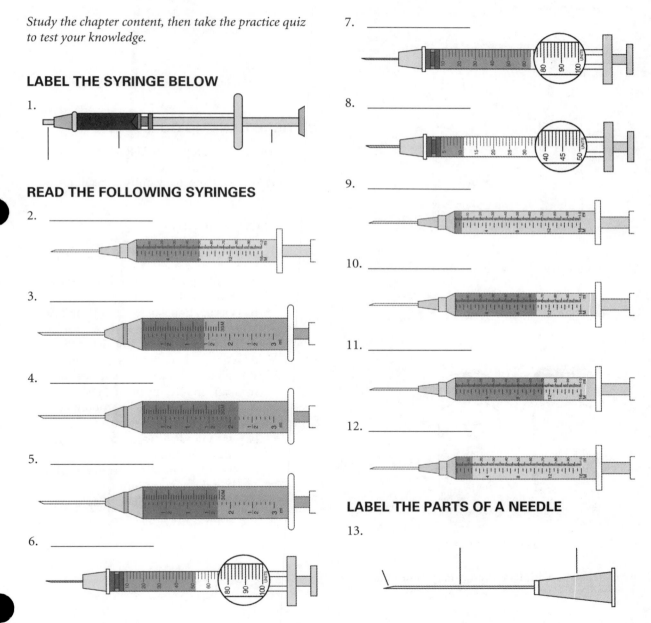

Copyright © 2004 Mosby Inc. All rights reserved.

COMPLETION

In the blanks provided, write the volume of a drug that can be injected at one site by the following methods.

14. Intradermal: _____ ml

15. Subcutaneous: _____ ml

16. Intramuscular: _____ ml

    Divided dose is: _____

17. Intravenous fluid: _____ ml

LABEL THE FOLLOWING

18. This is known as a(n) _____.

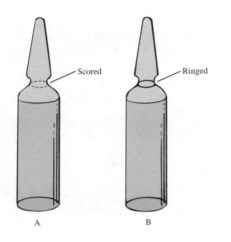

A   B

Explain how to withdraw fluid from this receptacle.

19. This is known as a(n) _____.

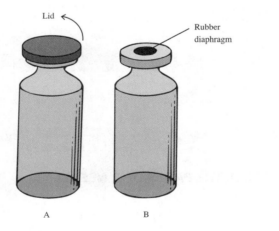

A   B

Explain how to withdraw fluid from this receptacle.

20. This is known as a(n) _____.

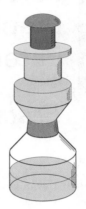

Explain how to withdraw fluid from this receptacle.

CRITICAL THINKING QUESTION

21. Explain how to prepare 22 U Regular and 15 U NPH insulin in a syringe.

    Note: Review: How many units of insulin = 1 cc?

REVIEW QUESTIONS

_____ 1. Proper disposal of "sharps" is controlled by:
   a. Joint Commission on Hospital Accreditation.
   b. Occupational Safety and Health Administration.
   c. Intravenous Nurses Society.
   d. American Medical Association.

_____ 2. When removing a parenteral medication from an ampule, the nurse must:
   a. inject air equal to the amount of medication to be removed.
   b. use a needleless spike for removing the medication.
   c. use a filter needle to ensure no glass is in the medication.
   d. depress the top rubber diaphragm to displace the stopper.

Copyright © 2004 Mosby Inc. All rights reserved.

Parenteral Administration: Intradermal, Subcutaneous, and Intramuscular Administration

Syllabus

CHAPTER CONTENT

Administration of Medication by the Intradermal Route (p. 149)
Administration of Medication by the Subcutaneous Route (p. 151)
Administration of Medication by the Intramuscular Route (p. 153)

CHAPTER OBJECTIVES

Administration of Medication by the Intradermal Route

1. Describe the technique used to administer a medication via the intradermal route.

Administration of Medication by the Subcutaneous (SC) Route

1. Identify the equipment needed and describe the technique used to administer a medication via the SC route.

Administration of Medication by the Intramuscular (IM) Route

1. Describe the technique used to administer medications in the vastus lateralis muscle, rectus femoris muscle, ventrogluteal area, dorsogluteal area, or the deltoid muscle.
2. For each anatomical site studied, describe the landmarks used to identify the site before administration of the medication.
3. Identify suitable sites for intramuscular administration of medication in an infant, a child, an adult, and an elderly person.

KEY TERMS

intradermal
wheal
erythema
anergic
subcutaneous
intramuscular

vastus lateralis
rectus femoris
ventrogluteal area
dorsogluteal area
deltoid muscle
Z-track method

ASSIGNMENTS

Read textbook, pp. 149-159.
Study Key Terms associated with chapter content.
Study Review Sheet for Chapter 11.
Complete Chapter 11 Practice Quiz.
Complete Chapter 11 Exam.

WEB RESEARCH ACTIVITY

Access: www.keepkidshealthy.com/welcome/commonproblems/allergy_testing.html
Research different types of skin and allergy testing that is done and bring articles to class for discussion.

Copyright © 2004 Mosby Inc. All rights reserved.

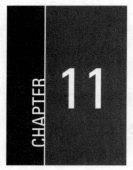

Parenteral Administration: Intradermal, Subcutaneous, and Intramuscular Administration

Review Sheet

The Question column and the Answer column have been offset so that you can cover the answer while reading the question, allowing you to assess your knowledge.

Question	Answer
1. Identify the layer of skin in which an intradermal injection is deposited.	
2. Name the common intradermal injection sites.	1. Intradermal injections are made into the dermal layer of skin below epidermis.
3. Prior to allergy sensitivity testing, what medications should be stopped for 24–48 hours?	2. Upper chest, scapular area of back, inner aspect of forearm.
4. What volume can safely be injected at one site for intradermal, SC, IM, and IV medications?	3. Antihistamines, anti-inflammatory agents, certain sleep medications, and immunosuppressants. (Always check with MD before discontinuing medications.)
5. What is the angle of the needle inserted for an intradermal injection?	4. Review Table 10-1, p. 137.
6. How do you "read" a skin test?	5. A 15 degree angle with the needle bevel upward.
7. List the terms associated with intradermal administration and reading of the reactions.	6. Positive reactions are measured, both the wheal and erythema, and by palpation and measurement of the size of any induration present.
8. Describe patient education that should be done in advance and at the time of performing intradermal testing.	7. See textbook, p. 150.
9. What types of SC injections do NOT require aspiration prior to injection of the medication?	8. See textbook, p. 149.
10. List the injection sites used for IM injections.	9. Heparin and insulin do not require aspiration prior to injection.
11. Why is the gluteal area NOT used for IM injections in children under 3 years of age?	10. See textbook, pp. 153-157.
12. When is the Z-track method of IM injection used?	11. The gluteal muscle is not adequately developed.
13. What is the purpose of performing a premedication assessment?	12. The Z-track method is used with medications that are particularly irritating or that will stain the skin (e.g., injectable iron).
	13. Premedication assessment is performed to prevent the administration of a medication to a patient whose diagnosis, symptoms, or other data indicate the medication should not be administered.

  Copyright © 2004 Mosby Inc. All rights reserved.

Student Name_____

Parenteral Administration: Intradermal, Subcutaneous, and Intramuscular Administration

Practice Quiz

Study the chapter content and then take the practice quiz to test your knowledge.

LABEL THE SYRINGE BELOW

1. _____

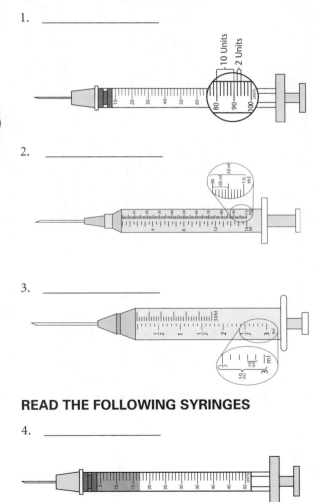

2. _____

3. _____

READ THE FOLLOWING SYRINGES

4. _____

5. _____

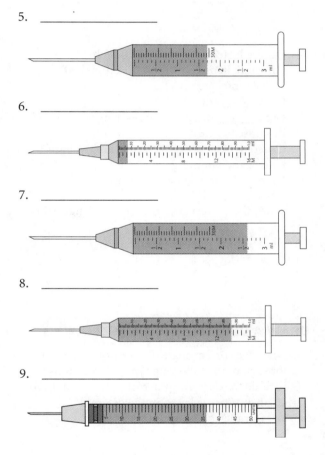

6. _____

7. _____

8. _____

9. _____

COMPLETION

In the blanks provided, write the volume of a drug that can be injected at one site by the following methods.

10. Intradermal: _____ ml

11. Subcutaneous: _____ ml

12. Intramuscular: _____ ml
    Divided dose is: _____

Copyright © 2004 Mosby Inc. All rights reserved.

PRACTICE SUBCUTANEOUS AND INTRAMUSCULAR CALCULATIONS:

13. Ordered: Ampicillin 500 mg q 6 h, IM
    Directions: For IM use, add 3.5 ml diluent. Resulting solution contains 250 mg ampicillin per ml
    Give: _____ ml
    Shade the correct amount on the syringe below.

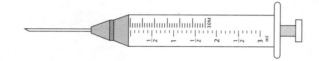

14. Ordered: Heparin 7000 U SC, q 8 h
    On hand: heparin sodium injection, USP 10,000 units per ml
    Give: _____ ml
    Use a _____ (what volume) syringe to measure this dose.

15. Ordered: Compazine 8.6 mg IM q 3–4 h for nausea and vomiting.
    On hand: Compazine 5 mg per ml
    Give: _____ ml
    Shade the correct amount on the syringe below.

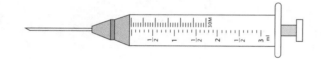

DRAW A DIAGRAM OF THE FOLLOWING

16. Draw the correct angle of insertion of a needle for each of the following types of injections. Include the dermis, epidermis, muscle, and subcutaneous tissue layers in the diagram.
    a. Intradermal drug administration:

    b. SC drug administration:

    c. IM drug administration:

17. Label the figure below with the injection sites used for SC drug administration.

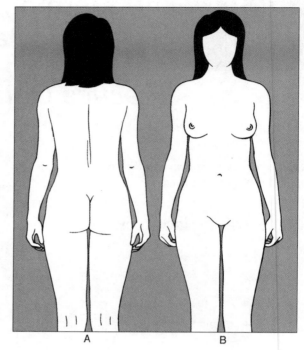

A   B

18. Draw a diagram to illustrate where an IM injection is given to an adult in the vastus lateralis muscle. Include the following structures in the drawing: greater trochanter, femoral artery and vein, sciatic nerve, patella, and vastus lateralis muscle.

19. Draw a diagram to illustrate where an IM injection is given to a child in the ventrogluteal site. Include the following structures in the drawing: iliac crest, anterior superior iliac spine, gluteus medius, and greater trochanter.

Copyright © 2004 Mosby Inc. All rights reserved.

20. Label the pictures below with the sites for intra-muscular injection in a child and an adult.

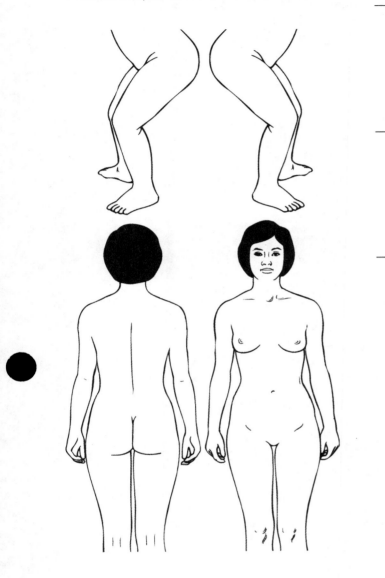

REVIEW QUESTIONS

_____ 1. The instructor requests you to gather the equipment needed to perform an intra-dermal injection. Which of the following would be appropriate?
   a. 3 ml syringe, 25-gauge 1" needle
   b. TB syringe, 26-gauge 3/8" needle
   c. 3 ml syringe, 21-gauge 1" needle
   d. TB syringe, 21-gauge 3/8" needle

_____ 2. When reading a reaction to an allergen you observe no wheal and a 3 mm flare. This would be recorded as a _____ reaction.
   a. 1+
   b. 2+
   c. 3+
   d. 4+

_____ 3. The American Diabetes Association (ADA) recommends insulin sites be rotated by rotating injections:
   a. within one area before going to the next site (arms, legs, abdomen, back).
   b. using a new site—arms, legs, abdomen, or back—each time.
   c. using the arm in the AM and the leg in the PM.
   d. using the abdomen and legs.

Copyright © 2004 Mosby Inc. All rights reserved.

CHAPTER 12
Parenteral Administration: Intravenous Route

Syllabus

CHAPTER CONTENT

Equipment Used for Intravenous Therapy (p. 160)
Intravenous Dose Forms (p. 165)
Administration of Medications by the Intravenous
    Route (p. 168)
Basic Guidelines of Intravenous Administration of
    Medicines (p. 172)
Monitoring Intravenous Therapy (p. 183)

CHAPTER OBJECTIVES

Intravenous Therapy
1. Define intravenous (IV) therapy.
2. Describe the processes used to establish guidelines for nurses to perform infusion therapy.

Equipment Used for Intravenous Therapy
1. Describe equipment used to perform intravenous therapy (e.g., winged or butterfly needle, over-the-needle catheter, administration sets, and intravenous access devices).
2. Differentiate among peripheral, midline, central venous, and implantable access devices used for intravenous therapy.

Intravenous Dose Forms
1. Differentiate among isotonic, hypotonic, and hypertonic intravenous solutions.
2. Explain the usual circumstances for administration of isotonic, hypotonic, and hypertonic intravenous solutions.
3. Describe the three intravascular compartments and the distribution of body water among them.
4. Describe the different types of large-volume containers available.

Administration of Medications by the Intravenous Route
1. Identify the dosage forms available, the types of sites of administration, and general principles of administering medications via the IV route.

2. List criteria used for the selection of an intravenous access site.
3. Describe the correct technique for administering medications by means of an established peripheral or central IV line, a heparin lock, an IV bag, a bottle or volume-control device, or through a secondary piggyback set.
4. Describe the recommended guidelines and procedures for IV catheter care (including proper maintenance of patency of IV lines and implanted access devices), IV line dressing changes, and for peripheral and central venous IV needle or catheter changes.

Monitoring Intravenous Therapy
1. Discuss the proper baseline patient assessments needed to evaluate the IV therapy.
2. Explain the signs, symptoms, and treatment of complications associated with intravenous therapy (e.g., phlebitis, thrombophlebitis, localized infection, septicemia, infiltration, extravasation, air in tubing, pulmonary edema, catheter embolism, and "speed" shock).

KEY TERMS

intravenous (IV)
Infusion Nurses
    Society (INS)
IV administration sets
nonvolumetric IV
    controllers
volumetric IV
    controllers
syringe pumps
peripheral devices
midline catheters
central devices

implantable infusion
    ports
winged, butterfly, or
    scalp needles
over-the-needle
    catheter
saline, heparin, or
    medlock
in-the-needle catheter
peripherally inserted
    central venous
    catheter (PICC)

Copyright © 2004 Mosby Inc. All rights reserved.

tunneled central
    venous catheters
intravenous solutions
electrolytes
intravascular
    compartment
isotonic
hypertonic
hypotonic
tandem setup,
    piggyback (IVPB),
    or IV rider
SASH guidelines

piggyback or secondary
    set
phlebitis
thrombophlebitis
septicemia
infiltration
extravasation
infiltration scale
air embolism
pulmonary edema
pulmonary embolus
speed shock

WEB RESEARCH ACTIVITY

Access: www.venousaccess.com and review the following content:

General Information/History
Access Site Anatomy
Types of Access
Choosing the Right Access
Procedures
Complications, Prevention & Treatment
Catheter Care

ASSIGNMENTS

Read textbook, pp. 160-188.
Study Key Terms associated with chapter content.
Study Review Sheet for Chapter 12.
Complete Chapter 12 Practice Quiz.
Complete Chapter 12 Exam.

Copyright © 2004 Mosby Inc. All rights reserved.

CHAPTER 12

Parenteral Administration: Intravenous Route

Review Sheet

The Question column and the Answer column have been offset so that you can cover the answer while reading the question, allowing you to assess your knowledge.

Question	Answer

Question

1. What does the term *intravenous* mean?
2. Nurses having certification for IV therapy can use the initials _____ in their title.

3. Name two agencies that are recommended resources for establishing standards relating to IV therapy.
4. What types of IV administration sets are available?
5. What types of controller clamps are commonly used on IV administration sets?
6. Differentiate between nonvolumetric and volumetric IV infusion controllers.
7. Differentiate among peripheral access devices, midline catheters, central devices, and implantable venous infusion ports. Identify their uses, sites of insertion, and what vessel the catheter tip should be in when placement is complete.
8. How frequently should peripheral catheters be changed?
9. Describe the flushing of Hickman, Broviac, and Groshong catheters.
10. What types of needles are used to access an implanted port and a CathLink 20 port?
11. What does it mean when an IV solution is *isotonic*, *hypotonic*, or *hypertonic*?

12. What criteria are used to select an isotonic, hypotonic, or hypertonic IV solution for administration to a patient?
13. Compare the preparation for administration of IV solutions delivered in glass bottles with those in plastic bags.

Answer

1. *Intravenous* means "in the vein." In the context of this chapter, it means administration of fluids directly into the bloodstream.
2. CRNI

3. Infusion Nurses Society (INS) and Centers for Disease Control and Prevention (CDC)
4. See textbook, p. 161.

5. Roller and slide clamps. *Note:* A dial-style controller is also available for use.
6. Nonvolumetric infusion devices only monitor the gravity-induced flow by counting drops that pass through the drip chamber; volumetric IV controllers apply external pressure to pump the IV fluid at a specified rate.
7. See textbook, pp. 163-165.

8. 72–96 hours (check policy manual where functioning).
9. See textbook, p. 164.

10. All ports except the CathLink 20 are accessed using a Huber needle. The CathLink 20 uses a standard over-the-needle IV catheter (pp. 165-166).
11. See textbook, pp. 166-167.

12. See textbook, pp. 166-167.

Copyright © 2004 Mosby Inc. All rights reserved.

14. When setting up an IV fluid or medication for administration as an IV piggyback, how should the piggyback bag be positioned?
15. Compare common peripheral access devices and the intended use of each.
16. Describe vein selection for the initiation of an IV.
17. Identify common veins used for initiating IV therapy in infants and children.
18. What are the most common veins used for central venous catheter access?
19. Study and practice IV-related procedures found throughout this chapter in the laboratory setting (e.g., venipuncture, spiking and hanging an IV, adding an IV piggyback to a primary line, giving IV drugs by bolus method, preparing an ADD-Vantage or similar prepackaged system of medication for administration IV, and operating syringe pumps and volumetric and nonvolumetric infusion control devices. Check with the instructor for details.)
20. Obtain copies of procedures used at the clinical site where you are assigned for:
    • frequency of changing IV tubing.
    • IV peripheral sites.
    • length of time IV solutions can remain hanging.
    • recording of IV fluids and IV medications on the MAR.
    • procedures for flushing and dressing of heparin, saline, or medlock.
    • central venous catheters and PICC lines.
21. Explain the SASH procedure used for IV therapy.
22. Which type of IV central catheter does not require flushing with heparin?
23. What is a commonly accepted rate for a TKO (to keep open) IV order?
24. What is the purpose of a premedication assessment?
25. What is the formula used to calculate an IV drip rate?

13. See Figure 12-1 A, B, and C, p. 172.
14. See Figure 12-11.
15. See Figures, 12-5, 12-6 A and B, and textbook, pp. 163-164.
16. See Figure 12-12, p. 169 and Figure 12-13, p. 170.
17. See Figure 12-14, p. 171.
18. The subclavian and jugular veins are most commonly used for central IV access.
19. Consult with your instructor to obtain detailed instructions for practicing and being "checked-off" on procedures relating to IV.
20. See general guidelines, textbook pp. 170-171. Guidelines of individual practice settings should always be consulted.
21. **S**= Saline
    A= Administer drug
    S= Saline
    H= Heparin (Not all types of vascular access devices require the use of heparin; check hospital policy.)
22. Groshong
23. A commonly accepted rate for TKO IV is 10 ml/hr.
24. Premedication assessment is performed to prevent the administration of a medication to a patient whose diagnosis, symptoms, or other data indicate the medication should not be administered. See details on textbook p. 132, p. 172.

Copyright © 2004 Mosby Inc. All rights reserved.

26. Describe the correct method of monitoring an infusing IV solution and site.

27. Describe how to assess for infiltration at an IV site.

28. If you see air in the tubing of a running IV, what should you do?

29. What are the signs and symptoms of circulatory overload and pulmonary edema?
30. How is a suspected pulmonary embolism verified?

31. Differentiate between the terms *infiltration* and *extravasation*.

25.

$$\frac{\text{ml of solution x number of drops/ml}}{\text{hrs of administration x 60 min/hr}} = \text{drops/min}$$

26. Apply a tourniquet proximal to the infusion site to restrict flow. Continued flow with the tourniquet in place confirms infiltration.

27. Check for limb's color, size, or skin integrity; compare with the opposite limb. See textbook for guidelines to follow and for the infiltration scale, Figure 12-19, p. 185.

28. Clamp the tubing; use a syringe to withdraw the air bubble.

29. Symptoms of circulatory overload include engorged neck veins; dyspnea; reduced urine output; edema; bounding pulse; and shallow, rapid respirations.
Symptoms of pulmonary edema include dyspnea, cough, anxiety, rales, rhonchi, possible cardiac arrhythmias, thready pulse, frothy sputum, and elevation or drop in blood pressure depending on the severity. Treatment: high-Fowler's position, oxygen, collect vital signs; summon help from other health care providers. Have medications ready (e.g., diuretics, vasodilators, and morphine sulfate).

30. A lung scan is done as well as drawing ABGs and baseline prothrombin times.

31. Infiltration is leakage of IV solution into the tissue surrounding the vein; extravasation is leakage of an irritant chemical into the tissue surrounding the vein.

Copyright © 2004 Mosby Inc. All rights reserved.

CHAPTER 12

Parenteral Administration: Intravenous Route

Practice Quiz

COMPLETION

Complete the following statements.

1. Based on drop volume, an IV administration set that delivers 20 gtt/ml is called a(n) _____ set.

2. A type of IV device that holds a pre-filled syringe is called a(n)_____.

3. A(n) _____-the-needle catheter is commonly inserted peripherally for routine peripheral infusion therapy.

4. This type of IV infusion device is designed for use over a 2–4-week period of use. It is known as a(n) _____.

5. A type of central venous catheter that a qualified nurse can insert is known as a(n) _____ catheter.

6. A type of tunneled venous catheter that does not require flushing with heparin is known as a(n) _____ catheter.

7. Name three types of vessels that comprise the intravascular compartment: 1. _____, 2. _____, and 3. _____.

8. Isotonic solutions have an osmolality range of _____ mOsm/L.

9. Hypertonic solutions (e.g., parenteral nutrition solutions) are administered through central infusion lines directly into the _____ vein.

10. Name an agency that is recognized as a recommended resource to be consulted when establishing guidelines relating to infectious diseases. _____

11. Are topical antibiotic ointments and creams used on routine IV sites? (Why or why not?) _____

12. What volume of routine flush solution would be used for a saline/heparin/medlock located in the lower arm? _____ ml

13. What information should be included on the label placed on an IV administration set tubing?

14. The usual time interval between tube changes on lipid solutions is _____ hours.

15. Describe how a volume chamber is operated when used to administer an IV medication.

PRACTICE CALCULATIONS

16. Give 100 ml/hr D_5W using a 20 gtt/ml administration set. Run at _____ gtt/min.

17. Give 125 ml/hr lactated Ringer's using a 15 gtt/ml administration set. Run at _____ gtt/min.

18. Give 1000 ml D_5W over 10 hours using a 10 gtt/ml administration set. Run at _____ gtt/min.

19. Give 250 ml 0.9% sodium chloride over 2 hours using a 15 gtt/ml administration set. Run at _____ gtt/min.

LABEL THE FOLLOWING

20. This is: _____

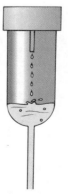

Copyright © 2004 Mosby Inc. All rights reserved.

21. Figure A is a(n): _____

A   B

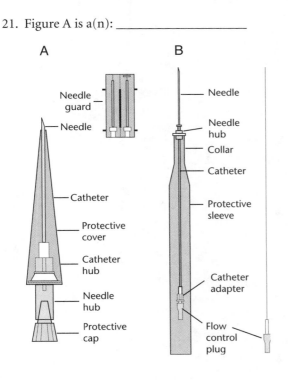

Needle guard

Needle

Catheter

Protective cover

Catheter hub

Needle hub

Protective cap

Needle

Needle hub

Collar

Catheter

Protective sleeve

Catheter adapter

Flow control plug

DRAW A DIAGRAM OF THE FOLLOWING

22. There are two bags of intravenous infusion solution to be hung for the patient. One is a 1000 ml D_5W; the second is 100 ml 0.9% sodium chloride containing a medication. Draw how these would be arranged on the IV pole.

REVIEW QUESTIONS

_____ 1. If air is seen in the IV tubing, the nurse should:
   a. immediately close the clamp on the tubing.
   b. notify the primary nurse.
   c. get the instructor.
   d. disregard it if less than 1–2 ml.

_____ 2. A patient's skin at the site of a running IV in a peripheral IV access site appears swollen, feels cool, and the patient complains of discomfort. The nurse should:
   a. apply a tourniquet and check patency.
   b. flush the site with saline.
   c. lower the IV bottle to check for blood return.
   d. notify the health care provider.

_____ 3. After changing a primary IV, it will not run. The nurse should first check for:
   a. type of IV solution hung.
   b. clamps not released.
   c. height of container.
   d. piggyback or rider set needed.

_____ 4. When initiating an intravenous access device for the first time in an extremity, it should be placed:
   a. near the antecubital space.
   b. in the biggest vein visible.
   c. in the dominant hand.
   d. in the metacarpal vein if large enough.

_____ 5. When planning to insert a Huber needle into a port, the nurse should:
   a. use aseptic technique throughout the procedure.
   b. use clean technique throughout the procedure.
   c. don latex examination gloves.
   d. use sterile technique with gloves, supplies, and put on a mask.

Copyright © 2004 Mosby Inc. All rights reserved.

Drugs Affecting the Autonomic Nervous System

Syllabus

CHAPTER CONTENT

CHAPTER OBJECTIVES

1. Differentiate between afferent and efferent nerve conduction within the central nervous system.
2. Explain the role of neurotransmitters at synaptic junctions.
3. Name the most common neurotransmitters known to affect central nervous system function.
4. Identify the two major neurotransmitters of the autonomic nervous system.
5. Cite the names of nerve endings that liberate acetylcholine and those that liberate norepinephrine.
6. Explain the action of drugs that inhibit the actions of the cholinergic and adrenergic fibers.
7. Identify two broad classes of drugs used to stimulate the adrenergic nervous system.
8. Name the neurotransmitters that are called catecholamines.
9. Review the actions of adrenergic agents to identify conditions that would be affected favorably and unfavorably by these medications.
10. Explain the rationale for use of adrenergic blocking agents for conditions that have vasoconstriction as part of the disease pathophysiology.
11. Describe the benefits of using beta-adrenergic blocking agents for hypertension, angina pectoris, cardiac arrhythmias, and hyperthyroidism.

12. Identify disease conditions that preclude the use of beta-adrenergic blocking agents.
13. List the neurotransmitters responsible for cholinergic activity.
14. List the predictable side effects of cholinergic agents.
15. List the predictable side effects of anticholinergic agents.
16. Describe the clinical uses of anticholinergic agents.

KEY TERMS

central nervous system
afferent nerves
efferent nerves
peripheral nervous
    system
motor nervous system
autonomic nervous
    system
neuron
synapse
neurotransmitters
norepinephrine

acetylcholine
cholinergic fiber
adrenergic fiber
anticholinergic agent
adrenergic blocking
    agent
catecholamine
alpha receptor
beta receptor
dopaminergic
    receptors

ASSIGNMENTS

Read textbook, pp. 189, 198.
Study Key Terms associated with chapter content.
Study Review Sheet for Chapter 13.
Complete Chapter 13 Practice Quiz.
Complete Chapter 13 Exam.

WEB RESEARCH ACTIVITY

Access an Internet search engine and type in "drugs affecting the autonomic nervous system" and additional resources available on the study of these agents will be available.

Copyright © 2004 Mosby Inc. All rights reserved.

Drugs Affecting the Autonomic Nervous System

Review Sheet

The QUESTION column and the ANSWER column have been offset so that you can cover the answer while reading the question, allowing you to assess your knowledge.

Question	Answer
1. The central nervous system is composed of _____.	
2. The autonomic nervous system relays information from the central nervous system to _____ _____.	1. The central nervous system (CNS) is composed of the brain and spinal cord.
3. The autonomic nervous system controls the functions of what types of tissue?	2. The autonomic nervous system (ANS) relays information from the CNS to the whole body.
4. What primary function is controlled by the motor nervous system?	3. The ANS controls the functions of all tissue except striated muscle.
5. What neurotransmitter is liberated by cholinergic fibers?	4. Skeletal muscle contractions are controlled by the motor nervous system.
6. What neurotransmitter is liberated by adrenergic fibers?	5. The cholinergic fibers secrete acetylcholine.
7. What three major types of receptors are found in the autonomic nervous system?	6. The adrenergic fibers secrete norepinephrine.
8. Stimulation of alpha$_1$ receptors causes what action on blood vessels?	7. The three major types of receptors found in the ANS are alpha-, beta-, and dopaminergic receptors.
9. Stimulation of beta$_1$ receptors produces what type of effect on the heart rate?	8. Stimulation of alpha$_1$ receptors causes vasoconstriction. This results in a rise in blood pressure; therefore, before giving alpha$_1$-type medications, the blood pressure should be checked. This action makes these drugs useful in the treatment of hypotension and shock.
10. Stimulation of beta$_2$ receptors produces what effects?	9. Stimulation of beta$_1$ receptors increases the heart rate. If excessive doses of a beta$_1$ agonist are administered, the patient may experience tachycardia and arrhythmias.
11. Define *adrenergic agent*.	10. Stimulation of beta$_2$ receptors relaxes the smooth muscle of the bronchi, uterus, and peripheral blood vessels. These actions make these drugs useful as bronchodilators and inhibitors of preterm labor.

Copyright © 2004 Mosby Inc. All rights reserved.

12. When beta-adrenergic agents are administered, what effects will be seen on blood vessels, bronchi, heart rate, blood pressure, respiration, lungs, gastric motility and tone, and blood glucose?

13. What premedication assessments should be completed prior to administering an adrenergic agent?

14. Giving an excessive dose of an adrenergic agent results in what adverse effects?

15. List the primary actions of alpha-adrenergic blocking agents and beta-adrenergic blocking agents.

16. Why/when are alpha- and beta-adrenergic blocking agents prescribed?

17. State the possible effects of administering beta blockers to a patient with a known respiratory disease such as asthma or emphysema.

18. Which portion of the autonomic nervous system do cholinergic agents affect?

19. What effect do beta blockers have on a patient with diabetes mellitus?

20. What pharmacologic effect may be expected when indomethacin and beta blocker therapy are combined?

21. What drug is a specific antidote for cholinergic agents?

22. Under what types of clinical conditions are cholinergic agents be used?

11. An adrenergic agent produces or mimics the effects of stimulation of the sympathetic nervous system. Therefore, these drugs are also known as "sympathomimetic" agents.

12. When adrenergic agents are administered, blood vessels dilate, bronchi dilate, heart rate increases, blood pressure may drop, GI peristalsis decreases, relaxation of the gastric smooth muscle occurs, and blood glucose increases.

13. Before administering an adrenergic agent, the following assessments should be completed: baseline vital signs (e.g., heart rate, blood pressure), screen for respiratory tract disease, and ascertain if the patient uses bronchodilators or decongestants.

14. Excessive doses of an adrenergic agent may result in arrhythmias, hypertension, nervousness, anxiety, and insomnia due to stimulation of the sympathetic nervous system.

15. Alpha-adrenergic blocking agents act by plugging the alpha receptors, preventing vasoconstriction of arterioles. Beta-adrenergic blocking agents act by plugging the beta-adrenergic receptors, preventing beta stimulation, especially from norepinephrine and epinephrine.

16. Alpha-adrenergic blocking agents are used to treat diseases with vasoconstriction (e.g., peripheral vascular disease, Buerger's disease, and Raynaud's disease). Beta blocking agents are used to treat hypertension, angina pectoris, cardiac arrhythmias, and hyperthyroidism.

17. Administering a beta blocker to a person with a known respiratory disease may cause bronchoconstriction and make the person experience respiratory distress.

18. Cholinergic agents affect the parasympathetic portion of the nervous system.

19. Beta blockers induce hypoglycemia; they decrease the release of insulin in response to hypoglycemia and mask the symptoms normally associated with hypoglycemia.

20. The combination of indomethacin and beta blocker therapy may cause loss of hypertensive control. The dosage of the beta blocker may need to be increased.

21. Atropine sulfate, an anticholinergic agent, is a specific antidote for cholinergic agents.

Copyright © 2004 Mosby Inc. All rights reserved.

23. What side effects can be anticipated when an anticholinergic agent is administered?

24. What actions of anticholinergic agents make them useful in the clinical treatment of gastrointestinal disorders?

25. Before administering any anticholinergic agent, the patient's history should be checked for the presence of what type of eye disorder?

26. Atropine is an example of an anticholinergic agent frequently used preoperatively. Which of the drug's anticholinergic properties make this drug useful preoperatively?

27. What premedication assessments should be completed before administering an anticholinergic agent?

28. The postoperative patient who has been given atropine sulfate needs to be monitored for

_____.

29. Describe the action(s) and side effects of the following drug classifications and/or drugs: alpha-adrenergic agents, beta-adrenergic agents, cholinergic agents, anticholinergic agents, beta-adrenergic blocking agents, physostigmine, epinephrine, and atropine.

22. Cholinergic agents can be used to treat glaucoma, urinary retention, myasthenia gravis, as a muscle relaxant to reverse nondepolarizing agents, and for gastrointestinal disorders such as paralytic ileus.

23. Anticholinergic agents produce the following side effects: dryness of mouth and tongue, blurring of vision, mild nausea, and nervousness. Other side effects include constipation, urinary hesitancy or retention, tachycardia, palpitations, mydriasis, muscle cramping, and mild transient postural hypotension.

24. Anticholinergic (also known as *antispasmodic*) agents' actions include decreased secretion of saliva, hydrochloric acid, pepsin, bile, and other enzymatic fluids necessary for digestion, along with relaxation of the sphincter muscles and decreased spasm, which allows peristalsis to move the contents of the stomach and bowel through the gastrointestinal tract.

25. All patients' charts should be screened for the presence of angle-closure glaucoma before any anticholinergic agent is administered.

26. Atropine sulfate is given preoperatively to dry secretions of the mouth, nose, throat, and bronchi, and decrease secretions during surgery. It also prevents vagal stimulation and bradycardia during the placement of the endotracheal tube.

27. Check for a history of angle-closure glaucoma or history of enlarged prostate and urinary hesitancy or retention before administering an anticholinergic agent.

28. The postoperative patient who received atropine sulfate needs to be monitored frequently for urinary retention. There may also be postoperative constipation.

29. See textbook, pp. 193-197. Examine drug monographs and drug classification explanations.

Copyright © 2004 Mosby Inc. All rights reserved.

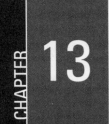

CHAPTER 13

Drugs Affecting the Autonomic Nervous System

Practice Quiz

COMPLETION

Complete the following statements.
1. Catecholamines that are secreted naturally in the body are _____, _____, and _____.
2. Dopamine is secreted at what three primary sites in the body? _____, _____, _____
3. The three types of sympathetic autonomic nervous system receptors are _____, _____, and _____.
4. Cholinergic agents are also known as _____.
5. Stimulation of the adrenergic receptors causes _____ of the bronchial muscles, which causes _____ of the airway.
6. Stimulation of the cholinergic receptors causes _____ of bronchial muscles, which causes _____ of the airway.
7. Prior to administration of an adrenergic agent, what premedication assessments should be done?
8. List two common side effects to expect with the administration of adrenergic agents.
9. When an anticholinergic agent is prescribed, what monitoring should be done?
10. The generic names of all beta$_1$ blocking agents end in "-_____."

Describe the action(s) of the following agents.
11. Cholinergics _____.
12. Beta-adrenergics _____.
13. Alpha-adrenergics _____.
14. Beta-adrenergic blockers _____.

END-OF-CHAPTER MATH REVIEW

1. Order: Benadryl 40 mg, PO, tid. Benadryl 12.5 mg/5 ml is available. Give: _____.
2. Order: propranolol 60 mg, PO, tid. Propranolol 40 mg tablets are available. Give: _____.
3. Ordered: atropine sulfate gr 1/150 SC preoperatively "on call." Atropine sulfate 0.3, 0.4, and 0.5 mg/ml are available. Give: _____.

CRITICAL THINKING QUESTIONS

1. Based on a review of this chapter, related to the actions, uses, and side effects of the primary drug classifications (adrenergic, adrenergic blocking agents, cholinergic, anticholinergic agents), develop a list of premedication assessments that should be made before using these drugs.
2. Summarize the actions of the cholinergic and anticholinergic agents. Arrange the summaries in columns to compare cholinergic and anticholinergic actions.
3. Examine the drug actions listed for adrenergic blocking agents. Explain the mechanisms by which these drugs are beneficial for the treatment of angina pectoris, cardiac arrhythmias, and hypertension.
4. Explain the effect of vasoconstriction and vasodilation of blood vessels on blood pressure.
5. What type of autonomic system drugs should not be used in patients with pulmonary disorders?

Copyright © 2004 Mosby Inc. All rights reserved.

Student Name_____

REVIEW QUESTIONS

_____ 1. Which of the following components in the history and physical would cause the nurse to verify a preoperative medication order for atropine sulfate and meperidine before administration?
   a. episodes of hypertension
   b. bradycardia
   c. increased gastric motility
   d. prostatic enlargement

_____ 2. Beta-adrenergic blocking drugs can cause:
   a. hypertension.
   b. angina pectoris.
   c. bronchoconstriction.
   d. cardiac arrhythmias.

Copyright © 2004 Mosby Inc. All rights reserved.

Sedative-Hypnotics

Syllabus

CHAPTER CONTENT

Sleep and Sleep Disturbances (p. 199)
    Sedative-Hypnotic Therapy (p. 200)
    Drug Therapy for Sleep Disturbances (p. 201)
        Drug Class: Barbiturates (p. 201)
        Drug Class: Benzodiazepines (p. 204)
        Drug Class: Miscellaneous Sedative-
           Hypnotic Agents (p. 206)

CHAPTER OBJECTIVES

1. Differentiate among the terms *sedative* and *hypnotic; initial, intermittent,* and *terminal insomnia;* and *rebound sleep* and *paradoxic excitement.*
2. Identify alterations found in the sleep pattern when hypnotics are discontinued.
3. Cite nursing interventions that can be implemented as alternatives to administering a sedative-hypnotic.
4. Compare the effects of barbiturates and benzodiazepines on the central nervous system.
5. Explain the major benefits of administering benzodiazepines rather than barbiturates.
6. Identify laboratory tests that should be monitored when benzodiazepines or barbiturates are administered over an extended period.
7. Develop a patient education plan for a patient receiving a hypnotic.

KEY TERMS

REM sleep
insomnia
hypnotic
sedative
rebound sleep

ASSIGNMENTS

Read textbook, pp. 199-206.
Study Key Terms associated with chapter content.
Complete Collaborative Activities as assigned.
Study Review Sheet for Chapter 14.
Complete End-of-Chapter Math Review and Critical Thinking Questions.
Complete Chapter 14 Practice Quiz.
Complete Chapter 14 Exam.

WEB RESEARCH ACTIVITIES

Access:
1. www.sleepapnea.org and research the diagnostic tests and treatments used for sleep apnea.
2. www.asda.org and read resource articles designed for professionals and for patients on the topic of sleep disorders. Bring an article relating to sleep disorders to class for discussion.

COLLABORATIVE ACTIVITIES

Complete the following activities to prepare for in-class discussion and group work that may be assigned by the instructor.
1. Perform an interview. Use information in "Nursing Process for Sedative-Hypnotics" to formulate a data assessment, develop questions, and interview a family member, neighbor, or friend who has complained about inability to sleep.
2. Read two articles on sleep disturbance or on the drug classes of the benzodiazepines or barbiturates and bring a copy of the article to a conference. Be prepared to summarize the article and discuss how it applies to the topic being studied.

Copyright © 2004 Mosby Inc. All rights reserved.

3. During the postinterview conference, answer the following questions:
   a. What type of sleep pattern disturbance is present?
   b. Is anxiety contributing to the problem?
   c. What type of sleeping environment is present?
   d. Does the individual use caffeine?

4. After examining the data collected, discuss possible interventions to help alleviate the problem without drugs.

(*Note:* Attend a follow-up conference with your instructor to discuss data or to seek guidance with this project.)

Copyright © 2004 Mosby Inc. All rights reserved.

Sedative-Hypnotics

Review Sheet

The QUESTION column and the ANSWER column have been offset so that you can cover the answer while reading the questions, allowing you to assess your knowledge.

Question	Answer
1. What are the four stages of sleep?	
2. What is another name for paradoxic sleep?	1. Sleep stages I-IV are explained in the textbook, p. 199.
3. What is insomnia?	2. Rapid eye movement (REM) sleep is also called paradoxic sleep.
4. What premedication assessments should be performed prior to administering any sedative-hypnotic agent?	3. Insomnia is the inability to sleep.
5. Differentiate between the actions of a sedative and a hypnotic.	4. Before administering a sedative-hypnotic agent, assess for level of alertness, orientation, and ability to perform motor functions, as well as current blood pressure, pulse, respirations, sleep pattern, anxiety level, and environmental and nutritional factors that might impede sleep.
6. What should a nursing history relating to a patient's complaints of insomnia include?	5. Hypnotics produce sleep. Sedatives relax the patient.
7. Name two classes of drugs used as sedative-hypnotics. What ending appears on the generic drug names?	6. A nursing history related to a patient's complaints of insomnia should include usual pattern of sleep, anxiety level, environmental factors, nutritional habits, and medications or actions tried before seeking current treatment.
8. State the effect of hypnotics on respiratory function.	7. Two classes of sedative-hypnotics are barbiturates (all end in "-tal") and benzodiazepines (all end in "-am", except chlordiazepoxide [Librium]).
9. What changes in REM sleep occur with the administration of barbiturates?	8. Hypnotics produce mild to marked respiratory depression, depending on dosage and pulmonary function.
10. What is a rebound effect associated with discontinuing barbiturates?	9. Barbiturates initially decrease REM sleep; however, as tolerance builds, REM sleep returns to normal.
11. What is meant by *morning hangover* associated with barbiturates, benzodiazepines, and miscellaneous agents used as sedative-hypnotics? State the associated health teaching that needs to be initiated.	10. A rebound effect associated with discontinuing barbiturates is increase in REM; it may take several weeks following barbiturate therapy for this to resolve.

Copyright © 2004 Mosby Inc. All rights reserved.

12. What is a paradoxical response to hypnotics and what nursing actions are required if this response occurs?

13. What laboratory studies are recommended with continued use of barbiturates and benzodiazepines?

14. List the generic and brand names of commonly prescribed barbiturates, benzodiazepines, and miscellaneous sedative-hypnotic agents as assigned by the instructor.

15. In addition to their use as sedative-hypnotics, for what other clinical uses are barbiturates prescribed?

16. What effect can the regular use of barbiturates have on oral contraceptive therapy?

17. What is the blood-brain barrier?

18. What side effects can be expected from the administration of sedative-hypnotics?

19. What are side effects to report when taking sedative-hypnotics?

20. What premedication assessments should be performed before administration of a benzodiazepine?

11. Morning hangover from sedative-hypnotics includes blurred vision, mental dullness, and mild hypotension. Health teaching about this effect should include directions to consult physician if these symptoms become too bothersome; instructions to rise slowly to sitting position, equilibrate, then stand; and a caution regarding use of machinery, etc.

12. Paradoxical response is a period of excitement prior to sedation induced by use of barbiturates and other sedative-hypnotics not usually associated with benzodiazepine therapy. Appropriate nursing actions include protecting patient from harm providing for channeling of energy.

13. RBC, WBC, and differential count lab studies should be done with continued use of barbiturates and benzodiazepines. Also immediately report sore throat, fever, progressive weakness, purpura, or jaundice.

14. Consult Tables 14-1, p. 203; 14-2, p. 205; and 14-3, p. 207.

15. Specific agents are used as anticonvulsants and induction anesthetics.

16. The client may need to use an alternative form of contraceptive therapy, particularly if spotting or breakthrough bleeding occurs.

17. The blood-brain barrier is a membrane that controls the passage of drugs into the central nervous system to the receptor sites on the cells within the central nervous system.

18. Side effects of sedative-hypnotics include hangover, sedation, lethargy, blurred vision, and transient hypotension.

19. Side effects of sedative-hypnotics to report are excessive use or abuse, paradoxical response, pruritus, rash, high fever, sore throat, purpura, and jaundice.

20. Before administering a benzodiazepine, assess vital signs, including blood pressure in lying and sitting positions. Check whether the client is in the first trimester of pregnancy, breast-feeding, or has a history of a blood dyscrasia or hepatic disease.

Copyright © 2004 Mosby Inc. All rights reserved.

Sedative-Hypnotics

CHAPTER 14

Practice Quiz

COMPLETION

Use the following vocabulary words to complete the statements: sedative, hypnotic, rebound sleep, paradoxic excitement, initial insomnia, intermittent insomnia, terminal insomnia.

S.C. has difficulty falling asleep and the physician he consults tells him this is (1) _____ insomnia. While at the sleep disorder clinic, S.C. tells another patient, W.S., about his difficulty sleeping. W.S. quickly explains this isn't the same as his problem. He falls asleep, but awakens about 4 AM and can't get back to sleep. W.S.'s insomnia pattern is called (2) _____ insomnia.

Prior to surgery, the physician prescribes a(n) (3) _____ to help J.T. to sleep. The next morning, a (4) _____ is ordered for 8 AM (0800) for the purpose of providing relaxation and rest while awaiting scheduled surgery at 10:30 AM (1030). Two days after surgery, J.T. asks the nurse if it would be OK to ask the doctor for a prescription for the "wonderful medication" she took prior to surgery because she had the best sleep that day. The nurse asked her about her sleep pattern. She described that she generally has difficulty sleeping all night at home. She sleeps a while, awakens, and sleeps in cycles several times nightly. The nurse tells her this is known as (5) _____ insomnia.

Develop a response to J.T.'s question regarding her intention to request a prescription for a (6) _____ from the physician for use at home. Include in the explanation why long-term use of sedative-hypnotics is not beneficial and explain rebound sleep in lay terms.

Based on the data given for J.T.'s situation, develop two nursing diagnosis statements appropriate for her case.

7.

8.

9. List the side effects that can be anticipated with the administration of barbiturates and benzodiazepines.

   Barbiturates:

   Benzodiazepines:

10. What is meant by the statement that a drug produces physical dependence?

11. What premedication assessments should be performed prior to the administration of ANY sedative-hypnotic? Which assessments should be completed prior to administering a benzodiazepine or a barbiturate?

END-OF-CHAPTER MATH REVIEW

1. Dr. Smith wrote orders to start J.H. on triazolam 0.5 mg at bedtime 4 days only. Triazolam is available in 0.125 and 0.25 mg tablets. What will you administer?

2. Dr. Jones wrote orders for J.S. to receive 400 mg of chloral hydrate 1 hour before a computed tomography scan. Chloral hydrate is available in 250 and 500 mg capsules and 250 and 500 mg/5 ml syrup. What will you administer?

3. L.H. is scheduled for an endoscopy at 9 AM tomorrow. He weighs 60 kg. A dose of midazolam 7.5 mg IV is scheduled to be administered a few minutes before the endoscopy. The normal midazolam dose is 0.1–0.15 mg/kg. Is the 7.5 mg dose a reasonable dose for this patient?

Copyright © 2004 Mosby Inc. All rights reserved.

Student Name_____

CRITICAL THINKING QUESTIONS

1. Three hours after being given a hypnotic, C.G. is still awake. She is having major surgery in the morning. Describe the actions you should initiate and the rationale for performing each.

2. Why should patients be cautioned against the use of alcohol when taking sedative-hypnotics?

3. Describe situations in which repeating a dose of a sedative-hypnotic would be appropriate.

REVIEW QUESTIONS

_____ 1. As individuals age, their sleep becomes:
   a. more fragmented.
   b. more sound.
   c. characterized by fewer nocturnal awakenings.
   d. both b and c.

_____ 2. A patient receiving a benzodiazepine who also ingests alcohol may:
   a. experience erratic sleep and need less of the prescribed medication.
   b. experience additive effects of the alcohol and sedative-hypnotic agent.
   c. experience antagonist effects of the alcohol and sedative-hypnotic agent.
   d. require a higher dose of benzodiazepine and frequent assessments.

_____ 3. Long-term administration of benzodiazepines may result in:
   a. nephrotoxicity.
   b. alcohol-like withdrawal symptoms if withdrawn rapidly.
   c. a rush of morning energy with repeated usage.
   d. seizures during the time it is being administered.

Copyright © 2004 Mosby Inc. All rights reserved.

CHAPTER 15

Drugs Used for Parkinson's Disease

Syllabus

CHAPTER CONTENT

Parkinson's Disease (p. 209)
> Drug Therapy for Treatment of Parkinson's
> Disease (p. 210)
> Drug Class: Dopamine Agonists (p. 213)
> Drug Class: COMT Inhibitors (p. 220)
> Drug Class: Anticholinergic Agents (p. 221)
> Drug Class: Miscellaneous Antiparkinson's
> Agents (p. 223)

CHAPTER OBJECTIVES

1. Prepare a list of signs and symptoms of Parkinson's disease and accurately define the vocabulary used for the pharmacologic agents prescribed and the disease state.
2. Name the neurotransmitter found in excess and the deficient neurotransmitter in persons with parkinsonism.
3. Describe reasonable expectations of medications prescribed for treatment of Parkinson's disease.
4. Identify the period of time necessary for a therapeutic response to be observed when drug therapy for parkinsonism is initiated.
5. Name the action of bromocriptine mesylate, carbidopa, levodopa, and tolcapone neurotransmitters involved in Parkinson's disease.
6. List symptoms that can be attributed to the cholinergic activity of pharmacologic agents.
7. Cite the specific symptoms that should show improvement when anticholinergic agents are administered to the patient with Parkinson's disease.
8. Develop a health teaching plan for an individual being treated with levodopa.

KEY TERMS

Parkinson's disease	akinesia
dopamine	propulsive movements
neurotransmitter	livedo reticularis
acetylcholine	anticholinergic agents
tremor	levodopa
dyskinesia	

ASSIGNMENTS

Read textbook, pp. 209-215.
Study Key Terms associated with chapter content.
Complete Collaborative Activities as assigned.
Study Review Sheet for Chapter 15.
Complete End-of-Chapter Math Review and Critical Thinking Questions.
Complete Chapter 15 Practice Quiz.
Complete Chapter 15 Exam.

WEB RESEARCH ACTIVITY

Access: www.apdaparkinson.com/ and research publications and videos available.
Locate the closest Parkinson's disease support group in your vicinity.
Retrieve a copy of the Unified Parkinson's Disease Rating Scale from the Internet.

COLLABORATIVE ACTIVITIES

Complete the following activities. Be prepared to share your responses during in-class discussion or group work that may be assigned by the instructor.

1. Select a patient with Parkinson's disease.
2. What medications, of those listed on the MAR (medication administration record), are specifically used to treat this disease?
3. List the desired action of each antiparkinsonian medication prescribed.

Copyright © 2004 Mosby Inc. All rights reserved.

4. Develop focused assessments that can be used to detect a positive or negative response to these drugs.

5. Discuss the findings in class, conference, or a seminar setting.

Copyright © 2004 Mosby Inc. All rights reserved.

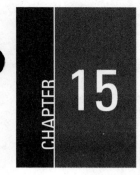

Drugs Used for Parkinson's Disease

Review Sheet

The QUESTION column and the ANSWER column have been offset so that you can cover the answer while reading the question, allowing you to assess your knowledge.

Question	Answer
1. Prepare a list of signs and symptoms of parkinsonism.	
2. Summarize the purpose of giving medications to treat Parkinson's disease.	1. Signs and symptoms of parkinsonism are expressionlessness; masklike face; tremors of hands, lips, tongue, and jaw; "pill-rolling" movements of fingers; excessive salivation; and dyskinesia.
3. Identify the basic components of a baseline assessment of a patient's neurologic function.	2. Medications are given to treat Parkinson's disease to provide maximum relief of symptoms and to optimize independence of movement and activity. See also Drug Therapy for Treatment of Parkinson's Disease, p. 210.
4. What are the monitoring parameters found on the Unified Parkinson's Disease Rating Scale?	3. Baseline neurologic assessment includes orientation to name, date, time, and place; degree of alertness; ability to comprehend and follow instructions; and degree of involvement in activities of daily life.
5. What are the meanings of the terms: *dyskinesia; propulsive, uncontrolled movement;* and *akinesia*?	4. See textbook, p. 211 and results of assigned web activity.
6. Persons taking amantadine hydrochloride may experience confusion, disorientation, and mental depression. What actions should the nurse take if/when this occurs?	5. Dyskinesia: inability to perform voluntary movements. Propulsive, uncontrolled movements: quick, short steps forward or backward that cannot be controlled. Akinesia: lack of movement.
7. Because of the many side effects known to occur with medications used to treat parkinsonism, what health teaching should be initiated?	6. The nurse should provide for patient safety, report alterations for evaluation by the physician, and continue to make regularly scheduled assessments of the individual's neurologic status.

Copyright © 2004 Mosby Inc. All rights reserved.

8. Compare the actions of amantadine hydrochloride, bromocriptine mesylate, carbidopa, levodopa, pergolide mesylate, selegiline, and tolcapone.

9. Summarize the side effects associated with medication therapy used in the treatment of parkinsonism. State nursing actions that could be used to alleviate and/or prevent the side effects.

10. What type of glaucoma prohibits the use of levodopa?

11. What specific type of vitamin preparation should be used by patients taking levodopa?

12. List three drugs used to treat parkinsonism.

13. What drugs may be combined with levodopa to improve its effectiveness?

14. Persons taking levodopa (Larodopa) for several months may develop what type of central nervous system side effects?

15. Why should a baseline neurologic assessment be done prior to and periodically during the administration of commonly prescribed drugs for treatment of Parkinson's disease?

16. What neurologic side effects are most often seen with pergolide?

7. Prepare a list of symptoms the patient has before starting therapy and involve the patient in keeping track of alterations (as the individual's abilities permit). Explain the need for continuing therapy for a period sufficient for the effectiveness of medications to be evaluated. Have patient report effects that are particularly bothersome; work cooperatively to plan approaches to alleviate the problems.

8. Amantadine hydrochloride slows destruction of dopamine and may aid in release of dopamine from storage sites. Bromocriptine mesylate stimulates dopamine receptors in basal ganglia of the brain. Carbidopa inhibits the metabolism of levodopa. Levodopa replaces dopamine deficiency in the basal ganglia of the brain. Pergolide mesylate stimulates postsynaptic dopamine receptors. Selegiline has an unknown mechanism of action. Tolcapone reduces the destruction of dopamine in peripheral tissue allowing significantly more to reach the brain.

9. See p. 215 (amantadine), p. 216 (bromocriptine), p. 217 (levodopa), p. 218 (pergolide), p. 220 (entacapone), and p. 221 (anticholinergic agents).

10. Angle-closure glaucoma prohibits the use of levodopa.

11. Pyridoxine-free multiple vitamin (Larobec) should be used by patients taking levodopa.

12. Drugs used to treat parkinsonism include bromocriptine mesylate (Parlodel), levodopa (Larodopa), amantadine (Symmetrel), carbidopa (Sinemet), pergolide mesylate (Permax), and ropinirole (Requip).

13. Carbidopa, an enzyme inhibitor that reduces the metabolism of levodopa, allowing a greater portion of the administered levodopa to reach the receptor sites in the basal ganglia. Entacapone inhibits the metabolism of dopamine, resulting in a more constant dopaminergic stimulation in the brain.

14. Long-term use of levodopa can cause abnormal movements (e.g., rocking, facial grimacing, chewing motions, head and neck bobbing).

15. Several of the drugs used to treat Parkinson's disease can cause adverse effects such as confusion and hallucinations. It is important to know which is a progression of the disease and which is due to an adverse effect of drug therapy.

Copyright © 2004 Mosby Inc. All rights reserved.

17. What is the primary mechanism of action of anticholinergic agents?

18. What are the therapeutic outcomes desired when an anticholinergic agent is prescribed for a Parkinson's patient?

19. When the ability to perform motor functions is impaired, what nursing diagnosis statement could be made?

16. Common neurologic side effects with pergolide include dyskinesia, hallucinations, somnolence, and insomnia.

17. The primary mechanism of action of anticholinergic agents is to reduce overstimulation caused by the excess of acetylcholine, a cholinergic neurotransmitter.

18. The desired effects are reduction in drooling, sweating, tremors, and depression.

19. Risk for injury related to Parkinson's disease; manifested by propulsive gait, unsteadiness, and progressive inability to walk unassisted.

Copyright © 2004 Mosby Inc. All rights reserved.

Student Name_____

CHAPTER 15
Drugs Used for Parkinson's Disease

Practice Quiz

COMPLETION

Complete the following statements.

1. With Parkinson's disease, the neurotransmitter _____ is deficient, leaving a relative excess of the neurotransmitter _____.

2. The primary goals of drug therapy for the treatment of Parkinson's disease are _____ and _____.

3. List five symptoms of Parkinson's disease.

4. State two nursing diagnoses that may apply when medicines are administered to treat Parkinson's disease (for example, levodopa-carbidopa, bromocriptine mesylate).

5. When a drug monograph lists orthostatic hypotension as a possible adverse effect, what nursing actions should be implemented?

6. How is a person's mental status assessed?

7. How soon after initiation of drug therapy for Parkinson's disease will a therapeutic response be seen?

8. To help reduce an excess amount of acetylcholine, _____ agents are prescribed.

9. All patients receiving levodopa should have the following premedication assessment:

10. The major action of the drug carbidopa is _____.

11. The major action of the drug levodopa is _____.

12. The major action of the drug entacapone is: _____.

13. The term used for the lack of ability to move is: _____.

14. _____ is an adverse dermatologic response to amantadine therapy.

15. _____ are a fairly new side effect to be reported associated with dopamine agonists.

END-OF-CHAPTER MATH REVIEW

1. Dr. Jones wrote orders to start a patient on Sinemet 25/100 mg at an initial dose of one tablet tid. Sinemet is available in ratios of 10/100, 25/100, 25/250, and 50/200 mg strengths. Which strength should be used and how many tablets should be administered for each individual dose?

2. Dr. Jones wrote orders to start a patient on levodopa 0.25 g qid. Levodopa is available in 100, 250, and 500 mg strengths. Which strength should be used and how many tablets should be administered at one time?

3. Dr. Jones wrote to start a patient on bromocriptine at an initial dose of 1.25 mg two times daily with meals. Bromocriptine is available in 2.5 mg tablets and 5 mg capsules. What will you administer?

CRITICAL THINKING QUESTIONS

1. What physiologic effect does stimulation of dopamine receptors have?

2. G.H.'s family asks you to explain the basic underlying problem that is causing the symptoms of Parkinson's disease in their mother. Give a simple explanation of the symptoms, appropriate for use with a lay person. Include an explanation of neurotransmitters and the basic imbalances found with Parkinson's disease.

3. Discuss the normal course of progression of Parkinson's disease and include the rationale for drug therapy to alleviate the symptoms.

4. Develop a teaching plan to be used with the patient and family of an individual being started on Sinemet for the treatment of Parkinson's disease.

Copyright © 2004 Mosby Inc. All rights reserved.

5. Explain baseline assessment of an individual's mental status and physical symptoms that are important before and periodically throughout the course of treatment of Parkinson's disease.

6. F.J. is being started on an anticholinergic drug as part of the treatment plan for Parkinson's disease. What symptoms could you anticipate improvement in and conversely, what problems could also arise from starting this medication?

REVIEW QUESTIONS

_____ 1. The use of selegiline (Eldepryl) in the early treatment of Parkinson's disease has the primary purpose of:
  a. reducing excessive acetylcholine stimulation.
  b. increasing dopamine in basal ganglia.
  c. slowing symptom progression; delaying initiation of levodopa therapy.
  d. reducing metabolism of levodopa, thereby making more available.

_____ 2. Essential patient education for an individual receiving levodopa includes:
  a. taking daily multivitamins.
  b. limiting daily intake of fluids.
  c. taking medication with food or milk.
  d. providing monthly gait training.

Copyright © 2004 Mosby Inc. All rights reserved.

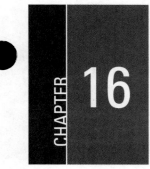

Drugs Used for Anxiety Disorders

Syllabus

CHAPTER CONTENT

Anxiety Disorders (p. 225)
    Drug Therapy for Anxiety Disorders (p. 226)
        Drug Class: Benzodiazepines (p. 229)
        Drug Class: Azapirones (p. 231)
        Drug Class: Selective Serotonin Reuptake
            Inhibitors (p. 231)
        Drug Class: Miscellaneous Agents (p. 232)

CHAPTER OBJECTIVES

1. Define terminology associated with anxiety states.
2. Describe the essential components of a baseline assessment of a patient's mental status.
3. Cite the side effects of hydroxyzine therapy and identify those effects requiring close monitoring when the drug is used preoperatively.
4. Develop a teaching plan for patient education of persons taking antianxiety medications.
5. Describe signs and symptoms indicating a positive therapeutic outcome in a patient being treated for a high-anxiety state.
6. Discuss psychologic and physiologic drug dependence.

KEY TERMS

generalized anxiety disorder
anxiety
panic disorder
phobias
obsession
compulsion
anxiolytics
tranquilizers

ASSIGNMENTS

Read textbook, pp. 225-234.
Study Key Terms associated with chapter content.
Complete Collaborative Activities as assigned.
Study Review Sheet for Chapter 16.
Complete Chapter 16 Practice Quiz.
Complete End-of-Chapter Math Review and Critical Thinking Questions.
Complete Chapter 16 Exam.

WEB RESEARCH ACTIVITY

Access: www.adaa.org/ and go to the Learn More About General Anxiety Disorder site and take the self-assessment test(s) found there.

COLLABORATIVE ACTIVITIES

Answer the following questions. Be prepared to share your responses during in-class discussion and group work that may be assigned by the instructor.
1. When hydroxyzine (Vistaril, Atarax) is used pre-operatively and postoperatively, what side effects can be expected and what assessments should be made to detect them? When side effects are present, what nursing actions are appropriate?
2. Explain how to prepare the following preoperative drug orders for administration:
    Hydroxyzine 50 mg, IM, on call to operating room.
    Demerol 75 mg, IM, on call to operating room.
3. What nursing assessments should be performed on a regular basis on a patient who has an anxiety disorder?
4. What premedication assessments should be performed before administering hydroxyzine?
5. Explain appropriate health teaching for a patient being started on meprobamate therapy.

Copyright © 2004 Mosby Inc. All rights reserved.

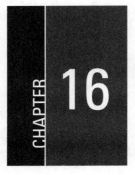

Drugs Used for Anxiety Disorders

Review Sheet

The QUESTION column and the ANSWER column have been offset so that you can cover the answers while reading the questions, allowing you to assess your knowledge.

Question	**Answer**
1. Define *anxiety disorder*.	
2. What is a *phobia*?	1. Patients are said to suffer from an anxiety disorder when their responses to stressful situations are abnormal, irrational, and impair normal daily functioning.
3. What is obsessive-compulsive disorder?	2. Phobias are irrational fears of a specific object, activity, or situation. The patient recognizes the fear as exaggerated or unrealistic. The fear persists, however, and the patient seeks to avoid the situation.
4. What is a panic disorder?	3. An obsession is an unwanted thought, idea, image, or urge that a patient recognizes as time-consuming and senseless but that repeatedly intrudes into the consciousness despite attempts to ignore, prevent, or counteract it. A compulsion is a repetitive, intentional, purposeful behavior performed to decrease the anxiety associated with an obsession.
5. State another common name for *tranquilizers*.	4. See textbook, p. 225.
6. Summarize nursing assessments and interventions that are used for the patient displaying anxiety.	5. Tranquilizers are also called *anxiolytic agents* or *antianxiety* medications.
7. State the action of benzodiazepines.	6. See textbook, pp. 226-229.
8. What is the ending spelling of all generic drug names of benzodiazepines except chlordiazepoxide?	7. Benzodiazepines stimulate an inhibitory neurotransmitter gamma amino benzoic acid (GABA).
9. Name three benzodiazepines that are relatively short acting and therefore most appropriate for an older adult or an individual with reduced hepatic function.	8. All generic drug names of benzodiazepines end in "-am."
10. What premedication assessments should be performed prior to administering a benzodiazepine?	9. Alprazolam, lorazepam, oxazepam are appropriate benzodiazepines for older adults or individuals with reduced hepatic function.

Copyright © 2004 Mosby Inc. All rights reserved.

11. State the desired therapeutic outcome for any drug prescribed for an anxiety disorder.

12. Why is the use of benzodiazepines avoided during the first trimester of pregnancy?

13. Describe side effects to expect with buspirone (BuSpar), hydroxyzine (Vistaril), and meprobamate (Equanil).

14. Based on the side effects of the drugs listed in question 13, what nursing diagnosis could be developed?

15. When you read a drug monograph that lists possible orthostatic hypotension as a side effect, what nursing actions would be appropriate, in addition to teaching the patient to rise slowly from a supine to sitting position?

16. What are additive effects associated with concurrent CNS system depressants?

17. What are symptoms of hepatotoxicity?

18. What are the side effects to expect with hydroxyzine?

19. What is the major advantage of buspirone, an azapirone agent, over other antianxiety agents?

20. What is the action of fluvoxamine (Luvox), an SSRI agent?

21. When used as a preoperative medication, what are the desired actions of hydroxyzine (Vistaril, Atarax)?

10. Before administering a benzodiazepine, assess for level of anxiety present; vital signs, especially blood pressure in sitting and supine positions; blood dyscrasias; hepatic disease; and whether the patient is in the first trimester of pregnancy or breast-feeding.

11. The desired outcome of drug therapy for anxiety disorders is a decreased level of anxiety so that the individual can function normally in life's daily activities.

12. Use of benzodiazepines in the first trimester of pregnancy is associated with increased incidence of birth defects.

13. Side effects to expect include sedation and lethargy with buspirone; blurred vision, constipation, dryness of mucous membranes, and sedation with hydroxyzine; and sedation, slurred speech, and dizziness with meprobamate.

14. A possible nursing diagnosis is: Injury, high risk for, related to antianxiety drug therapy (meprobamate, buspirone, hydroxyzine) manifested by lethargy, sedation, blurred vision, dizziness.

15. Monitor blood pressure in supine and standing positions every shift and provide for patient safety.

16. Combining more than one drug that depresses the CNS will cause exaggeration of the depressant effects and could reach potentially fatal levels.

17. Symptoms of hepatotoxicity include anorexia, nausea, vomiting, hepatomegaly, splenomegaly, and abnormal liver function tests (elevated bilirubin, AST, ALT, GGT, alkaline phosphatase, and prothrombin time).

18. Side effects to expect with hydroxyzine include blurred vision, constipation, dry mucosa (thirst), and sedation.

19. There is lower incidence of sedation with buspirone.

20. Luvox inhibits serotonin reuptake at the nerve endings, prolonging the serotonin activity. It is used to assist persons with obsessive-compulsive disorder to gain better control over obsessive actions.

21. Used preoperatively, hydroxyzine causes sedation, acts as an antiemetic and reduces the narcotic dose needed for analgesia.

Copyright © 2004 Mosby Inc. All rights reserved.

CHAPTER 16

Drugs Used for Anxiety Disorders

Practice Quiz

DEFINITIONS

Define the following terms:

1. Tranquilizer—
2. Compulsion—
3. Phobias—
4. Panic disorder—
5. Obsession—
6. Anxiety—

NURSING PROCESS

7. Summarize the nursing assessments used to collect data relating to:
   a. mood/affect
   b. clarity of thought
   c. psychomotor functions
   d. obsessions or compulsions
   e. sleep pattern
   f. dietary history
8. What is the nursing intervention with the highest priority for an individual suffering from a severe anxiety attack?

DRUG ACTIONS/SIDE EFFECTS

State the action and side effects of the following drug classes or drugs used in the treatment of anxiety disorders.

	Actions	**Side Effects**
9. Benzodiazepines		
10. Azapirones		
11. Hydroxyzine		
12. Meprobamate		

13. What premedication assessments should be performed prior to administering a benzodiazepine?

END-OF-CHAPTER MATH REVIEW

1. Ordered: hydroxyzine (Vistaril) 20 mg, IM, stat.
   On hand: hydroxyzine (Vistaril) 25 mg/ml.
   Give: _____ ml.
2. Ordered: meprobamate (Miltown) 1600 mg, PO daily in four divided doses.
   How many mg/dose will be administered?
3. Ordered: lorazepam (Ativan) 3 mg, IM, stat.
   On hand: lorazepam (Ativan) 4 mg/ml.
   Give: _____ ml.

CRITICAL THINKING QUESTIONS

Read the following situation and answer the questions.

J.H. enters the unit with symptoms of generalized anxiety disorder. During the admission interview the following information is obtained.

J.H. is so fearful of losing her job that she discusses the possibility several times a day. This has been an increasing concern over the past eight months. Her work performance was previously regarded as above average; however, over the past two months she has had increasing difficulty concentrating and completing her responsibilities. Finally, last week her employer suggested she take a brief vacation to "get it together." Since then her symptoms have escalated significantly.

She is having difficulty falling asleep and frequently awakens with palpitations and clammy hands.

When asked to describe her feelings she says, "I'm out of control, I'm going to lose my job. What am I ever going to do?"

1. What additional nursing assessments must be made? Research a typical data intake assessment sheet used with anxiety disorder.
2. J.H.'s admission orders include giving alprazolam 0.25 mg, tid. What time schedule would be used to administer these doses?

Copyright © 2004 Mosby Inc. All rights reserved.

Student Name_____

3. Describe premedication assessment data needed and what additional assessments should be made after initiation of drug therapy using benzodiazepines.

4. How soon after initiation of drug therapy is it reasonable to expect a therapeutic response from antianxiety medication?

5. Describe the behavior monitoring system and intervention flow records used to detect the side effects of anxiolytic drugs in the clinical setting where you are assigned.

6. What assessments and nursing interventions (including health teaching) need to be performed to deal with the possible physical dependence or tolerance known to occur with benzodiazepine therapy?

REVIEW QUESTIONS

_____ 1. The benzodiazepine drug monograph states hepatotoxicity as a side effect to report. Laboratory tests to be reviewed to assess this include:
   a. bilirubin, alkaline phosphatase, gamma glutamyltransferase (GGT), and prothrombin time.
   b. albumin, ferritin, and prothrombin time.
   c. aspirate aminotransferase (AST), GGT, and ferritin.
   d. creatinine, creatinine clearance, and albumin.

_____ 2. Side effect(s) to report from hydroxyzine (Vistaril), a commonly used drug for preoperative anxiety, include:
   a. blurred vision.
   b. sedation.
   c. constipation.
   d. slurred speech/dizziness.

Copyright © 2004 Mosby Inc. All rights reserved.

17 Drugs Used for Mood Disorders

Syllabus

CHAPTER CONTENT

Mood Disorders (p. 235)
Treatment of Mood Disorders (p. 237)
Drug Therapy for Mood Disorders (p. 237)
Drug Therapy for Depression (p. 240)
    Drug Class: Monoamine Oxidase Inhibitors
      (p. 240)
    Drug Class: Selective Serotonin Reuptake
      Inhibitors (p. 242)
    Drug Class: Tricyclic Antidepressants (p. 244)
    Drug Class: Miscellaneous Agents (p. 246)
    Drug Class: Antimanic Agents (p. 250)

CHAPTER OBJECTIVES

1. Describe the essential components of a baseline assessment of a patient with depression or bipolar disorder.
2. Discuss the mood swings associated with bipolar disorder.
3. Compare drug therapy used during the treatment of the manic phase and depressive phase of bipolar disorder.
4. Cite monitoring parameters used for patients taking monoamine oxidase inhibitors (MAOIs), selective serotonin reuptake inhibitors (SSRIs), or tricyclic antidepressants.
5. Prepare a teaching plan for an individual receiving tricyclic antidepressants.
6. Differentiate between the physiologic and psychologic therapeutic responses seen with antidepressant therapy.
7. Identify the premedication assessments necessary before administration of MAOIs, SSRIs, tricyclic antidepressants, and antimanic agents.
8. Compare the mechanism of action of SSRIs to that of other antidepressant agents.
9. Cite the advantages of SSRIs over other antidepressant agents.
10. Examine the monographs for SSRIs to identify significant drug interactions.

KEY TERMS

mood
mood disorder
neurotransmitter
depression
cognitive symptoms
psychomotor
   symptoms

bipolar disorder
mania
euphoria
labile mood
grandiose
suicide
antidepressant

ASSIGNMENTS

Read textbook, pp. 235-253.
Study Key Terms associated with chapter content.
Complete Collaborative Activities as assigned.
Study Review Sheet for Chapter 17.
Complete Chapter 17 Practice Quiz.
Complete End-of-Chapter Math Review and Critical
   Thinking Questions.
Complete Chapter 17 Exam.

WEB RESEARCH ACTIVITIES

Access: www.ndna.org
1. Find a support group located in your immediate vicinity.
2. Go to: Information on Mood Disorders , Depression, and read information available in two or more of the areas listed below:

Depression

Symptoms of
   Depression
Types of Depression
Depression in Late Life
Women and
   Depression
Depression in Children

Men and Depression
Helping a Friend
Treatments
Depression & Other
   Illnesses
Support Groups

Copyright © 2004 Mosby Inc. All rights reserved.

COLLABORATIVE ACTIVITIES

Complete the following research questions. Be prepared to share your findings during in-class discussion and group work that may be assigned by the instructor.

Research the type of monitoring that is performed to detect extrapyramidal symptoms (EPS) in the clinical site(s) where you are assigned.

1. What records and reports are used?
2. How often are the assessments performed and recorded?
3. When extrapyramidal symptoms are initially detected, what are the appropriate nursing actions?

Copyright © 2004 Mosby Inc. All rights reserved.

Drugs Used for Mood Disorders

Review Sheet

The QUESTION column and the ANSWER column have been offset so that you can cover the answers while reading the questions, allowing you to assess your knowledge.

Question	Answer
1. Define *mood disorders*.	
2. Which neurotransmitters are affected by depression?	1. Mood disorders are also known as *affective disorders*. The person's ability to function is impaired for a prolonged period of time going beyond brief periods of emotional upset from negative life experiences. Mood disorders are characterized by abnormal feelings of euphoria and/or depression.
3. What are characteristic symptoms found in a person experiencing depression?	2. Norepinephrine, serotonin, and dopamine are the neurotransmitters affected by depression.
4. Define *bipolar disorder*.	3. Characteristic symptoms of depression are: persistent, reduced ability to experience pleasure in life's usual activities, sometimes accompanied by personality change and sadness.
	4. Bipolar disorder is characterized by distinct episodes of mania (euphoria) and depression separated by intervals without mood disturbances.
5. Define *flight of ideas*.	5. Quick thoughts that rapidly change from one topic to another are called *flight of ideas*.
6. Cite the incidence of attempted suicide in individuals with mood disorders.	6. The frequency of suicide attempts in individuals with mood disorders is 15%, 30 times higher than general population.
7. Cite the three stages that patients with mood disorders experience as they strive for achievement of full functioning status.	7. The stages one goes through during treatment of a mood disorder are: acute, continuation, and maintenance. See textbook, p. 237, for definitions of each.
8. Give two examples of cognitive symptoms and psychomotor symptoms.	8. Cognitive symptoms involve the ability to concentrate, altered clarity of thought (e.g., confusion, poor short-term memory). Psychomotor symptoms include slowed or retarded movements, pacing, and outbursts of shouting.
9. Define *labile moods*.	9. Labile moods are rapid shifts in mood. A person may be happy, then rapidly switch to anger and irritability.
10. Define *grandiose thinking*.	

Copyright © 2004 Mosby Inc. All rights reserved.

11. List the drug classifications used in the treatment of depression.
12. Describe basic components of assessment for an individual with a mood disorder.

13. In general, what is the decision-making capacity of an individual with a mood disorder?

14. What are the basic actions of medicines used to treat depression?

15. Why is it necessary to closely monitor patients taking antidepressants?

16. What is the anticipated therapeutic outcome for antidepressant therapy?

17. Discuss premedication assessments needed for an individual who is to receive 1) MAOIs; 2) SSRIs; 3) tricyclic antidepressants; or 4) miscellaneous agents, including bupropion, maprotiline, mirtazapine, nefazodone, trazodone, and venlafaxine.
18. State appropriate nursing diagnoses as indicators of antidepressant therapy.

19. Name the drug used to treat manic episodes. List the important premedication assessments as well as assessments needed for long-term therapy.
20. List the normal serum level for lithium.

10. Grandiose thinking is overestimation of oneself and one's abilities or importance.
11. Drugs used in the treatment of depression include MAOIs, tricyclic antidepressants, SSRIs, and a miscellaneous group of monocyclic and tetracyclic agents.
12. Basic components of assessment for mood disorders include history of mood disorders, basic mental status, interpersonal relationships, mood/affect, clarity of thought, thoughts of death, psychomotor function, sleep pattern, and dietary history.
13. The decision-making capacity of an individual with a mood disorder is highly variable. The nurse must evaluate the individual's abilities and need to be protected from self-harm.
14. All antidepressants block the uptake and destruction of the neurotransmitters serotonin, norepinephrine, and/or dopamine.
15. Patients taking antidepressants may be suicidal. When drug therapy is initiated, it may take 1–4 weeks before a therapeutic response is evident. An early improvement in mood or other symptoms should not be used as an indicator that the depression is no longer present. Individuals may require 4–6 weeks to reach a full therapeutic level of the medicine.
16. The anticipated therapeutic outcome for individuals taking antidepressants is improvement of mood with a concurrent reduction in the feelings of depression.

17. MAOIs, textbook p. 240; SSRIs, textbook p. 242; tricyclic antidepressants, textbook p. 244; miscellaneous agents, textbook p. 246.
18. Risk for violence: self-inflicted—hopelessness—dysfunctional grieving—ineffective individual coping—social isolation, and disturbed perception.
19. Lithium carbonate (Eskalith, Lithane) is used to treat manic episodes. Before beginning lithium therapy, stress importance of the need for adequate hydration and sodium intake. Teach the patient the signs of lithium toxicity (e.g., nausea, vomiting, abdominal pain, diarrhea, lethargy, speech difficulty, mild dizziness, muscle twitching, and tremors).

Copyright © 2004 Mosby Inc. All rights reserved.

21. Describe teaching that should be completed about sodium intake while receiving lithium therapy.
22. Why is behavioral monitoring during antidepressant therapy done?

20. Normal serum lithium range is 0.4–1.5 mEq/L.

21. During lithium therapy, normal daily intake of sodium is essential, as is adequate hydration. Stress using salt in cooking and at the table. The person should also drink 10–12 8 oz glasses of water daily.
22. Behavioral monitoring during antidepressant therapy is done to detect development of extrapyramidal symptoms and to monitor for degree of therapeutic response to therapy.

Copyright © 2004 Mosby Inc. All rights reserved.

Drugs Used for Mood Disorders

CHAPTER 17

Practice Quiz

COMPLETION

Complete the following statements.

A patient has been diagnosed with bipolar disorder. This disorder is characterized by mood swings between

1. _____, and
2. _____ (abnormal degree of sadness)

Drug classes known as antidepressants include:

3. _____
4. _____
5. _____
6. _____

Premedication assessments for MAOIs should include:

7. _____
8. _____
9. _____
10. _____

Behavioral monitoring is used to detect:

11. _____
12. _____
13. What is the generally recognized mechanism of action of antidepressant medications?
14. Persons taking MAOIs must omit foods containing:
15. Which classification of antidepressants is most widely used today in the treatment of depression?
16. A major bothersome side effect of tricyclic antidepressant therapy is:

Two additional common side effects of tricyclic antidepressants are:

17. _____, and
18. _____

Premedication assessments prior to initiation of lithium therapy should include:

19. _____
20. _____
21. _____
22. _____
23. The normal therapeutic range for serum lithium is:
24. Three neurotransmitters found in the brain are: _____, _____, and _____.
25. Periods of elation or euphoria are known as:
26. Give an example of what is meant by "manipulative behavior": _____.
27. _____ is a pain medication that should be avoided when MAOIs are being taken.

END-OF-CHAPTER MATH REVIEW

1. Ordered: lithium carbonate 300 mg, PO, twice daily
   On hand: lithium carbonate 150 mg tablets
   Give: _____ tablets
2. Ordered: maprotiline 100 mg, PO, this AM
   On hand: None found in medication container; consult drug monograph for dosage availability. What strength tablets would most likely be dispensed and how would you administer the dose?

CRITICAL THINKING QUESTIONS

1. During her clinic visit, a patient complains to the nurse that since she started taking amitriptyline (Elavil) for depression, she has had a "terrible dry mouth" and she feels "sleepy all the time." What additional information would you elicit? What interventions could you suggest to alleviate these symptoms?

Copyright © 2004 Mosby Inc. All rights reserved.

2. A patient at the clinic is taking fluoxetine (Prozac) He is 5' 6" tall, weighs 120 lbs. and has been receiving the medication for 6 weeks. He reports that he feels like a "cloud has been lifted from my mind." What additional data would be appropriate to collect during this visit?

3. When a patient is starting therapy with an MAOI, what health teaching is important?

4. The drug monograph for MAOI therapy states that one major potential complication of this therapy is hypertensive crisis. Discuss hypertensive crisis, how to recognize it, and the interventions that should be implemented if it occurs.

5. Discuss the behavioral monitoring sheets used in the clinical setting where you are practicing to assess for the development of extrapyramidal symptoms. How often are the assessments made, how are they recorded, and when is the physician notified of changes in the patient's behavior?

Situation (for questions 6–8): A patient, age 34, is being treated for bipolar disorder with lithium 300 mg, PO, 4 times daily. She is being seen today in the clinic. During the intake interview she tells the nurse that her medicine "never works." Further exploration reveals that she has not taken the medication for the past 4 days.

6. When reviewing the patient's history, the nurse reads that her lithium level taken the month before was 2.0 mEq/L. As the nurse in this situation, how would you proceed?

7. What symptoms might you expect with this lithium level?

8. The history also notes that the importance of adequate intake of water and sodium was discussed with the patient. How does the sodium level within the body influence the metabolism of lithium?

REVIEW QUESTIONS

_____ 1. Fluoxetine (Sarafem), an SSRI used for mood disorders, is also approved for treatment of:
   a. hallucinations associated with psychosis.
   b. extrapyramidal symptoms.
   c. premenstrual dysphoric disorder (PMDD).
   d. neuroleptic malignant syndrome.

_____ 2. A patient taking an MAOI needs to be monitored for:
   a. blood dyscrasias.
   b. hyperglycemia.
   c. hypertension.
   d. hyperactivity.

_____ 3. Bupropion hydrochloride (Wellbutrin) may cause hypertension when combined with:
   a. nicotine.
   b. levodopa.
   c. anticholinergics.
   d. lithium carbonate.

Copyright © 2004 Mosby Inc. All rights reserved.

CHAPTER 18

CHAPTER

Drugs Used for Psychoses

Syllabus

CHAPTER CONTENT

Psychosis (p. 254)
Treatment of Psychoses (p. 255)
Drug Therapy for Psychoses (p. 257)
    Drug Class: Antipsychotic Agents (p. 260)

CHAPTER OBJECTIVES

1. Identify signs and symptoms of psychosis.
2. Describe major indications for the use of anti-psychotic agents.
3. Identify common adverse effects observed with antipsychotic medications.
4. Develop a teaching plan for a patient taking haloperidol and for a person receiving clozapine.

KEY TERMS

psychosis
delusions
hallucinations
disorganized thinking
loosening of
    associations
disorganized behavior
changes in affect
target symptoms
typical antipsychotic
    agents
atypical antipsychotic
    agents
equipotent doses
extrapyramidal
    symptoms

dystonia
pseudoparkinsonian
    symptoms
akathisia
tardive dyskinesia
abnormal involuntary
    movement scale
dyskinesia
    identification
    systems: condensed
    user scale
neuroleptic malignant
    syndrome
depot antipsychotic
    medicine

ASSIGNMENTS

Read textbook, pp. 254-263.
Study Key Terms associated with chapter content.
Complete Collaborative Activities as assigned.
Study Review Sheet for Chapter 18.
Complete Chapter 18 Practice Quiz.
Complete End-of-Chapter Math Review and Critical
    Thinking Questions.
Complete Chapter 18 Exam.

WEB RESEARCH ACTIVITIES

Access: www.mentalhelp.net
1. Review resource materials available on the Internet:

Resources
Community
News
Book Reviews
Psych Self-Help
Self-Help Groups
Tests
Symptoms
Medications
Videos
Glossary
Phone Numbers
Therapists/Clinics

2. Access two other online resources listed at the end of Chapter 18 and bring information on the use of rating scales to evaluate dystonia and tardive dyskinesia to class for discussion.

Copyright © 2004 Mosby Inc. All rights reserved.

COLLABORATIVE ACTIVITIES

Complete the following activity and questions. Be prepared to share your findings during in-class discussion and group work that may be assigned by the instructor.

Perform an assessment of a patient receiving an antipsychotic medication, such as clozapine.

1. What laboratory studies were completed on admission or prior to initiating therapy?

2. Compare the laboratory studies performed in question 1 with the most recent laboratory values. Are there significant changes, and if so, what nursing actions would be appropriate?

   Are the recommended laboratory studies listed in the drug monograph, textbook p. 261, being performed? If not, what nursing actions would be appropriate?

Copyright © 2004 Mosby Inc. All rights reserved.

Drugs Used for Psychoses

Review Sheet

The QUESTION column and the ANSWER column have been offset so that you can cover the answer while reading the questions, allowing you to assess your knowledge.

Question	Answer
1. Define *psychosis*.	
2. Differentiate among delusions, hallucinations, and disorganized thinking.	1. Psychosis does not have a single definition, but is a clinical descriptor that means that a person is out of touch with reality.
3. What is change in affect?	2. Delusions are false, irrational beliefs unchanged in the presence of data to the contrary. Hallucinations are false sensory perceptions experienced by an individual without external stimulus. Disorganized thinking is recognized when an individual switches rapidly from one idea or thought to another unrelated topic.
4. What is meant by *target symptoms*?	3. Change in affect is characterized by diminished emotional expression, reduced spontaneous movement, and poor eye contact. The individual withdraws from effective functioning in interpersonal relations, work, education, and self-care.
5. What rating scales have been developed for objective measurement of target symptoms due to psychotherapy and pharmacology?	4. Target symptoms are those symptoms to be assessed to evaluate therapeutic response to drug therapy and nonpharmacologic interventions.
6. What is another name for an antipsychotic agent?	5. Brief Psychiatric Rating Scale (BPRS), the Positive and Negative Scale for Schizophrenia (PANSS), the Clinical Global Impression (CGI) scale, and the Rating of Aggression Against People and/or Property (RAAPP) Scale are recently developed scales in use for objective measurement of target symptoms. (*Note:* Students could benefit from further online research of the scales listed.)
7. Differentiate between the terms *low-potency* and *high-potency* antipsychotic agents.	6. Neuroleptic agent—usually reserved for the typical antipsychotic agents.
8. What are typical and atypical antipsychotic agents?	7. These terms refer ONLY to the milligram doses and not to the difference in effectiveness of antipsychotic agents.

Copyright © 2004 Mosby Inc. All rights reserved.

9. Cite the desired therapeutic outcome(s) from antipsychotic therapy.

10. Define *extrapyramidal symptoms*, including dystonia, pseudoparkinsonian symptoms, akathisia, and tardive dyskinesia.

11. What causes pseudoparkinsonian symptoms?

12. What monitoring scales are used to rate dystonia?

13. What are the DISCUS or AIMS scales?

14. Describe common adverse effects associated with antipsychotic therapy.

15. What is neuroleptic malignant syndrome? What are the symptoms, and how is it treated?

16. Summarize nursing implementations and patient education used for patients being treated for psychoses.

8. Typical agents are listed in Table 18-1, p. 256. Atypical antipsychotic agents include clozapine, olanzapine, quetiapine, risperidone, and ziprasidone. These classifications are based on the drugs' mechanisms of action. See textbook, pp. 255-257, for an explanation of the actions of typical and atypical antipsychotic agents on dopamine receptors.

9. Calmed the individual, reduced psychomotor agitation and insomnia, reduced thought disorders so the individual is able to function with minimal exacerbation of psychotic symptoms.

10. Dystonia is spasmodic movements of muscle groups (e.g., tongue protrusion, rolling back of the eyes). Pseudoparkinsonian symptoms are tremors, muscular rigidity, masklike expression, shuffling gait, and loss or weakness of motor function. Akathisia is a feeling of anxiety, restlessness, pacing, rocking, and inability to sit still. Tardive dyskinesia is progressive symptoms of involuntary, hyperkinetic, abnormal movements.

11. Pseudoparkinsonian symptoms are caused by a relative deficiency of dopamine and an excess of acetylcholine, caused by antipsychotic agents.

12. Toronto Western Spasmodic Torticollis Rating Scale (TWSTRS), Global Dystonia Scale (GDS), Unified Dystonia Scale (UDRS), and the Fahn-Marsden Scale. (See also related web sites on documentation of dystonia.)

13. Both the DISCUS and AIMS scales are involuntary movement scales for rating dyskinetic movements. (See textbook Appendix H for the DISCUS scale.)

14. Adverse effects of antipsychotic therapy include sedation, drowsiness, appetite stimulation, postural hypotension, reflex tachycardia, lowering of seizure threshold, and development of symptoms of tardive dyskinesia.

15. See textbook, p. 258. Symptoms of neuroleptic malignant syndrome include fever, extrapyramidal symptoms, and lead-pipe rigidity, probably due to excessive dopamine depletion. It is treated with bromocriptine or amantadine as dopamine agonists and dantrolene, a muscle relaxant. Fever is treated with cooling blankets, adequate hydration, and antipyretics.

Copyright © 2004 Mosby Inc. All rights reserved.

17. Memorize the generic and brand names of these commonly prescribed antipsychotic agents: Thorazine, Trilafon, Compazine, Mellaril, Clozaril, Haldol, and Risperdal.

16. See textbook, pp. 255-260.

17. The generic and brand names of commonly prescribed antipsychotic agents are: chlorpromazine—Thorazine; perphenazine—Trilafon; prochlorperazine—Compazine; thioridazine—Mellaril; clozapine—Clozaril; haloperidol—Haldol; and risperidone—Risperdal.

Copyright © 2004 Mosby Inc. All rights reserved.

Student Name _____

Drugs Used for Psychoses

Practice Quiz

MATCHING

Select the definition that best describes the term(s) listed.

_____ 1. hallucinations
_____ 2. delusions
_____ 3. akathisia
_____ 4. tardive dyskinesia
_____ 5. dystonia

a. Syndrome demonstrated by anxiety, restlessness, pacing, and rocking
b. Alternating feelings of danger and elation
c. Involuntary hyperkinetic abnormal movements
d. False sensory perceptions experienced without external stimulus
e. Prolonged spasmodic movements of muscle groups
ab. A false, irrational belief that a patient embraces despite evidence to the contrary

List the generic or brand names of the following antipsychotic agents:

6. chlorpromazine
7. Trilafon
8. Mellaril
9. clozapine
10. Haldol
11. Compazine

CRITICAL THINKING QUESTIONS

J.S. is taking a high-potency antipsychotic medication.

1. What are high-potency antipsychotics and what drugs are included in this category?

2. What are extrapyramidal side effects? How often should the patient be monitored for these symptoms? When found, what nursing actions are appropriate?
3. It is decided that J.S. should receive clozapine. What are the side effects to expect and those to report with this medication?
4. Discuss monitoring for agranulocytosis.
5. Why is an anticholinergic agent frequently given in addition to haloperidol? What is its action?
6. State the usual anticipated side effects seen with antipsychotic therapy.
7. Explain the behavioral monitoring system used in your clinical site to detect dystonia extrapyramidal symptoms.

END-OF-CHAPTER MATH REVIEW

1. Ordered: chlorpromazine (Thorazine) 125 mg, PO
   On hand: chlorpromazine 100 mg per 5 ml
   Give _____ ml.
2. Order: benztropine mesylate (Cogentin) 1 mg, PO, at bedtime daily.
   On hand: benztropine mesylate 0.5 mg tablets.
   Give _____ tablets.
3. Ordered: trifluoperazine (Stelazine) 12 mg, IM.
   On hand: trifluoperazine 10 mg/ml and 20 mg/ml
   Which concentration would you use and what volume should be injected?

Copyright © 2004 Mosby Inc. All rights reserved.

REVIEW QUESTIONS

_____ 1. Four major side effects of antipsychotic medications are:
   a. nausea, vomiting, diarrhea, and sedation.
   b. orthostatic hypotension, blood dyscrasias, hepatotoxicity, and sedation.
   c. EPS, hypertension, mucosa dryness, and sedation.
   d. sedation, EPS, hypotension, and anticholinergic effects.

_____ 2. Premedication assessments for antipsychotic agents should include checking for:
   a. history of cardiovascular disorders.
   b. daily weights.
   c. positional blood pressure reading.
   d. history of diabetes mellitus.

Copyright © 2004 Mosby Inc. All rights reserved.

Drugs Used for Seizure Disorders

Syllabus

CHAPTER CONTENT

Seizure Disorders (p. 264)
Descriptions of Seizures (p. 265)
Anticonvulsant Therapy (p. 265)
Drug Therapy for Seizure Disorders (p. 268)
    Drug Class: Barbiturates (p. 268)
    Drug Class: Benzodiazepines (p. 268)
    Drug Class: Hydantoins (p. 271)
    Drug Class: Succinimides (p. 272)
    Drug Class: Miscellaneous Anticonvulsants
       (p. 273)

CHAPTER OBJECTIVES

1. Prepare a chart to be used as a study guide that includes the following information:
   - Seizure type
   - Description of seizure
   - Medications used to treat each type of seizure
   - Nursing interventions and monitoring parameters for seizures
2. Describe the effects of the hydantoins on patients with diabetes and on persons receiving oral contraceptives, theophylline, folic acid, or antacids.
3. Cite precautions needed when administering phenytoin or diazepam intravenously.
4. Explain the rationale for proper dental care for persons receiving hydantoin therapy.
5. Develop a teaching plan for persons diagnosed with a seizure disorder.
6. Cite the desired therapeutic outcomes for drug therapy for seizure disorders.
7. Identify the mechanisms of action thought to control seizure activity when anticonvulsants are administered.
8. Discuss the basic classification system used to describe types of epilepsy.

KEY TERMS

seizures
epilepsy
partial seizures
generalized seizures
anticonvulsants
tonic phase
clonic phase
postictal state
status epilepticus
atonic seizure

myoclonic seizures
absence (petit mal) epilepsy
seizure threshold
gamma-aminobutyric acid (GABA)
gingival hyperplasia
nystagmus
urticaria

ASSIGNMENTS

Read textbook, pp. 264-281.
Study Key Terms associated with chapter content.
Complete Collaborative Activity as assigned.
Study Review Sheet for Chapter 19.
Complete Chapter 19 Practice Quiz.
Complete End-of-Chapter Math Review and Critical Thinking Questions.
Complete Chapter 19 Exam.

WEB RESEARCH ACTIVITY

Access: www.ninds.nih.gov/health_and_medical/disorders/epilepsy.htm

View four or more articles found on this site to expand your knowledge of current treatments for epilepsy and resources available for professionals and lay persons.

Copyright © 2004 Mosby Inc. All rights reserved.

COLLABORATIVE ACTIVITY

Respond to the following case study. Be prepared to share your response during in-class discussion and group work that may be assigned by the instructor.

A patient is receiving ethotoin (Peganone) 500 mg, PO, qid. He is an insulin-dependent diabetic. What patient education should be performed when initiating this treatment and as the drug therapy progresses?

Copyright © 2004 Mosby Inc. All rights reserved.

CHAPTER 19 Drugs Used for Seizure Disorders

Review Sheet

The QUESTION column and the ANSWER column have been offset so that you can cover the answer while reading the question, allowing you to assess your knowledge.

Question

1. Define *seizures*.
2. Define *epilepsy*.

3. What are the most common types of generalized convulsive seizures?
4. Differentiate among the symptoms of each type of generalized convulsive seizure.
5. Define the types of partial seizures and differentiate among the symptoms of each.
6. Differentiate among tonic phase, clonic phase, and postictal state.
7. What is status epilepticus?

8. What is an atonic seizure or "drop attack"?

9. Define an *absence* or *petit mal seizure*.

10. What are first-line agents and how are they selected?

Answer

1. Seizures are brief periods of abnormal electrical activity in the brain that may or may not produce violent, involuntary muscle activity.
2. Epilepsy is diagnosed when a patient has chronic, recurrent seizures.
3. Tonic-clonic, atonic, and myoclonic seizures are the types of generalized seizures.
4. See textbook, p. 264.

5. See textbook, p. 265.

6. Tonic phase is when patient has intense muscle contractions, loss of consciousness, and rigidity of the body. The clonic phase is characterized by alternating jerking and relaxation of the muscles of the extremities. The patient may defecate or urinate during this phase. The postictal period is the period immediately following a seizure, during which the patient rests. The patient has no recollection of the attack after awakening.
7. Status epilepticus is a rapidly recurring generalized seizure that does not allow the individual to regain normal function between seizures.
8. Atonic seizures are characterized by a sudden loss of muscle tone, causing the head or limb to suddenly "drop." There is also loss of consciousness.
9. Petit mal seizures occur primarily in children. These seizures are characterized by a 5–20 second period of altered consciousness accompanied by a few rhythmic movements with no frank convulsive movements and no memory of events during the seizure. Partial seizures are localized convulsions of voluntary muscles. The person does not lose consciousness unless the

Copyright © 2004 Mosby Inc. All rights reserved.

11. What is the general action of all anticonvulsants?
12. What assessments should the nurse make during seizure activity?

13. What is meant by *postictal* behavior?

14. Identify components of the Glasgow Coma Scale.
15. What are the treatments used for status epilepticus?
16. What action should a patient requiring seizure medications take upon learning she is pregnant?
17. What actions do barbiturates have on seizure activity?

18. What three benzodiazepines are used as anticonvulsants?

19. What symptoms would be seen if benzodiazepines are suddenly stopped?
20. What time period should be used for the gradual withdrawal of benzodiazepines?

21. What precaution should be used when preparing diazepam or phenytoin for administration?
22. What precautions are required when giving IV diazepam or phenytoin?

23. Name the drugs known as hydantoins.

partial seizure progresses into generalized seizure.

10. See textbook, p. 265.

11. Anticonvulsants increase the seizure threshold and regulate neuronal firing with inhibiting excitatory processes or enhancing inhibitory processes. Medications can also prevent seizures from spreading to adjacent neurons.
12. During seizure activity, the nurse should note a description of the seizure, including onset, duration, body parts involved, any progression of symptoms, state of consciousness, respiratory pattern, salivation, pupil size and eye movement, and incontinence.
13. Postictal behavior is the person's state following a seizure. See textbook, p. 266.
14. Eye opening, best motor response, and verbal response. See textbook, p. 267.
15. Status epilepticus treatment is found on p. 268.

16. Do not discontinue medications; contact the health care provider immediately to discuss the medications being taken and appropriate actions for the well-being of the child and the mother.
17. Barbiturates elevate the seizure threshold and prevent spread of electrical seizure activity by the inhibitory effects of GABA.
18. Three benzodiazepines used as anticonvulsants are diazepam, clonazepam, and clorazepate.
19. Rapid withdrawal of benzodiazepines can result in symptoms similar to those seen with alcohol withdrawal.
20. Benzodiazepines require a 2–4-week period of gradual withdrawal.
21. Never mix diazepam or phenytoin in a syringe with another medication; either drug will form a precipitate in the syringe when combined with a second drug.
22. Do not administer diazepam IV at a rate of more than 5 mg per minute. Do not administer IV phenytoin at a rate over 25–50 mg per minute. Take the pulse before and periodically during IV administration of either drug—check for bradycardia. If this occurs, the rate of administration should be slowed until the pulse returns to normal. If possible, have an ECG in use when administering IV diazepam or IV phenytoin.

Copyright © 2004 Mosby Inc. All rights reserved.

24. What nursing action should be taken when a patient with diabetes is receiving phenytoin?

25. Explain health teaching that should be performed to reduce the severity of gingival hyperplasia.
26. What is the therapeutic range of a blood serum level for phenytoin?

27. List the signs and symptoms of phenytoin toxicity.
28. What is a brand name of phenytoin?

29. What over-the-counter drug decreases the therapeutic effects of hydantoins?
30. If a female patient receiving seizure medications tells the nurse that she has started spotting or bleeding between her regular menstrual cycles, what should the nurse advise?
31. In what way is the spelling of all succinimide anticonvulsants similar?

32. What are the uses of carbamazepine (Tegretol)? What laboratory studies are recommended with its use?
33. Access: www.aesnet.org and look up the nonapproved FDA uses of gabapentin.

34. What is the action of lamotrigine (Lamictal)?

35. Why is it necessary to check on whether a patient is already taking valproic acid before initiating therapy with lamotrigine?
36. Summarize the premedication assessments for each class of antiepileptics.

---

23. Hydantoins include phenytoin, ethotoin, fosphenytoin, and mephenytoin. (Note that these drug names all end in "-toin.")
24. Monitor the patient's blood sugar levels periodically because hyperglycemia may be caused by hydantoin therapy.
25. Provide for good oral hygiene that includes gum massage, proper brushing, and frequent dental care to prevent gum overgrowth (gingival hyperplasia).
26. Look up the therapeutic range of phenytoin in Appendix D.
27. Signs and symptoms of phenytoin toxicity include nystagmus, sedation, and lethargy.
28. Dilantin is the brand name of phenytoin.

29. Antacids decrease the therapeutic effects of hydantoins by interfering with their absorption.

30. The nurse should first check a drug reference to see if the seizure medication can reduce the effectiveness of an oral contraceptive; advise the patient appropriately to use an alternate form of contraceptive. This should also be documented in the chart and reported to the physician.
31. All succinimide medications end in "-suximide;" e.g., ethosuximide, methsuximide, and phensuximide.
32. Carbamazepine (Tegretol) may be used to treat seizures in combination with other anticonvulsant agents and to treat pain associated with trigeminal neuralgia. Blood studies to detect hepatotoxicity, nephrotoxicity, and/or blood dyscrasias should be performed.
33. Do research on the Internet to obtain the answer.
34. Lamotrigine blocks voltage-sensitive sodium channels in neuronal membranes.

35. Approximately 10% of patients receiving lamotrigine develop a skin rash and urticaria in the first 4–6 weeks of therapy. Combination therapy with valproic acid appears more likely to precipitate a serious rash. (See textbook, p. 275.)

Copyright © 2004 Mosby Inc. All rights reserved.

37. Review side effects to expect and report for seizure drugs.

36. Summary of premedication assessments for antiepileptics:
    - For the drug classes benzodiazepines, hydantoins, succinimides, and miscellaneous agents:
      — Baseline assessment of speech pattern, alertness, orientation and behavioral response to therapy.
    - For the drug classes hydantoins, succinimides, and for miscellaneous agent valproic acid:
      — Review blood reports to detect blood dyscrasias and hepatotoxicity.
    - Hydantoins:
      — Check blood sugar for diabetics (hyperglycemia with hydantoins).
    - Miscellaneous agents:
      — Carbamazepine (Tegretol)—CBC, liver and renal function tests, and ophthalmologic exam
      — Oxcarbazepine (Trileptal)—requires electrolyte studies periodically during this drugs use—review
      — Valproic acid (Depakene)—liver function tests, bleeding time, and platelet counts
      — Zonisamide (Zonegran)—check for allergy to sulfonamide medicines (do not administer drug until health care provider has approved its use). Check for history of skin rashes; if rash occurs notify health care provider immediately. Review baseline CBC, liver function, renal lab studies.

37. See individual monographs throughout chapter.

Copyright © 2004 Mosby Inc. All rights reserved.

CHAPTER 19

Drugs Used for Seizure Disorders

Practice Quiz

COMPLETION

Complete the following statements.

1. Name five classifications of drugs used to treat seizure disorders.
2. What is the mechanism of action of anticonvulsants?
3. Describe the tonic and clonic phases of seizure activity.
4. Diazepam, clonazepam, and clorazepate are anticonvulsants classified as _____.
5. Phenytoin can cause _____ in a diabetic patient.
6. Alternatives to oral contraceptives should be used when a patient takes _____, _____, or _____ as an anticonvulsant.
7. A decrease in therapeutic effectiveness of phenytoin can occur when an OTC _____ is taken concurrently.
8. Summarize patient education that should be completed when a patient receives anticonvulsant therapy.
9. Describe side effects to report when carbamazepine (Tegretol) is administered.
10. Which miscellaneous agent requires a premedication eye exam?
11. Which miscellaneous agent requires a premedication assessment for a skin rash?
12. What are the non-FDA–approved uses of gabapentin?

END-OF-CHAPTER MATH REVIEW

1. Dr. Frye wrote orders to start J.B. on Dilantin 100 mg, tid and hs. What is your interpretation of the order and how will you administer it?

2. Dr. Haycock wrote orders to start B.S., a 10-year-old patient, on Tegretol suspension 50 mg, qid. The suspension is 100 mg/5ml. How will you administer this dose?
3. Dr. Tindall wrote orders for J.S., a 12-year-old newly diagnosed epileptic patient, weighing 110 lbs, to be started on valproic acid (Depakene) syrup 5 ml, tid. The normal starting dose is 15 mg/kg daily. Is Dr. Tindall's order reasonable, and if so, how would you administer it?

CRITICAL THINKING QUESTIONS

1. Both Valium and Dilantin have very specific administration precautions when these agents are administered intravenously. What are these precautions?
2. R.C. suddenly had a tonic-clonic seizure while attending a class at college. When his family was notified of this and his need for transportation home, his wife tells you he has not been taking his medications regularly. Describe how you would address this situation.
3. While you are working in the emergency room, the rescue squad notifies the ER desk that a patient in status epilepticus is being transported. What medicines and equipment should you have ready for the patient's arrival?
4. What health teaching should be done for an individual recently diagnosed with epilepsy?

Copyright © 2004 Mosby Inc. All rights reserved.

Student Name_____

REVIEW QUESTIONS

_____ 1. While administering intravenous phenytoin, the nurse should watch the patient for symptoms of which of the following adverse responses?
a. bradycardia
b. increased seizure activity
c. confusion
d. sedation

_____ 2. An infant is brought into the emergency department with observable twitching of the extremities and a temperature of 104.2° F reported by the parents. The priority action is to:
a. take vital signs.
b. call a health care provider.
c. check the airway.
d. take a history.

Copyright © 2004 Mosby Inc. All rights reserved.

CHAPTER 20

Drugs Used for Pain Management

Syllabus

CHAPTER CONTENT

Pain (p. 282)
Drug Therapy for Pain Management (p. 283)
    Drug Class: Opiate Agonists (p. 292)
    Drug Class: Opiate Partial Agonists (p. 294)
    Drug Class: Opiate Antagonists (p. 296)
    Drug Class: Anti-inflammatory Agents (p. 299)
    Drug Class: Nonsteroidal Anti-inflammatory
        Agents (p. 303)
    Drug Class: Miscellaneous Analgesics (p. 304)

CHAPTER OBJECTIVES

1. Differentiate among opiate agonists, opiate partial agonists, and opiate antagonists.
2. Describe monitoring parameters necessary for patients receiving opiate agonists.
3. Cite the side effects to expect when opiate agonists are administered.
4. Compare the analgesic effectiveness of opiate partial agonists when administered before or after opiate agonists.
5. Explain when naloxone can be used effectively to treat respiratory depression.
6. State the three pharmacologic effects of salicylates.
7. Prepare a list of side effects to expect, side effects to report, and drug interactions that are associated with salicylates.
8. Explain why synthetic nonopiate analgesics are not used for inflammatory disorders.
9. Prepare a patient education plan for a person being discharged with a continuing prescription for an analgesic.
10. Examine Table 20-5 and identify the active ingredients in commonly prescribed analgesic combination products. List products containing aspirin and compare the analgesic properties of agents available in different strengths.

KEY TERMS

pain experience
pain perception
pain threshold
pain tolerance
acute pain
chronic pain
nociceptive pain
somatic pain
visceral pain
neuropathic pain
idiopathic pain
analgesics
opiate agonists
opiate partial agonists
opiate antagonists
salicylates
nonsteroidal anti-inflammatory agents
nociceptors
opiate receptors
addiction
drug tolerance
ceiling effect

ASSIGNMENTS

Read textbook, pp. 282-307.
Study Key Terms associated with chapter content.
Complete Collaborative Activities as assigned.
Study Review Sheet for Chapter 20.
Complete Chapter 20 Practice Quiz.
Complete End-of-Chapter Math Review and Critical Thinking Questions.
Complete Chapter 20 Exam.

WEB RESEARCH ACTIVITIES

Access: www.halcyon.com/iasp
1. Open New Drugs/Indications and view information available, and
2. In the search box, type in "pain medications" and view information available on this topic.
Access: www.painmed.org
Compare the definitions relating to addiction, physical dependence, and tolerance.

Copyright © 2004 Mosby Inc. All rights reserved.

COLLABORATIVE ACTIVITIES

Complete the following activities and questions to prepare for in-class discussion and group work that may be assigned by the instructor.

1. Use a *PDR* or similar drug information reference available in the classroom or library to answer the following questions related to analgesics.

    a. What are the active ingredients of Empirin with Codeine?

    b. How does Empirin with Codeine No. 3 differ from Empirin with Codeine No. 4?

    c. What are the active ingredients in Tylenol with Codeine Nos. 2, 3, and 4?

    d. Compare the ingredients of Phenaphen with Tylenol with Codeine Nos. 3 and 4.

    e. What active ingredient does Percodan-Demi have that Percodan does not have?

    f. State the difference between the ingredients of Darvon Compound 65 and Darvon N.

    g. If a patient is allergic to aspirin, which analgesic preparations can be used safely?

2. Develop charting for analgesic recording on inventory control sheet and prn medication record. Do all charting associated with administration of:

    a. MS Contin 30 mg, PO, at 8:15 AM today to:
    T.G., Rm. 611
    012-12-1234
    Dr. Martin
    Dx: Prostatic cancer with metastasis

    b. Give T.G. Percodan, 1 tablet, at 10:15 AM today.

Copyright © 2004 Mosby Inc. All rights reserved.

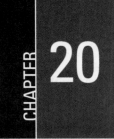

Drugs Used for Pain Management

Review Sheet

The QUESTION column and the ANSWER column have been offset so that you can cover the answer while reading the questions, allowing you to assess your knowledge.

Question	Answer
1. Define *pain perception*, *pain threshold*, and *pain tolerance*.	
2. Compare nociceptive pain, somatic pain, visceral pain, neuropathic pain, and idiopathic pain.	1. Pain perception is awareness of the pain sensation. Pain threshold is the point at which pain is felt. Pain tolerance is an individual's ability to withstand the pain experience.
3. Define *analgesic*.	2. Nociceptive pain is a result of stimulus to pain receptors (dull, aching); somatic pain originates in the skin, bone, or muscle; visceral pain originates in the organs of the thorax or abdomen; neuropathic pain results from injury to the peripheral or central nervous systems; and idiopathic pain is of unknown origin.
4. Name the classes of analgesics.	3. Analgesics are drugs that relieve pain.
5. What neurotransmitters are known to stimulate nociceptors?	4. Opiate agonists, opiate partial agonists, opiate antagonists, anti-inflammatory, nonsteroidal anti-inflammatory, and miscellaneous agents
6. What are the four types of opiate receptors?	5. The neurotransmitters bradykinin, prostaglandins, leukotrienes, histamines, and serotonin sensitize nociceptors.
7. What drug is usually prescribed for severe, chronic pain?	6. The four types of opiate receptors are mu, delta, kappa, and sigma receptors.
8. Summarize nursing process for pain management.	7. Morphine sulfate is usually prescribed for severe, chronic pain. It may also be combined with other drugs such as antidepressants.
9. Discuss the World Health Organization stepwise approach to pain management.	8. See textbook, pp. 284-291.
10. What are the primary therapeutic outcomes appropriate for pain management therapy?	9. See textbook, p. 292.
11. Read the Pain Care Bill of Rights.	10. See textbook, p. 284.
12. Obtain a copy of the pain assessment tools used in local clinical sites and discuss the appropriate assessments and recording of pain events using the tools assembled.	11. See Table 20-1, p. 284.

Copyright © 2004 Mosby Inc. All rights reserved.

13. What is the most effective route for administering an analgesic when immediate relief is needed?
14. Explain the benefits of patient-controlled analgesia (PCA).
15. What is meant by "on demand" in relation to the use of a PCA pump?

16. After completing the assigned web activity, differentiate among addiction, physical dependence, and tolerance.

17. Define *agonists, antagonists,* and *partial agonists.*

18. Opiate agonists are subdivided into what four groups?

19. Identify pain assessment data needed to establish a baseline for monitoring therapy before initiating treatment for pain.

20. For what type(s) of pain are opiate agonists used?

21. What premedication assessments should be performed before administering an opiate agonist?
22. Will naloxone reverse CNS depression caused by sedative/hypnotics or tranquilizers?

23. When is naloxone effective?

24. What three drugs are antidotes for opiate agonists and opiate partial agonists?
25. Do opiate partial agonists relieve pain effectively in persons who have recently taken opiate agonists?
26. Give an example of an opiate partial agonist.

27. What is the most common drug used as an analgesic for relief of mild to moderate pain?

12. Individualize to local clinical facilities.

13. The intravenous route gives the most immediate pain relief.
14. With PCA, the patient can initiate the administration of analgesics, allowing pain relief to be obtained rapidly. Most important is the sense of control a patient feels toward the pain and scheduling daily activities. The PCA system monitors the total dose(s) administered and limits can be set on the total amount that can be self-administered during a specified period.
15. "On demand" means the patient can self-administer a dosage of pain medication when needed. There is a "lock-out" safety device that limits the number of administrations over a specific period of time.
16. Research on the Internet definitions of *addiction, physical dependence,* and *tolerance.*
17. Agonists interact with receptors to stimulate response. Antagonists attach to a receptor but do not stimulate a response or block a response. Partial agonists are drugs that interact with a receptor to stimulate a response, but may inhibit other responses.
18. Opiate agonists are divided into four groups: morphine-like derivatives, meperidine-like derivatives, methadone-like derivatives, and other opiate agonists.
19. Baseline vital signs, neurologic exam, prior analgesics administered, and degree of pain control; voiding and bowel pattern.
20. Opiate agonists are used for moderate to severe pain.
21. Baseline vital signs, neurologic exam, prior analgesics administered, degree of pain control; voiding and bowel pattern.
22. Naloxone will not reverse CNS depression caused by sedative/hypnotics or tranquilizers.
23. Naloxone reverses the CNS depressant effects of the opiate agonists.
24. Nalmefene, naloxone, and naltrexone are antidotes for opiate agonists and opiate partial agonists.
25. Opiate partial agonists usually do not alleviate pain in persons who have recently taken opiate agonists.
26. See Table 20-3, p. 295.

Copyright © 2004 Mosby Inc. All rights reserved.

28. What three pharmacologic effects are associated with the salicylates?
29. When is ASA (aspirin) indicated?

30. What is salicylism?

31. What is the antidote for salicylism?

32. What are premedication assessments to perform before administering nonsteroidal anti-inflammatory drugs (NSAIDs)?
33. What are NSAIDs?
34. How do NSAIDs act?

35. Do NSAIDs control fever?

36. What is the major adverse effect of NSAIDs?

37. Name five commonly used NSAIDs.

38. Name the synthetic nonopiate analgesic used frequently for mild to moderate pain.
39. Compare the action of the drug in question 34 with the action of aspirin.

40. What are early indications of acetaminophen toxicity?

41. What premedication assessments are required for each classification of drug used to treat pain?

42. What effect does aspirin have on phenytoin, valproic acid, and oral hypoglycemic agents?

27. Aspirin is the most common drug used to relieve mild to moderate pain.
28. Three pharmacologic effects of salicylates are analgesic, antipyretic, and anti-inflammatory.
29. ASA is indicated for analgesic effect, fever reduction, and anti-inflammatory effects. Do not give aspirin to children who may be developing a viral infection. Salicylates have been associated with Reye's syndrome.
30. Salicylism is seen with high doses of salicylates. Symptoms include tinnitus, impaired hearing, sweating, dizziness, mental confusion, and nausea and vomiting.
31. There is no antidote for salicylism. Use gastric lavage, force IV fluids, and alkalization of urine with IV sodium bicarbonate; stop salicylates.
32. See textbook, p. 303.
33. NSAIDs are a relatively new class of analgesics that includes aspirin.
34. NSAIDs are prostaglandin inhibitors that have analgesic, anti-inflammatory, and in some cases (e.g., ibuprofen), antipyretic activity.
35. The antipyretic activity of most NSAIDs is low enough that they are not used clinically for fever control. Ibuprofen, however, is a good antipyretic agent and approved as such.
36. The major adverse effect of NSAID therapy is gastrointestinal (GI) complaints, which can develop into ulcers and GI bleeding.
37. See Table 20-4, pp. 300-302.
38. Acetaminophen (Tylenol, Datril, Tempra) is a synthetic nonopiate analgesic used frequently for mild to moderate pain.
39. Acetaminophen has no anti-inflammatory effect. However, it is a very good antipyretic and analgesic.
40. Early indications of acetaminophen toxicity include nausea, anorexia, vomiting, and jaundice accompanied by an elevation in liver function tests.
41. This information can be found in sections listed as premedication assessments in the drug monographs throughout Chapter 20.
42. When taken with aspirin, phenytoin levels are increased, causing toxicity: nystagmus, lethargy, sedation. Dosage adjustment may be required. Valproic acid levels are increased when taken with aspirin; dose adjustment may be needed. With oral hypoglycemics, aspirin increases potential for hypoglycemia.

Copyright © 2004 Mosby Inc. All rights reserved.

CHAPTER 20

Drugs Used for Pain Management

Practice Quiz

DEFINITIONS

Define the following terms.

1. Pain perception:
2. Pain threshold:
3. Analgesic:
4. List data needed prior to administering an analgesic:
5. List premedication assessments needed for an individual receiving an opiate agonist:
6. Are opiate partial agonists effective for pain management in an individual who has recently received an opiate agonist?
7. What are the side effects to expect with the administration of opiate agonists?
8. When should the drug naloxone (Narcan) be available?
9. List common side effects associated with salicylates.
10. Is acetaminophen (Tylenol) recommended for its anti-inflammatory properties?

Ordered: 1000 ml D$_5$W to run IV over the next 12 hours using a 15 gtt/ml administration set.

11. The IV should be adjusted to _____ gtt/min or
12. _____ ml/ hr.
13. When can acetaminophen be harmful to a patient?
14. What is salicylate overdose called and what are its signs and symptoms?
15. What drugs are used as antidotes for opiate agonists and opiate partial agonists?
16. What common medications interact with NSAIDs?

END-OF-CHAPTER MATH REVIEW

1. Ordered: aspirin 650 mg qid.
   On hand: aspirin 325 mg tablets.
   Give _____ tablets.

2. The pediatrician orders a 75 mg dose of ibuprofen suspension for a child. On hand is 100 mg/5 ml. Give _____ ml.
3. Morphine 15 mg IV every 6 hours has been ordered. Concentrations of 3, 4, 5, 8, 10, and 15 mg/ml are available. Which concentration would you use and what volume should be injected?
4. Dr. Sandmann wrote orders to start K.P. on codeine 30 mg, qid after her wisdom tooth extraction. What is your interpretation of the order and how will you administer it?

CRITICAL THINKING QUESTIONS

1. F.C., a terminal cancer patient, returns to the unit with a morphine PCA pump going. His daughter comes to you alarmed that her father may "overuse" the morphine and become addicted. How would you respond to her? Give the rationale for your answer.
2. What is the difference between an order for morphine sulfate immediate release (MSIR) and an order for MS Contin?
3. P.T., age 86, is taking enteric-coated aspirin for her arthritis. She reports to the nurse that she thinks she saw a whole tablet in her stools. What follow-up would you do? She has been on continuous aspirin therapy for 2 years. Explain assessments needed.
4. The head nurse sends the student nurse to evaluate M.S.'s postoperative pain. Upon entering the patient's room, the student observes M.S. conversing and joking with her friends. The student decides not to further investigate the question of postoperative pain. Evaluate the correctness of the student's decision and give your rationale.

Copyright © 2004 Mosby Inc. All rights reserved.

REVIEW QUESTIONS

_____ 1. The length of time required for a transdermal fentanyl (Duragesic) to reach a
steady blood level is _____ hours.
  a. 4
  b. 4–7
  c. 8–11
  d. 12–24

_____ 2. The management of respiratory depression (below 8 breaths/min) in a patient
receiving an epidural analgesic would
include the administration of:
  a. propoxyphene (Darvon).
  b. naloxone (Narcan).
  c. naltrexone (ReVia).
  d. bupivacaine (Marcaine).

_____ 3. Drug tolerance occurs when the patient
requires:
  a. increased doses of same analgesic to
     obtain the same relief.
  b. increased doses of a different analge-
     sic to obtain the same relief.
  c. monitoring for respiratory depres-
     sion.
  d. vital signs assessment at least q 4 h.

_____ 4. Opiate partial agonists such as butorpha-
nol (Stadol) and nalbuphine (Nubain)
are effective analgesics when:
  a. prior opiate antagonists have not
     been administered.
  b. dosages are increased following the
     use of prior opiate antagonists.
  c. prior NSAIDs have been adminis-
     tered.
  d. dosages are decreased following the
     use of prior opiate antagonists.

_____ 5. Which of the following medications contain codeine?
  a. Percogesic
  b. Tylenol #2, #3, #4
  c. Fioricet
  d. Darvon-N

Copyright © 2004 Mosby Inc. All rights reserved.

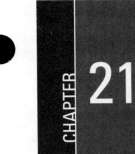

Drugs Used to Treat Hyperlipidemias

Syllabus

CHAPTER CONTENT

Atherosclerosis (p. 308)
Treatment of Hyperlipidemias (p. 308)
Drug Therapy for Hyperlipidemias (p. 309)
    Drug Class: Bile Acid-Binding Resins (p. 311)
    Drug Class: Niacin (p. 312)
    Drug Class: HMG-CoA Reductase Inhibitors
       (p. 313)
    Drug Class: Fibric Acids (p. 314)
    Miscellaneous Antilipemic Agents (p. 314)

CHAPTER OBJECTIVES

1. Identify the four major types of lipoproteins.
2. Describe the primary treatment modalities for lipid disorders.
3. State specific oral administration instructions needed with antilipemic agents.

KEY TERMS

atherosclerosis
hyperlipidemia
triglycerides
lipoproteins
chylomicrons
metabolic syndrome

ASSIGNMENTS

Read textbook, pp. 308-316.
Study Key Terms associated with chapter content.
Study Review Sheet for Chapter 21.
Complete Chapter 21 Practice Quiz.
Complete End-of-Chapter Math Review and Critical
    Thinking Questions.
Complete Chapter 21 Exam.

WEB RESEARCH ACTIVITIES

Access: www.heartinfo.com and click on Library.
    For classroom discussion, read *Exercise Cuts
Cholesterol Regardless of Weight.*
1. What specific changes occur in the reduction of the LDL cholesterol as a result of the different exercise criteria used for each of the four groups of participants?
2. As a result of this added information, what health teaching could be implemented for patients?

Copyright © 2004 Mosby Inc. All rights reserved.

Review Sheet

The QUESTION column and the ANSWER column have been offset so that you can cover the answer while reading the questions, allowing you to assess your knowledge.

Question	Answer
1. Define *atherosclerosis, hyperlipidemia, chylomicrons, triglycerides,* and *lipoproteins.*	
2. List the key characteristics of metabolic syndrome.	1. See textbook, p. 308.
3. What lifestyle changes should be used to treat hyperlipidemia prior to starting drug therapy?	2. Metabolic syndrome, also known as *syndrome X*, includes type II diabetes mellitus, abdominal obesity, hypertriglyceridemia, low HDL cholesterol, and hypertension.
4. What are the primary drugs for lowering serum cholesterol levels?	3. Lifestyle changes should be attempted for treatment of hyperlipidemia before starting drug therapy, including dietary changes (e.g., fat intake less than 30% of calories, decreased cholesterol and saturated fat intake, increased polyunsaturated and monounsaturated fats), weight reduction, and regular exercise.
5. Why aren't fibric acid agents used as first-line drugs for the treatment of hyperlipidemias?	4. Bile acid resins, niacin, and HMG-CoA are the primary classes of lipid-lowering drugs. Ezetimibe (Zetia) represents a new class of drugs whose clinical role is yet to be determined.
6. Which class of drugs used to treat hyperlipidemia is the most expensive?	5. Fibric acid agents do not result in substantial reduction of LDL-C, but are effective in lowering triglycerides.
7. Summarize nursing assessments needed for a patient with hyperlipidemia.	6. HMG-CoA drugs, known as *statins*, are the most expensive.
8. Why are supplemental vitamins required with bile acid-binding resins?	7. Nursing assessments needed for patients with hyperlipidemia include risk factors (e.g., family history of increased cholesterol and lipids), smoking, dietary habits, glucose intolerance, elevated serum lipids, obesity, and sedentary lifestyle.
9. What are the signs and symptoms of a vitamin K deficiency?	8. Bile acid-binding resins may deplete the body of its needed supply of fat-soluble vitamins (DEAK).
10. Describe the proper preparation of cholestyramine for administration.	9. Bruising; bleeding gums; dark, tarry stools; and "coffee ground" emesis are signs and symptoms of a vitamin K deficiency.

Copyright © 2004 Mosby Inc. All rights reserved.

11. What drug interactions can occur with the use of bile acid-binding resins?

12. Discuss patient teaching needed to minimize the common side effects to expect with antilipemic therapy such as constipation, bloating, fullness, nausea, and flatulence.

13. What is the primary desired therapeutic outcome from niacin?
14. What premedication assessments should be performed before administration of niacin?

15. Why is niacin not used with diabetic patients?

16. What suggestions can be given to patients taking niacin to minimize the side effects of flushing, itching, rash, tingling, and headache?
17. Cite the premedication assessments that should be done prior to niacin therapy.

18. Name three statin drugs.
19. How long is the trial period used to evaluate the use of statins for hyperlipidemias?

20. What are common side effects to expect from antilipemic therapy?

21. What is the effect on triglycerides of fibric acid agents?

22. What anticipated alterations may occur in the blood glucose level with gemfibrozil?
23. What is the mechanism of action of ezetimibe (Zetia)?

10. To prepare cholestyramine for administration, mix powdered resin with 2–6 oz water, soup, juice, or crushed pineapple; allow to stand until drug is absorbed and dispersed. Follow with an additional glass of water.
11. Bile acid-binding resins bind to drugs such as warfarin, thyroxine, thiazide diuretics, NSAIDs, and beta blockers, and therefore reduce absorption of these drugs. Minimize this effect by administering 1 hour before or 4 hours after giving a resin. (See also textbook pp. 311-312.)
12. See drug monograph, textbook p. 314.

13. The primary desired therapeutic outcome of niacin is decreased LDL and total cholesterol, decreased triglycerides, and increased HDL levels.
14. Before administering niacin, assess serum triglyceride and cholesterol levels, liver function, baseline uric acid and blood glucose levels, and vital signs. Document existing gastrointestinal symptoms.
15. Niacin is not recommended for diabetics because of glucose intolerance.

16. Take niacin with food, take aspirin 30 minutes before each dose of niacin (unless contraindicated). Tell the patient that tolerance develops quickly.
17. See textbook, p. 312.
18. The statin drugs include atorvastatin, fluvastatin, lovastatin, pravastatin, and simvastatin.
19. The trial period used to evaluate the therapeutic success of statins for hyperlipidemias is a period of up to 3 months.
20. Nausea, diarrhea, flatulence, bloating, and abdominal distress are side effects to expect with antilipemic therapy.
21. Fibrates are the most effective triglyceride-lowering agents.
22. Gemfibrozil may cause moderate hyperglycemia.

23. Ezetimibe (Zetia) acts by blocking the absorption of cholesterol by the small intestines. Note that it also does not elevate triglycerides.

Copyright © 2004 Mosby Inc. All rights reserved.

CHAPTER 21

Drugs Used to Treat Hyperlipidemias

Practice Quiz

ESSAY

1. Name two statins used to treat hyperlipidemia.
2. What four primary therapeutic outcomes are expected from drug therapy for hyperlipidemia?
3. What effect does gemfibrozil have on blood glucose?
4. What premedication assessments should be completed prior to starting hyperlipidemia therapy?
5. What vitamins are affected by the administration of bile acid-binding drugs?
6. Knowing that thyroxine and warfarin medications may be bound to bile acid-binding resins, what signs and symptoms should be assessed in the patient?

TRUE OR FALSE

Mark "T" for true and "F" for false next to each of the following statements. <u>*Correct all false statements.*</u>

_____ 7. HDLs (high-density lipoproteins) are also referred to as "good cholesterol" because they are beneficial in preventing coronary heart disease.

_____ 8 Niacin is effective in lowering triglycerides and cholesterol and raises LDL cholesterol levels.

_____ 9. Smoking contributes to the development and progression of coronary heart disease.

_____ 10. Bile acid-binding resins could potentially result in the development of a bleeding disorder if vitamins or a balanced diet are not taken regularly.

_____ 11. Bile acid-binding resins may bind with warfarin, NSAIDs, tetracycline, and beta blockers, thereby enhancing the drugs' effectiveness.

_____ 12. Common side effects of niacin administration are headache and flushing.

_____ 13. Gemfibrozil may cause hypoglycemia.

_____ 14. Vitamins A, C, and B are significantly affected by bile acid-binding resin drugs.

CALCULATION

15. Order: gemfibrozil 1200 mg, PO, daily in two divided doses 30 minutes ac breakfast and supper.
    On hand: gemfibrozil 300 mg capsules.
    Give: _____ capsules per dose

END-OF-CHAPTER MATH REVIEW

1. Order: nicotinic acid (niacin) 1.5 g, PO, in three divided doses daily.
   On hand: nicotinic acid (niacin) 500 mg tablets
   Give: _____ tablets per dose
   A total of _____ mg daily

2. Order: lovastatin (Mevacor) 80 mg, PO, daily
   On hand: lovastatin (Mevacor) 20 mg tablets
   Give: _____ tablets

CRITICAL THINKING QUESTIONS

1. Why is it essential to monitor a patient taking a bile acid-binding medication for a fat-soluble vitamin deficiency?

2. Why would bleeding problems be a potential side effect of bile acid-binding hypolipidemic drugs?

3. What effect do HMG-CoA reductase inhibitors have on LDL, HDL, VLDL cholesterol, and plasma triglycerides?

   When initiating therapy with a bile acid-binding resin, what assessments would be essential with regard to medications already prescribed?

Copyright © 2004 Mosby Inc. All rights reserved.

REVIEW QUESTIONS

_____ 1. A common side effect of niacin that the patient should be educated on how to avoid is:
   a. headache and hypertension.
   b. nausea, diarrhea, and flatulence.
   c. flushing, itching, and headache.
   d. constipation.

_____ 2. Fibric acids are used to lower:
   a. triglycerides.
   b. cholesterol.
   c. fatty acids.
   d. insulin resistance.

_____ 3. HMG-CoA reductase drugs are also known as:
   a. nicotinic acid.
   b. statins.
   c. hypoglycemics.
   d. cholesterol potentiators.

_____ 4. Liver function studies are not required/recommended prior to initiating:
   a. fibric acids.
   b. HMG-CoA reductase inhibitors.
   c. niacin.
   d. bile acid-binding resins.

_____ 5. Grapefruit juice should not be taken with:
   a. fibric acids.
   b. HMG-CoA reductase inhibitors.
   c. niacin.
   d. bile acid-binding resins.

Copyright © 2004 Mosby Inc. All rights reserved.

CHAPTER 22

Drugs Used to Treat Hypertension

Syllabus

CHAPTER CONTENT

Hypertension (p. 317)
  Prevention and Management of Hypertension
    (p. 320)
  Drug Therapy for Hypertension (p. 320)
    Drug Class: Diuretics (p. 324)
    Drug Class: Beta-Adrenergic Blocking
      Agents (p. 325)
    Drug Class: Angiotensin-Converting
      Enzyme Inhibitors (p. 326)
    Drug Class: Angiotensin II Receptor
      Antagonists (p. 328)
    Drug Class: Aldosterone Receptor
      Antagonists (p. 329)
    Drug Class: Calcium Ion Antagonists
      (p. 331)
    Drug Class: Alpha$_1$-Adrenergic Blocking
      Agents (p. 332)
    Drug Class: Centrally Acting Alpha$_2$
      Agonists (p. 334)
    Drug Class: Peripheral-Acting Adrenergic
      Antagonists (p. 335)
    Drug Class: Direct Vasodilators (p. 337)

CHAPTER OBJECTIVES

1. Summarize nursing assessments and interventions used during the treatment of hypertension.
2. State lifestyle modifications that should be implemented when a diagnosis of hypertension is made.
3. Identify the 10 classes of drugs used to treat hypertension.
4. Review Figure 22-1 to identify options for, and progression of, treatment for hypertension.
5. Identify specific factors the hypertensive patient can use to assist in the management of the disease.
6. Develop objectives for patient education for patients with hypertension.

7. Summarize the mechanism of action of each drug class used to treat hypertension.

KEY TERMS

arterial blood pressure
systolic blood pressure
diastolic blood
  pressure
pulse pressure
mean arterial pressure

cardiac output
hypertension
primary hypertension
secondary
  hypertension
systolic hypertension

ASSIGNMENTS

Read textbook, pp. 317-340.
Study Key Terms associated with chapter content.
Complete Collaborative Activity as assigned.
Study Review Sheet for Chapter 22.
Complete Chapter 22 Practice Quiz.
Complete End-of-Chapter Math Review and Critical
  Thinking Questions.
Complete Chapter 22 Exam.

WEB RESEARCH ACTIVITIES

Access: www.bloodpressure.com/
1. Explore this site to review the type of information that is available to patients. Note the brief, concise, simple explanations used throughout the patient-focused subjects on hypertension.
2. Select "medication reference tool" and research the drug hydrochlorothiazide (HCTZ).
   • What information should the health care professional be aware of before HCTZ is prescribed?
   • What does it tell the patient to do if a dose of HCTZ is missed?

Copyright © 2004 Mosby Inc. All rights reserved.

COLLABORATIVE ACTIVITY

Answer the following questions. Be prepared to share your responses during in-class discussion and group work that may be assigned by the instructor.

1. The nurse's aide asks you to explain why it is necessary to check a patient's blood pressure in the sitting, lying, and standing positions. What explanation is appropriate?

2. The next day, the nurse examines the blood pressures of a patient monitored q shift in sitting, lying, and standing positions yesterday. They are listed as:

BP	Sitting	Lying	Standing
7–3	140/90	140/90	140/90
3–11	156/96	160/94	164/92
11–7	156/84	142/80	158/86

What actions are appropriate based on this data?

Copyright © 2004 Mosby Inc. All rights reserved.

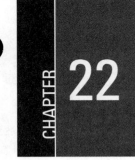

Drugs Used to Treat Hypertension

Review Sheet

The QUESTION column and the ANSWER column have been offset so that you can cover the answer while reading the questions, allowing you to assess your knowledge.

Question

1. What are systolic and diastolic blood pressure?
2. How is the mean arterial pressure or average pressure calculated?

3. What are the primary determinants of systolic and diastolic blood pressure?
4. What is the definition of *hypertension*?

5. Differentiate among prehypertension, primary hypertension, and secondary hypertension.

6. State the procedure for measuring blood pressure as recommended by JNC 7 guidelines.

7. Identify the goals of blood pressure therapy.

Answer

1. Systolic blood pressure is pressure exerted as blood is pumped from the heart; diastolic blood pressure is the pressure present during the resting phase of the heartbeat.
2. See textbook, p. 317.

3. The primary determinant of systolic blood pressure is cardiac output, and the determinant for diastolic blood pressure is peripheral vascular resistance.
4. Hypertension is an elevation in either the systolic or diastolic blood pressure or both. See textbook, pp. 318-319, for discussion of recommended screening in adults.
5. Prehypertension is a range of blood pressure readings that indicates a high probability of developing a heart attack, heart failure, stroke, or renal disease.
   Primary hypertension is a controllable but not curable form of hypertension of unknown etiology. There are known risk factors that contribute to the development of primary hypertension.
   Secondary hypertension occurs following the development of another disorder in the body (e.g., renal disease, head trauma).
6. Sit the patient in a chair with feet on the floor and the arm supported at heart level for at least 5 minutes. Use an appropriate size cuff (cuff bladder encircles at least 80 percent of the arm). Verify readings in the opposite arm. The person needs two or more readings on separate occasions to be classified as having hypertension. When readings of the systolic and diastolic fall into two different stages, the higher of the two

Copyright © 2004 Mosby Inc. All rights reserved.

8. List the drug classifications used in the treatment of hypertension.

9. What is therapeutic outcome for antihypertensive therapy?

10. Describe significant nursing processes for persons with hypertension.

11. How does JNC 7 classify antihypertensive agents in current use?

12. What class of drugs is used initially in the treatment of uncomplicated hypertension when lifestyle changes are not effective?

13. What is the treatment algorithm used for hypertension?

14. What are the nutritional goals for the treatment of hypertension?

15. Summarize the premedication assessments used prior to administration of antihypertensive drugs. (Examine differences among the various types of agents usually prescribed.)

16. What are the four classes of diuretic agents used to treat hypertension?

17. What laboratory test is used as a guide to indicate when a patient needs to switch from a thiazide-type to a loop diuretic?

18. What are the major side effects to expect and report with beta-adrenergic blocking agents?

19. What types of patients should avoid the use of beta-blocking agents?

stages is used to classify the degree of hypertension present.

7. Reduction and maintenance of BP below 140/90 mm Hg. Patients with concurrent conditions—e.g., diabetes mellitus, heart failure, and renal disease—less than 130/80. Weight reduction, DASH diet, dietary sodium reduction, physical activity, and moderation of alcohol consumption are recommended. Smoking cessation and stress reduction are also recommended.

8. Hypertension is treated primarily with preferred agents: diuretics and beta-adrenergic blockers; alternative agents: angiotensin-converting enzyme (ACE) inhibitors, angiotensin II receptor antagonists, calcium ion antagonists, alpha$_1$ adrenergic blockers; and adjunctive agents: centrally acting alpha$_2$ agonists, peripheral-acting adrenergic antagonists, and direct vasodilators.

9. The therapeutic outcome for antihypertensive therapy is to lower blood pressure by reducing peripheral resistance.

10. See textbook, pp. 320-324.

11. See textbook, p. 321, Fig. 22-1.

12. If lifestyle changes do not sufficiently reduce blood pressure, a diuretic or a beta-blocker are generally the initial treatment of choice.

13. See textbook, p. 321, Fig 22-1.

14. See textbook, pp. 320-321.

15. See sections labeled "premedication assessments" in the drug monographs throughout Chapter 22; e.g., pp. 324-338.

16. The four classes of diuretic agents used to treat hypertension are carbonic anhydrase inhibitors, thiazide and thiazide-like agents, loop diuretics, and potassium-sparing diuretics. Thiazide diuretics are most often used. Carbonic anhydrase inhibitors are rarely used to treat hypertension.

17. The creatinine clearance test is used when a patient needs to switch from a thiazide-like to a loop diuretic.

18. The major side effects to expect and report with beta-adrenergic agents include bradycardia, peripheral vasoconstriction, bronchospasm,

Copyright © 2004 Mosby Inc. All rights reserved.

20. What precautions should be instituted when beta-blocker therapy is to be discontinued?

21. What effect does angiotensin II have on blood vessels?

22. What effect does an increase in aldosterone secretion have on blood pressure?

23. Summarize the side effects to expect and to report with the use of ACE inhibitors.

24. What is the action of angiotensin II receptor antagonists?

25. What is the action of eplerenone, the aldosterone receptor blocking agent?

26. What are contraindications to the administration of the aldosterone receptor blocking agent eplerenone (Inspira)?

27. Review the side effects to report with use of eplerenone (Inspira), the aldosterone receptor blocking agent.

28. Which herbal product and fruit juice slows the absorption of eplerenone?

29. What is the action of calcium ion antagonists on the blood pressure?

30. What are side effects to expect with alpha$_1$-adrenergic blockers?

wheezing, hypoglycemia in diabetic patients, and heart failure.

19. Beta-blocking agents are not as effective in African-American patients and should be avoided in patients with asthma, type 1 diabetes mellitus, heart failure with an etiology of systolic dysfunction, and in patients with peripheral vascular disease.

20. After long-term treatment with beta-blockers, discontinue gradually over 1–2 weeks and monitor for anginal symptoms.

21. Angiotensin II produces vasoconstriction, which results in an increase in blood pressure.

22. Aldosterone results in sodium retention, which causes water retention and increased cardiac output, thereby increasing blood pressure.

23. Side effects to expect with ACE inhibitors include nausea, fatigue, headache, diarrhea, and orthostatic hypotension. Side effects to report include swelling face, eyes, lips; dyspnea; neutropenia; nephrotoxicity; hyperkalemia; chronic cough; and can cause fetal and neonatal harm during pregnancy.

24. Angiotensin II receptor inhibitors block the angiotensin II from binding to receptor sites in vascular smooth muscle and the adrenal glands. This prevents elevation of pressure and sodium-retaining properties of angiotensin II.

25. Eplerenone (Inspira), an aldosterone receptor blocking agent, blocks the stimulation of the mineralocorticoid receptors by aldosterone, thereby preventing sodium reabsorption.

26. Eplerenone (Inspira) is contraindicated in patients with serum potassium greater than 5.5 mEq/L, type 2 diabetes with microalbuminuria, serum creatinine greater than 2.0 mg/dl in males or 1.8 mg/dl in females; creatinine clearance less than 50 ml/min, patients taking potassium-sparing diuretics (e.g., amiloride, triamterene), and patients taking strong metabolic enzyme inhibitors (e.g., ketoconazole, cimetidine, others).

27. See textbook , p. 330.

28. Grapefruit juice and St. John's wort.

29. Calcium ion antagonists inhibit the movement of calcium ions across cell membranes. This causes slower rate of heart contraction and relaxation of smooth muscles of blood vessels, resulting in vasodilation and reduction of the blood pressure.

Copyright © 2004 Mosby Inc. All rights reserved.

31. Why should centrally acting alpha$_2$-agonists (e.g., clonidine, guanabenz, guanfacine, methyldopa) be discontinued gradually?

32. What is an anticipated side effect seen with minoxidil (Loniten, Minodyl)?

33. To what drug class does guanadrel (Hylorel) belong?

34. What is the ending of generic drug names belonging to the class of ACE inhibitors?

35. What is the ending of generic drug names belonging to the class of angiotensin II receptor antagonists?

36. What is the ending of generic drug names belonging to the class of calcium ion antagonists?

37. What is the ending of generic drug names belonging to the class of alpha$_1$-adrenergic blocking agents?

30. Side effects to expect with alpha$_1$-adrenergic blockers include drowsiness, headache, dizziness, weakness, tachycardia, and fainting.

31. Sudden discontinuation of centrally acting alpha$_2$-agonists can produce a rebound effect with sudden increase in blood pressure.

32. The anticipated side effect seen with minoxidil is hair growth on the body.

33. Guanadrel is a peripheral-acting adrenergic antagonist.

34. Generic drug names of ACE inhibitors end in "-pril" (enalapril, captopril, etc.).

35. Generic drug names of angiotensin II receptor antagonists end in "-sartan" (e.g., candesartan, losartan).

36. Generic drug names of calcium ion antagonists end in "-pine," with the exceptions of diltiazem and verapamil.

37. Generic drug names of alpha$_1$-adrenergic blocking agents end in "-azosin."

Copyright © 2004 Mosby Inc. All rights reserved.

CHAPTER

22

Drugs Used to Treat Hypertension

Practice Quiz

MATCHING

Select the correct statement associated with the terms.

_____ 1. diuretics
_____ 2. beta-adrenergic blockers
_____ 3. angiotensin-converting enzyme (ACE) inhibitors
_____ 4. calcium antagonists
   a. block beta receptors to inhibit cardiac response to sympathetic nerve stimulation
   b. block flow of calcium ions across cell membranes
   c. may produce swelling lips and tongue, dyspnea, neutropenia, nephrotoxicity, and/or chronic cough
   d. depletes norepinephrine from adrenergic nerve endings
   e. enhances fluid volume excretion, sodium excretion, and vasodilation of peripheral arterioles

Select the correct drug class associated with the drug names.

_____ 5. thiazide diuretic
_____ 6. beta-adrenergic blocker
_____ 7. angiotensin-converting enzyme (ACE) inhibitor
_____ 8. angiotensin II receptor antagonist
_____ 9. calcium ion antagonist
   a. atenolol
   b. hydrochlorothiazide
   c. nifedipine
   d. doxazosin
   e. clonidine
   ab. captopril
   ac. losartan

TRUE OR FALSE

Mark "T" for true and "F" for false next to each of the following statements. <u>Correct all false statements.</u>

_____ 10. Orthostatic hypotension is a possible side effect seen with most antihypertensive drugs.
_____ 11. Primary hypertension is caused by such disorders as renal disease or head trauma.
_____ 12. The primary goal of antihypertensive therapy is to reduce morbidity and mortality.
_____ 13. Angiotensin-converting enzyme (ACE) inhibitors and diuretics are the preferred agents for initiating treatment of hypertension.
_____ 14. The lifestyle changes required to reduce blood pressure are increased exercise, diet, and weight reduction.
_____ 15. The action of smoking on the blood vessels is vasodilation.
_____ 16. An order stating "take orthostatic blood pressure readings" means to take blood pressure every shift without fail.
_____ 17. An important nursing diagnosis when initiating antihypertensive therapy would be Injury, risk for, r/t antihypertensive therapy.
_____ 18. Drowsiness and fatigue are common during the first 2 weeks of antihypertensive therapy.
_____ 19. Potassium-sparing and loop diuretics are commonly used for initiating the step approach to antihypertensive therapy.
_____ 20. Blood pressure readings in supine and standing positions are all the data needed to initiate antihypertensive therapy with a diuretic.

Copyright © 2004 Mosby Inc. All rights reserved.

COMPLETION

Complete the following statements.

21. _____ pressure is the difference between the systolic and diastolic pressure.
22. The physiologic goal of antihypertensive therapy is a decrease in blood pressure through reduction in _____.
23. Smoking causes _____ of blood vessels and results in_____.

COMPUTATION

24. Ordered: IV of 1000 ml lactated Ringer's solution to run at 60 ml/hour. Using a microdrip administration set, how many gtt/min will be infused?

END-OF-CHAPTER MATH REVIEW

1. Ordered: clonidine hydrochloride (Catapres) 0.6 mg, daily in two divided doses.
   On hand: clonidine hydrochloride (Catapres) 0.1, 0.2 mg tablets
   Give: _____ tablets of _____ mg, and _____ tablets of _____ mg.
   Catapres is available in 0.3 mg tablets. What nursing action would be appropriate?
2. Ordered: methyldopa (Aldomet) 3 g, daily in three divided doses.
   On hand: methyldopa (Aldomet) 500 mg tablets
   Give: _____ tablets per dose.
   What time schedule should be established for this order?

CRITICAL THINKING QUESTIONS

1. A patient is receiving methyldopa 3 g per day. A possible nursing diagnosis is Sexual dysfunction related to methyldopa therapy manifested by impotence and/or failure to ejaculate. Address the health teaching needed and how the nurse might approach this subject.
2. Discuss the essential patient education needed regarding the initiation of prazosin therapy.
3. State the nursing assessments needed to monitor therapeutic response to, and/or side effects to expect or report with, beta-adrenergic blocking agents and calcium antagonists.

4. Review the beta-adrenergic blocking agent information in the monograph and develop patient education objectives for a patient receiving this class of drugs for treatment of hypertension.
5. A patient is being started on a drug regimen for hypertension that includes the use of reserpine. Initially her BP is 160/100, pulse is 64, respirations are 20/minute, weight 148 lb. She seems quiet, introspective, and contributes little information other than "yes" or "no" responses during an initial assessment. What further nursing actions would be appropriate?
6. E.S., age 56, is receiving guanethidine and a diuretic for treatment of hypertension that has not previously been controlled by other antihypertensive therapy. His weight is 168 lb, BP is 190/110, pulse is 78, and respirations are 18/minute. He has type I diabetes mellitus. Design a specific plan for nursing assessments needed for E.S. before and during his antihypertensive regimen.

REVIEW QUESTIONS

_____ 1. Which type of antihypertensive agent requires that the premedication assessment include checking for respiratory conditions that are present because this class of drug may cause a chronic cough?
   a. angiotensin II receptor antagonists
   b. diuretics
   c. angiotensin-converting enzyme inhibitors
   d. beta-adrenergic blocking agents

_____ 2. The generic drug names of all but one drug in which classification end in "-pril"?
   a. angiotensin II receptor antagonists
   b. diuretics
   c. angiotensin-converting enzyme inhibitors
   d. beta-adrenergic blocking agents

Copyright © 2004 Mosby Inc. All rights reserved.

_____ 3. Angiotensin II receptor antagonists act by:
  a. binding to angiotensin I receptors sites.
  b. binding to angiotensin II receptor sites.
  c. altering renal function.
  d. altering calcium ion movement across the cells.

_____ 4. Initial therapy for hypertension is most often:
  a. diuretics and alpha blockers.
  b. beta-blockers and calcium antagonists.
  c. diuretics and angiotensin II receptor blockers.
  d. diuretics or beta-adrenergic blocking agents.

_____ 5. A drug that reduces peripheral vascular resistance will:
  a. decrease the heart rate.
  b. decrease cardiac output.
  c. reduce blood pressure.
  d. increase blood pressure.

_____ 6. All antihypertensive agents in which class end in "-sartan"?
  a. angiotensin II receptor antagonists
  b. diuretics
  c. angiotensin-converting enzyme inhibitors
  d. beta-adrenergic blocking agents

_____ 7. The aldosterone receptor blocker eplerone acts by:
  a. blocking conversion of angiotensin I to angiotensin II.
  b. reducing sodium reabsorption.
  c. volume depletion, sodium excretion, and vasodilation of peripheral arterioles.
  d. blocking calcium ion movement across the cell membrane.

Copyright © 2004 Mosby Inc. All rights reserved.

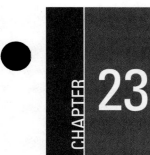

Drugs Used to Treat Heart Failure

Syllabus

CHAPTER CONTENT

Heart Failure (p. 341)
    Treatment of Heart Failure (p. 342)
    Drug Therapy for Heart Failure (p. 342)
        Drug Class: Digitalis Glycosides (p. 345)
        Drug Class: Phosphodiesterase Inhibitors
           (p. 348)
        Drug Class: Angiotensin-Converting
           Enzyme Inhibitors (p. 350)
        Drug Class: Naturetic Peptides (p. 350)

CHAPTER OBJECTIVES

1. Summarize the pathophysiology of heart failure, including the body's compensatory mechanisms.
2. Identify the goals of treatment of heart failure.
3. Explain the process of digitalizing a patient, including the initial dosage, preparation and administration of the medication, and nursing assessments needed to monitor therapeutic response and digitalis toxicity.
4. Describe safety precautions associated with the preparation and administration of digitalis glycosides.
5. State the primary actions on cardiac output of digoxin, angiotensin-converting enzyme inhibitors, nitrates, and calcium channel blockers.
6. Identify essential assessment data, nursing interventions, and health teaching needed for a patient with heart failure.

KEY TERMS

systolic dysfunction
diastolic dysfunction
inotropic agents
digitalis toxicity

positive inotropy
negative chronotropy
digitalization

ASSIGNMENTS

Read textbook, pp. 341-351.
Study Key Terms associated with chapter content.
Complete Collaborative Activity as assigned.
Study Review Sheet for Chapter 23.
Complete Chapter 23 Practice Quiz.
Complete End-of-Chapter Math Review and Critical Thinking Questions.
Complete Chapter 23 Exam.

WEB RESEARCH ACTIVITIES

Access: www.nhlbi.nih.gov/
Click on: For Health Care Professionals; read *Heart and Vascular Diseases.*
Print the sections in Facts about Heart Failure:

1. Making the Most of Your Doctor Visit
2. A Question for Your Pharmacist
3. Readying a Q & A for Your Doctor Visit

Review the Patient Self-Monitoring Form found in Chapter 23 of the textbook and add the above information from the articles to your folder for doing health teaching with the patient.

COLLABORATIVE ACTIVITY

Complete the following activity. Be prepared to share your responses during in-class discussion and group work that may be assigned by the instructor.

Transcribe the following initial order to a medication administration record (MAR) and the patient Kardex. Use the MAR and Kardex records distributed by the instructor or use the records provided on the next page.

    A patient, No. 123469, age 66, Dx: heart failure, Rm. 622-2, Dr. Bryce

Copyright © 2004 Mosby Inc. All rights reserved.

Physician's Order Sheet:

Meds:
      Captopril 50 mg, tid
      Furosemide 120 mg, PO, daily in the AM
      Isosorbide dinitrate 20 mg, q 6 hr
      Colace 100 mg, bid
ABGs, CBC, and electrolytes, stat
BUN, creatinine clearance, total protein, UA
ECG stat
O_2 @ 2 L/minute via nasal cannula
Admission weight, daily weights thereafter
Accurate I & O; report hourly output less than 30 ml/hr
to cardiac resident on duty (pager # 555-1356)

2 g sodium, soft, low-cholesterol, low-fat diet
Oral fluids restricted to 1200 ml per 24 hours, including on trays
Bed rest with BRP, HOB elevated 45° or above as comfortable
Vital signs q 1 h x 12, then q 2 h, if stable
Record neurologic status on admission and q 2 h x 24 hrs
Skin assessment per protocol
Alternating mattress

MEDICATION ADMINISTRATION RECORD

NAME:		RM-BD:		Init	Signature	Title
ID NO.:		AGE:				
DIAGNOSIS:		SEX:				

PHYSICIAN:		Ht:		Wt:	

SCHEDULED MEDICATIONS

DATE	MEDICATION-STRENGTH-FORM-ROUTE	0030-0729	0730-1529	1530-0029

** PRN MEDICATIONS**

Copyright © 2004 Mosby Inc. All rights reserved.

Drugs Used to Treat Heart Failure

Review Sheet

The QUESTION column and the ANSWER column have been offset so that you can cover the answers while reading the questions, allowing you to assess your knowledge.

Question	Answer
1. What are the results of systolic dysfunction of the heart?	
2. What is the ultimate problem associated with diastolic dysfunction of the heart?	1. The result of systolic dysfunction of the heart is inability of the heart to contract with sufficient force to pump all the blood from the heart to maintain sufficient cardiac output to meet the body's oxygenation needs.
3. What effect does the sympathetic nervous system's release of epinephrine and norepinephrine have on heart function?	2. Due to diastolic dysfunction of the heart, residual volume remains from the previous contraction and the left ventricle does not fill adequately prior to next contraction. Back-pressure builds up in the lungs and peripheral vasculature that results in symptoms of pulmonary congestion and peripheral edema.
4. What occurs when kidney perfusion is diminished?	3. Epinephrine and norepinephrine produce tachycardia and an increase in cardiac contractility, thereby increasing cardiac output.
5. Define the action of inotropic agents.	4. With reduced perfusion, the kidneys conserve sodium, which increases circulating blood volume. As this progresses, there is an increase in capillary pressure and edema results.
6. What is the action of intravenous nitroglycerin, nitroprusside, and nesiritide?	5. Inotropic agents increase the force of contraction of the heart as it beats, resulting in increased cardiac output to meet the body's oxygenation needs.
7. Why are diuretics used in the treatment of heart failure?	6. These drugs are vasodilators that reduce cardiac preload and afterload.
8. Name two common loop diuretics used in the treatment of heart failure.	7. Diuretics are used in the treatment of heart failure to reduce sodium and fluid overload associated with heart failure.
9. List the six cardinal signs of heart disease and give a rationale for their occurrence.	8. Loop diuretics used for heart failure include furosemide (Lasix), bumetanide (Bumex), and torsemide (Demadex).

Copyright © 2004 Mosby Inc. All rights reserved.

10. What classes of drugs are used to treat heart failure and what are the desired actions of each?

11. What nursing assessments should be performed at regular intervals to assess cardiac function?

12. Describe essential patient education and health promotion for patients being treated for heart failure.

13. List the nursing assessments that should be performed on a regular basis for a cardiac patient.

14. What is the desired therapeutic outcome of administering digoxin?

9. The six cardinal signs of heart disease are dyspnea, associated with inadequate tissue perfusion and diastolic dysfunction; chest pain, resulting from inadequate oxygen to support myocardium function; fatigue, due to depleted oxygen to body tissue; edema, because the left ventricle is not pumping adequate volumes of blood and a back-pressure builds up in the lungs (causing dyspnea) and the peripheral blood vessels, causing interstitial edema; syncope, due to insufficient oxygen to meet the brain's needs; and palpitations, caused by sympathetic nervous system's release of epinephrine and norepinephrine that produces tachycardia and arrhythmias.

10. The drug classes used to treat heart failure and their desired actions include vasodilator drugs, which decrease peripheral resistance the heart has to pump against; inotropic drugs, which increase force of each heart contraction resulting in increased cardiac output; and diuretics, which reduce fluid volume, sodium, and peripheral resistance. ACE inhibitors reduce circulating blood volume by inhibiting secretion of aldosterone. They also promote vasodilation and minimize cellular aggregation, preventing thrombus formation.

11. Mental status, vital signs (T, P, R), blood pressure, heart and lung sounds, skin color, neck vein status, presence of clubbing, CVP, abdomen size, fluid volume status, nutrition, activity and exercise tolerance, anxiety level, and laboratory tests should be checked regularly to assess cardiac function.

12. See textbook, pp. 344-345.

13. For cardiac patients, regular assessment of the respiratory rate, level of dyspnea seen in relation to exertional effort, and the degree of fatigue being experienced should be performed. Monitor for the occurrence of syncope and frequency of palpitations. Check for skin color, neck vein distention, pulse rate and rhythm, and blood pressure on a regularly scheduled basis. Perform auscultation and percussion of the lungs and heart. Check for the presence or absence of edema and for clubbing.

Copyright © 2004 Mosby Inc. All rights reserved.

15. Explain why a "loading dose" or digitalization is done.

16. List the common symptoms of digoxin toxicity.

17. What data should be gathered *before* administering a dose of digoxin?

18. Under what conditions should two qualified nurses check a dose of digoxin?

19. When should a blood sample be drawn to measure the level of digoxin in the blood?

20. Why should a patient taking digoxin be cautioned not to take an antacid within 2 hours of taking the digitalis without first consulting the physician?

21. What effect can the concurrent use of a digoxin and a diuretic have?

22. What is treatment for digoxin toxicity?

23. What is the action of phosphodiesterase inhibitors in the treatment of heart failure?

24. Name two phosphodiesterase inhibitors used to treat heart failure.

25. What is the action of ACE inhibitors in the treatment of heart failure?

14. Digoxin slows and strengthens the heartbeat, allowing the heart to empty and fill more completely, thereby improving circulation.

15. The process of digitalization allows the blood level of digoxin to be raised rapidly so the therapeutic effects can occur more rapidly. Once a therapeutic level [for digoxin (Lanoxin), 0.9–2.0 ng/ml] is achieved, the patient can be switched to a daily maintenance dose.

16. Common symptoms of digoxin toxicity include anorexia, nausea, extreme fatigue, weakness of arms and legs, visual disturbances, and psychiatric disturbances.

17. Before administering digoxin, apical pulse should be taken for one full minute. Consult the physician before administering the prescribed dose if the apical rate is below 60 beats per minute in an adult, or below 90 beats per minute in a child. When functioning in a nursing home environment, it may be permissible to take a radial pulse for one minute. Always check the clinical site's policies; if in doubt, take by the apical method.

18. Any time the dose requires calculation, two qualified nurses should check the dose.

19. Draw blood to measure the level of digoxin before the daily dose or at least 6–8 hours after administration of the last dose of digoxin.

20. An antacid taken with digoxin reduces the absorption of digoxin.

21. Diuretics may induce hypokalemia, which may result in signs of digoxin toxicity.

22. To treat for digoxin toxicity, stop digoxin, stop potassium-depleting diuretics and check potassium level and administer prescribed potassium if deficient. If signs of toxicity are severe and life-threatening, the antidote for digoxin, digoxin immune Fab (Digibind), may be administered.

23. Phosphodiesterase inhibitors increase the force of contraction of the myocardium, thereby increasing cardiac output (CO). They also cause relaxation of vascular smooth muscle, resulting in vasodilation that reduces preload and afterload.

24. Two phosphodiesterase inhibitors used to treat heart failure are inamrinone and milrinone (Primacor).

Copyright © 2004 Mosby Inc. All rights reserved.

26. Describe the premedication assessments needed for digoxin, phosphodiesterase inhibitors, and ACE inhibitors.

25. ACE inhibitors reduce afterload by blocking angiotensin II-mediated peripheral vasoconstriction promoting vasodilation; they also reduce circulating blood volume by inhibiting aldosterone, allowing excretion of excess water. They also minimize cellular aggregation, preventing thrombus formation.
26. See individual drug monographs, textbook pp. 347-349.

Copyright © 2004 Mosby Inc. All rights reserved.

Student Name_____

Drugs Used to Treat Heart Failure

Practice Quiz

COMPLETION

Complete the following statements.

1. _____ is the slowing of the heart rate.
2. _____ agents increase the force of contraction of the heart as it beats.
3. _____ is another term for administering a loading dose of digoxin.
4. The _____ pulse should be taken for _____ minute before administering digoxin in a hospital setting.
5. Digoxin should be scheduled (before, after) meals to prevent _____.
6. The overall action of diuretics on heart failure is to: _____.
7. Name the primary cardiac sign that occurs with stimulation of the sympathetic nervous system. _____
8. The action of angiotensin-converting enzyme (ACE) inhibitors during heart failure is to _____.
9. The desired action on the kidney in relation to heart failure is _____.
10. During the critical initial period of acute therapy of cardiac failure, drugs are usually administered _____.
11. The action of digoxin is to _____.

END-OF-CHAPTER MATH REVIEW

1. A 64-year-old man, weight 165 lbs, is in the emergency room with stat orders:
   Order: digoxin 6 mcg/kg, IV, stat
   On hand: digoxin 0.1 mg/ml
   165 lbs = _____ kg

   Based on this order, how many mcg of digoxin would be given stat? _____ mcg or _____ mg

   Use any drug reference to determine the following:
   Is digoxin given IV diluted or undiluted?
   What rate of IV injection is recommended?
   What IV solution(s) is digoxin compatible with?
2. The patient is transferred from the emergency room to the coronary unit for 24 hours. The following orders exist for medications:
   Order: digoxin 0.125 mg, IV, q 6 hours after stat dose
   On hand: digoxin 0.1 mg/ml and digoxin 0.25 mg/ml
   Give: digoxin _____ ml of _____ mg/ml
3. Following digitalization, the patient is placed on a maintenance dose as follows:
   Order: digoxin 0.375 mg, daily
   On hand: digoxin 0.125 mg and 0.25 mg tablets
   Give: _____ tablets of _____ mg tablet(s)

CRITICAL THINKING QUESTIONS

1. During the digitalization process what assessments should be made on a continuum? Discuss the rationale for these observations.
2. In addition to the medications listed above, the patient is started on furosemide 60 mg daily. What is the action of furosemide? Explain the nursing assessments that should be made to evaluate the effectiveness of the diuretic therapy.
3. Describe the purpose of drug therapy for heart failure when administering vasodilator drugs such as nitroprusside or nifedipine, a calcium channel blocker.

Copyright © 2004 Mosby Inc. All rights reserved.

REVIEW QUESTIONS

_____ 1. When an explanation of heart failure says that the sympathetic nervous system is activated, what actions occur?
   a. hypertrophy of cardiac wall
   b. dilation of chambers of the heart
   c. increased heart rate, contractility, and peripheral vascular resistance
   d. blood flow to kidneys decreases; kidneys increase release of renin

_____ 2. Inamrinone should be mixed for IV administration with:
   a. 5% dextrose/0.9% saline.
   b. 5% dextrose/0.2% water.
   c. 0.9% saline.
   d. 5% dextrose/0.2% sodium chloride + 20 mEq potassium chloride.

_____ 3. ACE inhibitors:
   a. reduce blood pressure (afterload).
   b. decrease renal flow.
   c. increase peripheral vascular resistance.
   d. cause vasoconstriction.

_____ 4. Digitalis toxicity symptoms are:
   a. increased renal output.
   b. anorexia, nausea, vomiting, blurred vision.
   c. increased potassium level.
   d. peripheral edema, pulse deficit, nocturnal leg cramps.

Copyright © 2004 Mosby Inc. All rights reserved.

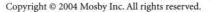

Drugs Used to Treat Arrhythmias

Syllabus

CHAPTER CONTENT

Arrhythmias (p. 352)
Treatment for Arrhythmias (p. 353)
Drug Therapy for Arrhythmias (p. 355)
    Drug Class: Antiarrhythmic Agents (p. 355)
    Drug Class: Beta-Adrenergic Blocking Agents
       (p. 357)

CHAPTER OBJECTIVES

1. Describe the therapeutic response that should
   be observable when an antiarrhythmic drug is
   administered.
2. Identify baseline nursing assessments that
   should be implemented during the treatment of
   arrhythmias.
3. List the dosage forms and precautions needed
   when preparing IV lidocaine for the treatment
   of arrhythmias.
4. Cite common side effects that may be observed
   with the administration of amiodarone,
   bretylium tosylate, disopyramide, lidocaine,
   flecainide, mexiletine, phenytoin, procainamide,
   quinidine, and tocainide.
5. Identify the potential effects of muscle relaxants
   used during surgical intervention when
   combined with antiarrhythmic drugs.

KEY TERMS

electrical system
arrhythmias
atrial flutter
atrial fibrillation
paroxysmal supraventricular tachycardia
atrioventricular block
tinnitus

ASSIGNMENTS

Read textbook, pp. 352-367.
Study Key Terms associated with chapter content.
Study Review Sheet for Chapter 24.
Complete Chapter 24 Practice Quiz.
Complete End-of-Chapter Math Review and Critical
    Thinking Questions.
Complete Chapter 24 Exam.

WEB RESEARCH ACTIVITY

Access: www.americanheart.org
Go to: Heart and Stroke Encyclopedia
    Access: AED (Automated External Defibrilla-
tor)—see Arrhythmias, Cardiac Arrest, Cardiopul-
monary Resuscitation (CPR) Statistics, Defibrilla-
tion, Operation Heartbeat, Sudden Cardiac Death,
Ventricular Fibrillation
- Review the following information: Arrhythmias
- Read: Evaluating Patients for Cardiac
  Arrhythmias
- What symptoms do patients with an
  arrhythmias have?
- What are common circumstances that might
  trigger the arrhythmia event?

Copyright © 2004 Mosby Inc. All rights reserved.

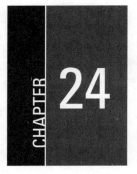

Drugs Used to Treat Arrhythmias

Review Sheet

The QUESTION column and the ANSWER column have been offset so that you can cover the answer while reading the question, allowing you to assess your knowledge.

Question	Answer
1. Define *arrhythmia*.	
2. What function does the electrical system of the heart have on heart action?	1. Any heart rate or rhythm other than normal sinus rhythm is an arrhythmia.
3. Review the sequence of the heart's conduction system.	2. The electrical system of the heart sequences the muscle contractions of the heart to provide an optimal volume of blood per beat of the heart.
4. How are arrhythmias produced?	3. The heart's conduction system goes from SA node to AV node to Bundle of His to Purkinje fibers to ventricular muscle tissue.
5. Define *sinus arrhythmia, sinus tachycardia, sinus bradycardia*, and *premature ventricular contraction*.	4. Arrhythmias are produced by the abnormal firing of the pacemaker cells and/or the blockage of the normal electrical system pathway.
6. What is a "pulse deficit"?	5. Sinus arrhythmia is a variable increase in heart rate originating from the SA node. The increase in rate may parallel the inspiratory phase of respirations. Sinus tachycardia is a regular rhythm of the heartbeat with a rate greater than 120 beats per minute. Sinus bradycardia is a regular rhythm of the heartbeat, but the rate is slower than 60 beats per minute. In premature ventricular contractions, the contraction occurs before the regular ventricular contraction as a result of an electrical impulse arising in the ventricular muscle outside the normal conduction pathway.
7. What electrolyte is responsible for electrical system conduction for the SA and AV nodes?	6. "Pulse deficit" is the difference between the apical and radial pulse rates; radial is generally lower than apical. For example: apical pulse = 74, radial pulse = 64, pulse deficit = 10.
	7. Calcium ions are responsible for electrical system conduction for the SA and AV nodes.
8. What electrolyte is responsible for electrical system conduction for the atrial muscle, the His-Purkinje system, and the ventricular muscle?	
9. What is the goal of treatment for arrhythmias?	8. Sodium is responsible for electrical system conduction for the atrial muscle, the His-Purkinje system, and the ventricular muscle.

Copyright © 2004 Mosby Inc. All rights reserved.

10. What effect do Class I, Ia, Ib, and Ic agents have on the electrical conduction system of the heart?

11. What methods are used to assess arrhythmias?

12. Review the six cardinal signs of cardiovascular disease.

13. Why can mental status/level of consciousness (LOC) be important when assessing a cardiac patient?

14. What type of changes in the vital signs should be reported to the HCP?

15. Why is it important to monitor hourly urine output in a patient with arrhythmias?

16. When is the use of adenosine (Adenocard) indicated?

17. Review the drug monograph, p. 356, for amiodarone hydrochloride (Cordarone) and identify uses, actions, side effects, and premedication assessments for this drug.

18. When beta-adrenergic blocking agents are administered, what cardiac response can be anticipated?

19. Bretylium tosylate (Bretylol) belongs to which class of antiarrhythmic agents?

20. When lidocaine (Xylocaine) is ordered for an arrhythmia, what should the nurse check on the bottle BEFORE using the medication for IV administration?

21. In general, what agent is the drug of choice for treatment of ventricular arrhythmias associated with acute myocardial infarction and ventricular tachycardia?

22. Describe the initial manifestations of mexiletine neurotoxicity.

9. The goal of treatment for arrhythmias is to restore normal sinus rhythm and maintain adequate cardiac output to maintain tissue perfusion.

10. The effects of Class I, Ia, Ib, and Ic agents are as follows: I is a myocardial depressant (inhibits sodium ion movement); Ia causes prolonged duration of electrical stimulation on cells and refractory time between electrical impulses; Ib shortens duration of electrical stimulation and time interval between electrical impulses; Ic is the most potent antiarrhythmic, causing myocardial depression and slowing conduction rate through the atria and the ventricles.

11. ECG monitoring, EPS (electrophysiologic studies), exercise electrocardiography, and laboratory values are used to assess for cardiac arrhythmias.

12. The six cardinal signs of cardiac disease are dyspnea, chest pain, fatigue, edema, syncope, and palpitations.

13. Mental status/LOC indicates whether there is adequate cerebral tissue perfusion.

14. See textbook, p. 354.

15. Hourly outputs reflect whether the kidney tissues are being adequately perfused.

16. Adenosine is indicated in treatment of paroxysmal supraventricular tachycardia that involves conduction in the SA node, atrium, or AV node.

17. See textbook, pp. 356-357.

18. Reduction in heart rate, systolic blood pressure, and cardiac output result from use of beta-adrenergic blocking agents.

19. Bretylium tosylate is an adrenergic blocking agent, class III antiarrhythmic agent.

20. The bottle must be labeled "Xylocaine for Arrhythmia" or "Lidocaine Without Preservatives."

21. Lidocaine (Xylocaine) is generally the drug of choice.

Copyright © 2004 Mosby Inc. All rights reserved.

23. What drug, also used for seizure disorders, may be used to treat paroxysmal atrial tachycardia and ventricular arrhythmias, particularly those induced by digoxin toxicity?

24. Explain the dosage conversion from lidocaine to tocainide.
25. What action does quinidine have on the heart?
26. When should blood samples for quinidine sulfate levels be drawn in relationship to doses being administered?
27. What is cinchonism?

28. What initial assessments of the heart disorder should be performed when an arrhythmia is suspected?

29. Review assessments performed for an individual with a heart disorder and compare these with premedication assessments listed throughout this chapter.
30. Why is physical activity curtailed in a patient having arrhythmias?
31. Why is O_2 administration required prn when an arrhythmia occurs?

32. What are the drawbacks of using amiodarone hydrochloride (Cordarone)?

22. Mexiletine has dose-related effects on the CNS. Serum levels greater than 2.0 mcg/ml may precipitate neurologic toxicity and occasionally paradoxic seizure activity. Fine hand tremor is often the first indication, but ataxia, dizziness, light-headedness, nystagmus, paresthesia, blurred vision, diplopia, dysarthria, confusion, and drowsiness are also signs of impending toxicity.
23. Phenytoin may be used to treat some cardiac arrhythmias, as well as seizure disorders.
24. See textbook, p. 366.
25. Quinidine stabilizes the rate of conduction resulting in a slow, regular pulse rate.

26. Blood samples for quinidine sulfate levels should be drawn before the daily dose or at least 6 hours after administration.
27. The signs and symptoms associated with quinidine toxicity (known as cinchonism) include salivation, tinnitus, headache, visual disturbances, and mental confusion.
28. Electrocardiogram should be performed when an arrhythmia is suspected.

29. See textbook, pp. 354-355, and see individual monographs throughout the chapter.
30. To conserve oxygen use so that the available oxygen can be used to meet the body's basic needs, physical activity is curtailed in patients with arrhythmias. Reduced oxygen levels (hypoxia) induce arrhythmias.
31. To prevent hypoxia and the development of arrhythmias, O_2 is administered prn.
32. Amiodarone hydrochloride requires hospitalization during loading dose and the maintenance dose is difficult to establish. Life-threatening arrhythmias may recur at unpredictable intervals. Once the drug is used, switching to a different antiarrhythmic is difficult because the body may store the drug; therefore, a drug interaction with the newly prescribed antiarrhythmic may occur.

Copyright © 2004 Mosby Inc. All rights reserved.

CHAPTER 24

Drugs Used to Treat Arrhythmias

Practice Quiz

COMPLETION

Complete the following statements.

The therapeutic goals of antiarrhythmic therapy are:

1.

2.

3.

4. Basic mental status function may be impaired with insufficient cardiac output that causes _____.

5. The action of Class I antiarrhythmic agents is:

6. The action of Class Ia antiarrhythmic agents is:

The actions of beta-adrenergic blocking agents are:

7.

8.

9.

10. Why should the label on a lidocaine container used for arrhythmias be different from the lidocaine used as a local anesthetic agent?

11. Cinchonism is _____.

12. State the sequence of the heart's conduction system.

13. The initial assessment for a suspected arrhythmia is:

List the six cardinal signs of heart disease that should be monitored on a continuum whenever a heart disorder is suspected.

14.

15.

16.

17.

18.

19.

TRUE OR FALSE

Mark "T" for true and "F" for false next to each of the following statements. Correct all false statements.

_____ 20. With amiodarone hydrochloride therapy it is difficult to predict the degree and duration of antiarrhythmic response.

_____ 21. When beta-adrenergic blockers are being taken, the diabetic patient needs to be monitored for hyperglycemia due to masking of the symptoms by the drug.

_____ 22. The basic causes of arrhythmias are the abnormal firing of pacemaker cells, blockage of normal electrical pathways, or a combination of the two.

_____ 23. The most potent antiarrhythmic agents that act as myocardial depressants and slow conduction rate through the atria and ventricles are Class Ia antiarrhythmic agents.

_____ 24. The nursing assessment of a patient should cite specifically whether dyspnea is present with or without exertion.

_____ 25. A narrowing pulse pressure is the difference between the apical and radial pulse rates.

_____ 26. The most frequently used drug for treatment of ventricular arrhythmias associated with an acute myocardial infarction is digitalis.

Copyright © 2004 Mosby Inc. All rights reserved.

Student Name _____

END-OF-CHAPTER MATH REVIEW

1. Order: quinidine 0.8 grams, PO, tid.
   On hand: quinidine 200 mg tablets
   Give: _____ tablets per dose
   Give: _____ total grams in 24 hours
2. Order: procainamide hydrochloride (Pronestyl)
   1 g, q 6 h.
   On hand: procainamide hydrochloride
   (Pronestyl) 250 mg capsules
   Give: _____ capsules per dose

CRITICAL THINKING QUESTIONS

Adenosine (Adenocard) 6 mg IV bolus was given
stat to a patient in the emergency room being
treated for paroxysmal supraventricular tachycardia.
At postconference the instructor discusses this case
with the student nurses.

Answer the following questions using any reference books:

1. What is paroxysmal supraventricular
   tachycardia and why is this dangerous to the
   patient?
2. What is the normal conduction of impulses
   through the heart?
3. Look up the following information for the drug
   adenosine:

Drug action:
Dosage:
Preparation of drug for IV use:
Dilution: Yes   No
Solutions that can be used to dilute the IV medica-
tion:
Rate of administration:
Incompatibility:
Side effects to expect:

Doctor's order: Quinidine sulfate 200 mg, PO, qid.

1. What time schedule would be used to fulfill this
   order? When a quinidine serum level is ordered,
   based on the time schedule established, when
   would the laboratory draw the blood sample?
2. What nursing assessments should be made
   during the administration of quinidine sulfate?
   What health teaching should be done?

The doctor orders disopyramide (Norpace) 150 mg,
q 6 h.

1. What time schedule would be used to
   administer the drug?
2. After a week of therapy, the therapeutic blood
   level report from the laboratory is 8 mg/L. What
   nursing action(s) would be initiated?

REVIEW QUESTIONS

_____ 1. A patient taking disopyramide (Norpace)
   develops a productive cough. The nurse
   should:
   a. disregard the symptom.
   b. perform a respiratory assessment.
   c. call the physician for an increase in
      dosage.
   d. check daily laboratory clotting test
      results.
_____ 2. When researching quinidine sulfate, a
   side effect listed is cinchonism. This term
   means the nurse would assess for:
   a. nocturnal leg cramps.
   b. rash, chills, fever, ringing in the ears.
   c. severe bradycardia.
   d. urinary retention, weight gain.
_____ 3. Adenosine (Adenocard) is ordered for the
   patient. The nurse knows this drug must
   be administered with _____ only.
   a. 1.5% dextrose and water
   b. 5% dextrose and 0.9% sodium
      chloride
   c. 0.9% sodium chloride
   d. May be given with any other drug or
      IV solution.
_____ 4. The health care provider asks you to
   get lidocaine for use in the treatment of
   a patient with a heart irregularity. You
   would select:
   a. 1% lidocaine with epinephrine.
   b. 2% lidocaine with epinephrine.
   c. 1% lidocaine.
   d. lidocaine for cardiac arrhythmias.

Copyright © 2004 Mosby Inc. All rights reserved.

Drugs Used to Treat Angina Pectoris

Syllabus

CHAPTER CONTENT

Angina Pectoris (p. 368)
Treatment of Angina Pectoris (p. 368)
Drug Therapy for Angina Pectoris (p. 369)
    Drug Class: Nitrates (p. 371)
    Drug Class: Beta-Adrenergic Blocking Agents
       (p. 373)
    Drug Class: Calcium Ion Antagonists (p. 374)
    Drug Class: Angiotensin-Converting Enzyme
       Inhibitors (p. 374)

CHAPTER OBJECTIVES

1. Describe the actions of nitrates, beta-adrenergic
    blockers, calcium channel blockers, and
    angiotensin-converting enzyme inhibitors on
    the myocardial tissue of the heart.
2. Explain the rationale for the use of HMG-CoA
    reductase inhibitors (statins) to treat anginal
    attacks.
3   Identify assessment data needed to evaluate an
    anginal attack.
4. Implement medication therapy health teaching
    to an anginal patient in the clinical setting.

KEY TERMS

angina pectoris
ischemic heart disease
chronic stable angina
unstable angina
variant angina

ASSIGNMENTS

Read textbook, pp. 368-376.
Study Key Terms associated with chapter content.
Complete Collaborative Activity as assigned.
Study Review Sheet for Chapter 25.
Complete Chapter 25 Practice Quiz.
Complete End-of-Chapter Math Review and Critical
    Thinking Questions.
Complete Chapter 25 Exam.

WEB RESEARCH ACTIVITIES

Access: www.americanheart.org
In the search box, type: *ACC/AHA 2002 Guideline
Update for the Management of Patients with Chronic
Stable Angina*
Read: Pharmacology Therapy, Overview of
Treatment
Bring answers to the following questions to class for
discussion:
1. What antiplatelet agents are recommended to
    prevent myocardial infarction and death?
2. What is the correlation in the reduction of
    cholesterol to the percent of reduction in
    coronary events?
3. What were the results of the HOPE study and
    why is this study unique?

COLLABORATIVE ACTIVITY

Prepare a teaching plan for an individual who
takes nitroglycerin sublingual prn, and nifedipine
(Procardia), 30 mg sustained-release capsules once
daily.

Copyright © 2004 Mosby Inc. All rights reserved.

Drugs Used to Treat Angina Pectoris

Review Sheet

The QUESTION column and the ANSWER column have been offset so that you can cover the answer while reading the questions, allowing you to assess your knowledge.

Question	Answer
1. Explain the underlying cause of anginal pain.	
2. Review the various presenting symptoms of angina.	1. The pain and discomfort of angina is caused by the lack of an adequate oxygen supply to the cells in the heart (ischemic heart disease). The underlying etiology is vasospasm of a coronary artery that reduces blood flow through the coronary arteries to the heart tissue.
3. Compare the precipitating factors associated with chronic stable angina, unstable angina, and variant angina.	2. See textbook, p. 369.
4. What are the desired therapeutic outcomes during treatment of angina?	3. Chronic stable angina is precipitated by physical exertion or stress. Unstable angina is precipitated by unpredictable factors such as atherosclerotic narrowing, vasospasm, or thrombus formation. Variant angina occurs at rest. The underlying etiology is vasospasm of a coronary artery that reduces blood flow through the coronary arteries to the heart tissue.
5. What questions should be asked during a nursing assessment related to an angina attack?	4. The goals in treatment of angina pectoris are to prevent myocardial infarction and death, thereby prolonging life, and to relieve anginal pain symptoms, thereby improving the quality of life. The pharmacologic treatment of angina is aimed at decreasing oxygen demand by decreasing heart rate, myocardial contractility, and ventricular volume without inducing heart failure. Because platelet aggregation, blood flow turbulence, and blood viscosity also play a role, especially in unstable angina, platelet-active agents are also prescribed to prevent anginal attacks (see Chapter 28). Since atherosclerosis causes narrowing and closure of coronary arteries inducing angina and myocardial infarction, the use of the HMG-CoA reductase inhibitors (statins) has also become standard therapy in

Copyright © 2004 Mosby Inc. All rights reserved.

6. What are the actions of nitrates, beta-adrenergic blockers, calcium channel blockers, and angiotensin-converting enzyme inhibitors on the myocardial tissue of the heart? Name two examples of each drug class used to treat angina pectoris.

7. Compare the premedication assessments required for nitrates, beta-adrenergic blockers, calcium channel blockers, and angiotensin-converting enzyme inhibitors.

8. What is the drug of choice for acute attacks of angina pectoris?

9. Why is it important to teach patients taking nitroglycerin not to use alcohol?

10. What dose forms are available for nitroglycerin?

11. What side effects can be expected when rapid-acting nitrates (e.g., nitroglycerin, amyl nitrite) are used?

the treatment of angina pectoris when the LDL cholesterol is elevated (see Chapter 21).

5. See textbook, pp. 369-371.

6. Nitrates do not increase total coronary artery blood flow. They cause relaxation of peripheral vascular smooth muscle that results in dilation of arteries and veins, reducing preload and leading to decreased oxygen demands on the heart. They dilate large coronary arteries and redistribute blood flow within the heart.

   Beta-adrenergic blocking agents decrease myocardial oxygen demands by blocking beta-adrenergic receptors in the heart, reducing stimulation by norepinephrine and epinephrine, which normally increases heart rate. Beta blockers also reduce blood pressure.

   Calcium channel blockers decrease myocardial oxygen demands and increase myocardial blood supply by coronary artery dilation. These agents block movement of calcium ions across the cell membrane, resulting in 1) inhibition of smooth muscle contraction; 2) dilation of blood vessels, including coronary arteries; and 3) decreased resistance to blood flow as a result of dilation of peripheral vessels.

   The angiotensin-converting enzymes inhibit the enzyme's action on the endothelial wall of coronary arteries promoting vasodilation and minimizing cellular aggregation, preventing further thrombus formation.

   Select two drugs from each classification from Tables 13-3, 22-5, 25-1, and 25-2 in textbook.

7. See textbook, pp. 371-374.

8. Nitroglycerin, administered sublingually, is the drug of choice for acute attacks of angina pectoris.

9. Alcohol use results in vasodilation and may lead to postural hypotension.

10. Sublingual tablets, transmucosal tablets, translingual spray, topical disks, sustained-release capsules, topical ointment, and intravenous forms of nitroglycerin are available.

Copyright © 2004 Mosby Inc. All rights reserved.

12. What premedication assessments should be performed prior to therapy with nitrates?

13. Describe the procedure for administering nitroglycerin sublingually, via translingual spray, topical ointment, transmucosal tablets, and topical disk.

14. How does one evaluate anginal attacks and what health teaching is needed for an individual who has anginal attacks?

15. What are some guidelines used during the preparation and administration of IV nitroglycerin?

16. What are the desired therapeutic outcomes of the use of beta blocker therapy for treatment of anginal pain?

17. What is the desired result of the use of calcium ion antagonists to treat angina?

18. What are common side effects associated with angiotensin-converting enzyme inhibitors?

11. Headache and hypotension caused by the vasodilation of blood vessels are side effects of nitroglycerin and amyl nitrite treatment.

12. Assess for pain level, location, duration, intensity, and pattern, and obtain a history of most recent nitrate use before beginning amyl nitrate therapy.

13. Procedure for administration of the various forms of nitroglycerin: textbook pp. 103-107 and pp. 371-373.

14. See textbook, pp. 369-371.

15. See textbook, p. 373.

16. The desired therapeutic outcomes of beta blocker therapy are decreased frequency and severity of anginal attacks, increased tolerance of activities, and decreased use of nitroglycerin for acute anginal attacks. Before administering beta blockers, take BP in supine and standing position, check for history of respiratory disorders such as COPD, and check for history of diabetes. If patient is a diabetic, determine whether the physician wants baseline blood glucose studies before initiating the medication.

17. The desired action of calcium ion antagonists in the treatment of angina is to decrease myocardial oxygen demands by increasing myocardial blood supply via coronary arteries and decrease resistance to blood flow and dilate peripheral vessels, resulting in decreased workload of the heart.

18. ACE inhibitors cause hypotension with dizziness, tachycardia, fainting, and nonproductive cough.

Copyright © 2004 Mosby Inc. All rights reserved.

25 Drugs Used to Treat Angina Pectoris

CHAPTER

Practice Quiz

ESSAY

1. List a minimum of four symptoms of an angina attack.
2. What nursing assessments are appropriate for an individual who arrives at the emergency room complaining of chest pain? What if the person has a history of angina pectoris?
3. Explain the lifestyle modifications needed as part of the treatment of angina pectoris.
4. How often should sublingual nitrates be administered when ordered prn?
5. How often are sustained-release tablets of nitroglycerin administered?
6. How are transmucosal tablets administered and how often is this form of a nitrate administered daily?
7. State the procedure for administering translingual nitrate spray, topical ointment, transdermal disks, and IV nitroglycerin.
8. State the mechanism of action of nitrates, calcium channel blockers, beta-adrenergic blockers, and angiotensin-converting enzyme inhibitor agents in the treatment of anginal pain.
9. Name two calcium channel blockers, two beta-adrenergic blockers, and two angiotensin-converting enzyme inhibitors used to treat angina.
10. Explain the premedication assessments that should be performed before administering nitrates, beta blockers, calcium channel blockers, and angiotensin-converting enzyme inhibitor agents.

END-OF-CHAPTER MATH REVIEW

1. Order: nitroglycerin 0.3 mg, SL, prn for chest pain
   On hand: nitroglycerin 0.15 mg, SL tablets.
   Give: _____ tablets

2. Order: nifedipine (Procardia) 10 mg, SL, for acute pain
   On hand: nifedipine (Procardia) 10 mg capsules
   Give: _____ capsules.
3. Order: propranolol hydrochloride (Inderal), 160 mg, qd
   On hand: propranolol hydrochloride (Inderal) concentrated oral solution 80 mg/ml
   Give: _____ ml.

CRITICAL THINKING QUESTIONS

A 64-year-old man comes to the emergency room with acute chest pain. He is holding his chest with his fist directly over the sternum. He appears diaphoretic. He is in work clothes and has been mowing the lawn. It is 98° F outside.

1. What nursing actions would be appropriate immediately?
2. What drug(s) would likely be ordered if this is acute angina pectoris?
3. Describe the correct procedure for administering nitroglycerin SL.
4. If a stat dose of nitroglycerin sublingual spray is ordered, explain how you would instruct the patient to give it.
5. When giving AM medications in the nursing home, the nurse comes to an order to apply Nitro-Dur patch 2.5 mg. The MAR (medication administration record) indicates the prior patch was applied to the right scapula area. The patch is not there. How would you proceed to execute the order?

Copyright © 2004 Mosby Inc. All rights reserved.

REVIEW QUESTIONS

_____ 1. Premedication assessments for calcium ion antagonist drugs include checking:
   a. the laboratory values for nephrotoxicity.
   b. the laboratory values for hepatotoxicity.
   c. potassium level.
   d. for respiratory disease/disorders.

_____ 2. Transmucosal tablets administered for angina release nitroglycerin over the next:
   a. 3–5 hours.
   b. 6–10 hours.
   c. 10–12 hours.
   d. 12–18 hours.

_____ 3. Following administration of a nitrate the patient may experience:
   a. bradycardia.
   b. tachycardia.
   c. hypotension.
   d. prolonged palpitations.

_____ 4. Patients using Nitro-Dur patches should wait _____ hours after removing an old patch before applying a new patch.
   a. 3–5 hours
   b. 6–10 hours
   c. 8–12 hours
   d. 12–24 hours

_____ 5. The most effective agents for relieving ischemia and angina are:
   a. beta blockers, calcium antagonists, and nitrates.
   b. HMG-CoA reductase inhibitors and nitrates.
   c. nitrates and antiplatelet agents.
   d. beta blockers and HMG-CoA reductase inhibitors.

Copyright © 2004 Mosby Inc. All rights reserved.

Drugs Used to Treat Peripheral Vascular Disease

Syllabus

CHAPTER CONTENT

Peripheral Vascular Disease (p. 377)
Treatment of Peripheral Vascular Disease (p. 378)
Drug Therapy for Peripheral Vascular Disease
    (p. 378)
    Drug Class: Hemorrheologic Agents (p. 380)
    Drug Class: Vasodilators (p. 381)
    Drug Class: Platelet Aggregation Inhibitors
      (p. 383)

CHAPTER OBJECTIVES

1. List the baseline assessments used to evaluate a patient with peripheral vascular disease (PVD).
2. Identify specific measures the patient can use to improve peripheral circulation and prevent complications from PVD.
3. Identify the systemic effects to expect when peripheral vasodilators are administered.
4. Explain why hypotension and tachycardia occur frequently with the use of peripheral vasodilators.
5. Develop measurable objectives/outcomes for patient education for patients with peripheral vascular disease.
6. State both pharmacologic and nonpharmacologic goals of treatment for PVD.

KEY TERMS

arteriosclerosis obliterans
intermittent claudication
paresthesias
Raynaud's disease
vasospasm

ASSIGNMENTS

Read textbook, pp. 377-385.
Study Key Terms associated with chapter content.
Study Review Sheet for Chapter 26.
Complete Chapter 26 Practice Quiz.
Complete End-of-Chapter Math Review and Critical
    Thinking Questions.
Complete Chapter 26 Exam.

WEB RESEARCH ACTIVITIES

Access: www.americanheart.org and research
Raynaud's disease and PVD.
After reading the sections on Raynaud's disease and
PVD, write and submit to the instructor the answers
to the following:
1. When is an attack of Raynaud's disease likely to occur? What class of drugs is used to treat Raynaud's disease?
2. Cite drugs used to treat peripheral arterial disease (PAD).

Copyright © 2004 Mosby Inc. All rights reserved.

Drugs Used to Treat Peripheral Vascular Disease

Review Sheet

The QUESTION column and the ANSWER column have been offset so that you can cover the answer before reading the questions, thus allowing you to assess your knowledge.

Question	**Answer**
1. Explain the pathophysiology of intermittent claudication, vasospasm, paresthesia, arteriosclerosis obliterans, and Raynaud's disease.	
2. What are the goals of treatment of arteriosclerosis obliterans?	1. See textbook, pp. 377-378.
3. List the agents specifically approved by the FDA to treat chronic occlusive arterial disease.	2. Improve blood flow, relieve pain, and prevent skin ulcerations and/or gangrene.
4. Name the three calcium ion antagonists used in the treatment of Raynaud's disease.	3. pentoxifylline and cilostazol
5. What is the action of an ACE inhibitor in the treatment of PVD?	4. Diltiazem, verapamil, and nifedipine
6. What preventative actions can be taken by a patient with Raynaud's disease to reduce or stop vasospastic attacks?	5. Vasodilation
7. What nursing assessments should be made on a regular basis when peripheral vasodilators are prescribed?	6. Avoid cold temperature, emotional stress, tobacco, and drugs known to induce attacks.
8. Describe the health teaching needed when PVD is diagnosed that would promote improved tissue perfusion.	7. Assess for color and temperature of the hands, fingers, legs, and feet. Check for signs and symptoms of skin breakdown, presence of limb pain, or a reduction in sensation in the extremities. Pedal pulses and radial pulse rates should be taken and recorded q 4 h during hospitalization and bid upon discharge.
9. What is the action of pentoxifylline (Trental) and cilostazol (Pletal)?	8. See textbook, pp. 379-380.
10. What type of vascular conditions may be treated using peripheral vasodilating agents?	9. Trental increases RBC (red blood cell) flexibility, decreases concentration of fibrinogen in the blood, and prevents aggregation of RBCs and platelets, thus preventing blood clotting. Cilostazol inhibits platelet aggregation and promotes vasodilation.

Copyright © 2004 Mosby Inc. All rights reserved.

11. What is the mechanism of action of vasodilators used to treat PVD?

12. What are the side effects to expect with the administration of vasodilating agents?

13. List the premedication assessments required for all prescribed medications for PVD.

10. Intermittent claudication, arteriosclerosis obliterans, vasospasms associated with thrombophlebitis, nocturnal leg cramps, and Raynaud's disease.

11. Relaxation of peripheral arterial blood vessels, thereby increasing blood flow to the extremities.

12. Flushing, tingling, sweating. May also produce orthostatic hypotension and tachycardia. Also may cause possible nervousness and weakness as therapy progresses.

13. Baseline assessment of symptoms of PVD and degree of pain present; take baseline vital signs.

Copyright © 2004 Mosby Inc. All rights reserved.

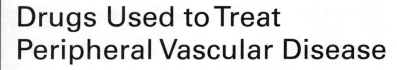

CHAPTER 26
Drugs Used to Treat Peripheral Vascular Disease

Practice Quiz

TRUE OR FALSE

Mark "T" for true and "F" for false next to each of the following statements. <u>*Correct all false statements.*</u>

_____ 1. Part of the assessment process for PVD includes reviewing laboratory data relating to serum glucose levels and serum lipids.

_____ 2. Foot care for an individual with PVD should include regular trimming of toenails and corns.

_____ 3. Improvement in the symptoms of PVD includes reduction in frequency and degree of pain, intolerance to exercise, and an overall improvement in quality of the peripheral pulses.

_____ 4. Vasodilating agents have the potential for initiating orthostatic hypotension.

_____ 5. Flushing of the face, neck, and chest are expected side effects of vasodilators.

ESSAY

6. Explain why hemorrheologic agents and vasodilators may relieve the symptoms of PVD.

7. What nonpharmacologic measures can improve peripheral circulation?

8. Explain how to assess tissue that is affected by PVD.

9. What is the desired therapeutic outcome to expect from the use of vasodilators to treat PVD?

10. How do platelet aggregation inhibitors relieve the symptoms of PVD?

END-OF-CHAPTER MATH REVIEW

1. Ordered: pentoxifylline (Trental) 400 mg, PO, qd, for 4 days, then 400 mg per day, bid.
   On hand: pentoxifylline (Trental) 400 mg tablets.
   How many 400 mg tablets would be needed to administer the first 4 days of dosages?
   _____ tablets
   How many 400 mg tablets would be needed to administer the next 5 days of dosages?
   _____ tablets

2. Ordered: papaverine hydrochloride (Pavabid) 300 mg, q 12 h
   On hand: papaverine hydrochloride (Pavabid) 150 mg timed-release capsules
   Give: _____ capsules per dose

CRITICAL THINKING QUESTIONS

1. A patient tells you when she and her husband go for their daily walks she can only go two blocks and then has to sit down because of pain in the calves of her legs. They rest a while, walk another two blocks, and the pain is back. The patient asks your advice. What would you say?

   Two days later, the patient is assigned to you for nursing care. The patient's primary nursing diagnosis is: Ineffective tissue perfusion related to insufficient oxygenation of the lower limbs manifested by pain on walking two blocks, diminished popliteal pulses, bilaterally. What nursing assessments would you plan to make?

   The health care provider prescribes cilostazol (Pletal) 100 mg, bid. Review the drug monograph and discuss the drug's action and side effects to anticipate. What health teaching would be needed in relation to the prescribed drug?

Copyright © 2004 Mosby Inc. All rights reserved.

2. A 76-year-old patient has been suffering from arteriosclerosis obliterans with intermittent claudication and refuses to give up smoking. At the last office visit, a prescription for pentoxifyl-line (Trental) 400 mg, tid, PO with meals was written. After leaving the examination room, the patient tells the office nurse that the health care provider did not explain how this would work to improve his "leg pain."

Give a simple explanation of what is thought to be the mechanism of action of Trental and draw a diagram that depicts "erythrocyte flexibility" as a visual aid to assist in understanding how the drug could improve his "leg pain."

A week later, the patient calls the office: "That new medication you gave me for my leg pain isn't working." How should you respond?

REVIEW QUESTIONS

_____ 1. The health care provider orders phenoxy-benzamine hydrochloride and the patient asks you what side effects to expect from this medication. The main point to make when responding is:
   a. that the side effects are a rapid pulse, nasal congestion, and episodes of low blood pressure.
   b. that most of the side effects you've explained will resolve with continued therapy.
   c. if the side effects occur, the drug should be stopped immediately.
   d. to decrease the dose when the side effects explained occur.

_____ 2. Pentoxyfylline (Trental) acts:
   a. to increase the flexibility of erythro-cytes.
   b. as an anticoagulant.
   c. to increase the viscosity of blood flow.
   d. to break down the plaque in blood vessels.

_____ 3. Premedication assessments with periph-eral vascular disease should include:
   a. checking for renal disease.
   b. obtaining a pain rating.
   c. checking mentation.
   d. assessment of respiratory function.

Copyright © 2004 Mosby Inc. All rights reserved.

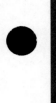

Drugs Used for Diuresis

Syllabus

CHAPTER CONTENT

Diuretic Therapy (p. 386)
>Drug Therapy with Diuretics (p. 389)
>>Drug Class: Carbonic Anhydrase Inhibitors (p. 389)
>>Drug Class: Methylxanthines (p. 389)
>>Drug Class: Loop Diuretics (p. 391)
>>Drug Class: Thiazide Diuretics (p. 395)
>>Drug Class: Potassium-Sparing Diuretics (p. 397)
>>Drug Class: Combination Diuretic Products (p. 399)

CHAPTER OBJECTIVES

1. Cite nursing assessments used to evaluate a patient's state of hydration.
2. Review possible underlying pathology that may contribute to the development of excess fluid volume in the body.
3. State which electrolytes may be altered by diuretic therapy.
4. Cite nursing assessments used to evaluate renal function.
5. Identify the effects of diuretics on blood pressure, electrolytes, and diabetic or prediabetic patients.
6. Review the signs and symptoms of electrolyte imbalance and normal laboratory values of potassium, sodium, and chloride.
7. Identify the action of diuretics.
8. Explain the rationale for administering diuretics cautiously to older adults and individuals with impaired renal function, cirrhosis of the liver, or diabetes mellitus.
9. Describe the goal of administering diuretics to treat hypertension, heart failure, increased intraocular pressure, or before vascular surgery in the brain.
10. List side effects that can be anticipated whenever a diuretic is administered.
11. Cite alterations in diet that may be prescribed concurrently with loop, thiazide, or potassium-sparing diuretic therapy.
12. State the nursing assessments needed to monitor therapeutic response or development of side effects to expect or report from diuretic therapy.
13. Develop objectives for patient education for patients taking loop, thiazide, and potassium-sparing diuretics.

KEY TERMS

aldosterone
tubule
loop of Henle
orthostatic hypotension
electrolyte imbalance
hyperuricemia

ASSIGNMENTS

Read textbook, pp. 386-400.
Study Key Terms associated with chapter content.
Complete Collaborative Activity as assigned.
Study Review Sheet for Chapter 27.
Complete Chapter 27 Practice Quiz.
Complete End-of-Chapter Math Review and Critical Thinking Questions.
Complete Chapter 27 Exam.

WEB RESEARCH ACTIVITY

Access the web using an available search engine. Type in "diuretic therapy" and then research articles that explain precautions when using diuretic therapy. Bring two articles to class for group discussion.

Copyright © 2004 Mosby Inc. All rights reserved.

COLLABORATIVE ACTIVITY

Complete the following as preparation for in-class discussion and group work that may be assigned by the instructor.

The doctor orders furosemide (Lasix) 40 mg IV stat. Refer to the drug monograph and any other drug resources necessary, then explain how the nurse would prepare and administer the dose via a saline lock that is in place. Explain how to calculate the rate of administration when the drug is given IV push.

If administering a stat dose of furosemide to a patient with a Foley catheter, why should the nurse empty the catheter bag and record the amount of urine in the bag immediately before administering the stat dose of medication?

Copyright © 2004 Mosby Inc. All rights reserved.

Drugs Used for Diuresis

Review Sheet

The QUESTION column and the ANSWER column have been offset so you can cover the answer while reading the question, allowing you to assess your knowledge.

Question	**Answer**
1. Explain the therapeutic outcomes associated with diuretic therapy.	
2. What laboratory tests should be performed to determine if kidney function is impaired?	1. The therapeutic outcomes of diuretic therapy are diuresis with reduction of edema and improvement in the symptoms of fluid overload and reduced blood pressure.
3. What laboratory studies should be performed whenever a diuretic is prescribed?	2. Check for elevated BUN and serum creatinine; also check for decreased creatinine clearance, decreased urine output, and increasing edema.
4. What patient assessments should be performed on a regular basis when diuretics are being taken?	3. Check Hct, serum electrolytes, blood glucose, uric acid, BUN, and serum creatinine.
5. What is the action of a diuretic?	4. Assess intake and output of fluids, state of hydration, presence of edema, heart rate and rhythm, blood pressure bid or qid, and daily weights. Check for signs and symptoms of electrolyte imbalance, gastric irritation, rash, hyperuricemia, and hyperglycemia. Monitor for drug interactions (e.g., digitalis glycosides, corticosteroids, lithium).
6. What are the six classes of diuretics?	5. Diuretics inhibit the reabsorption of sodium, increasing the loss of water.
7. Which class of diuretic has the most rapid onset of action? (List the four drugs.) What three routes of administration can be used for loop diuretics?	6. The six classes of diuretic are thiazide, loop, potassium-sparing, osmotic, methylxanthine, and carbonic anhydrase inhibitors. Thiazides and potassium-sparing diuretics are also available as combination products.
8. After administration of a loop diuretic using each of these routes, how soon will diuresis occur and how long will it last?	7. Loop diuretics are furosemide (Lasix), ethacrynic acid (Edecrin), bumetanide (Bumex), and torsemide (Demadex). Oral (PO), intramuscular (IM), or intravenous (IV) routes.
9. When would loop diuretics be prescribed?	8. Oral: onset, 30–60 minutes; peak, 1–2 hours; duration, 6–8 hours. IM: onset, 30–40 minutes; peak, 1–2 hours; duration, 5–6 hours. IV: onset, 5 minutes; peak 15–45 minutes; duration, 2 hours.

Copyright © 2004 Mosby Inc. All rights reserved.

10. Of the four loop diuretics, which is most frequently prescribed?

11. Would thiazide or loop diuretics be used when renal function is impaired?

12. What classes of diuretics can cause a loss of serum potassium (hypokalemia)?

13. What class(es) of diuretic(s) can cause an increase in serum potassium (hyperkalemia)?

14. What type(s) of diuretic(s) are used to reduce intraocular and intracranial pressure?

15. Why would a potassium-sparing and another type of diuretic be prescribed simultaneously?

16. What actions can be taken to prevent and/or treat hypokalemia?

17. What actions can be taken to prevent hyperkalemia when potassium-sparing diuretics are prescribed?

18. Are diuretics useful for edema that occurs during pregnancy?

19. What medicine may need to be ordered for patients who have gouty arthritis who require diuretics?

20. Which type of diuretic has been associated with hearing loss when used concurrently with aminoglycoside antibiotics or cisplatin?

21. What class of antibiotics can cause hearing loss and, if combined with loop diuretics, may increase the possibility of ototoxicity?

22. After reading that diuretics can interact with digoxin to produce digoxin toxicity, what signs and symptoms would you monitor when therapy is combined?

23. What are the normal values for sodium, potassium, and chloride?

24. List six foods that are good sources of potassium.

25. Why should salicylates not be taken with furosemide for prolonged periods?

26. Describe the signs and symptoms of salicylate toxicity.

9. When rapid diuresis is needed (e.g., in pulmonary edema) or when renal function is diminished.

10. Furosemide

11. Loop diuretics are more effective than other classes of diuretics when renal function is impaired (decreased creatinine clearance).

12. Thiazide, loop, and osmotic diuretics

13. Potassium-sparing diuretics

14. Osmotic diuretics

15. To prevent hypokalemia, improve diuresis, and lower blood pressure.

16. Give potassium supplements and/or increase dietary intake of foods rich in potassium.

17. Do not use salt substitutes that contain potassium. Maintain an adequate fluid intake. Do not administer potassium supplements. Use ACE inhibitors, angiotensin II receptor blockers, eplerenone, and NSAIDs with extreme caution to prevent hyperkalemia.

18. Diuretics are rarely used for edema associated with pregnancy. Diuretics cross the placental barrier and may be harmful to the fetus. Consult a physician before taking any medication during pregnancy or while breastfeeding.

19. Allopurinol

20. Loop diuretics

21. Aminoglycosides: gentamicin, tobramycin, kanamycin, amikacin, neomycin, streptomycin, netilmicin.

22. Anorexia, nausea, fatigue, blurred or colored vision, bradycardia, arrhythmias.

23. Sodium: 135–145 mEq/L; potassium: 3.5–4.7 mEq/L; chloride: 95–105 mEq/L

24. Dried almonds; apricots, raw; avocados, raw; bananas, raw; beans, lima (cooked, boiled); carrots, raw; cocoa, plain; potatoes (cooked, boiled)

25. The potential for salicylate toxicity may be increased if taken concurrently for several days.

Copyright © 2004 Mosby Inc. All rights reserved.

27. Which class of diuretics can affect the male libido?

28. Why are potassium-sparing diuretics not used in patients with renal failure?

29. What are the signs and symptoms of circulatory overload?

30. Why must the IV site be checked frequently when osmotic agents are administered IV?

31. How do carbonic anhydrase inhibitors decrease intraocular pressure?

32. What premedication assessments should be made before administering any type of diuretic?

26. Nausea, tinnitus, fever, sweating, dizziness, mental confusion, lethargy, and impaired hearing

27. Potassium-sparing diuretics [e.g., amiloride (Midamor), spironolactone (Aldactone)]

28. They are usually not effective as diuretics in moderate to severe renal failure and may cause hyperkalemia.

29. Bounding, full pulse; jugular vein distention; dyspnea; frothy sputum; cough

30. If the drug leaks into tissue surrounding the blood vessel (infiltration, extravasation) it can cause tissue necrosis.

31. Carbonic anhydrase inhibitors decrease production of aqueous humor; thus, they are used to treat both closed-angle and open-angle glaucoma.

32. Baseline vital signs, lung sounds, weight, assessment of degree of edema, level of consciousness (LOC), muscle strength, tremors, general appearance; blood glucose levels for patients with diabetes. Baseline laboratory studies as prescribed by physician.

Copyright © 2004 Mosby Inc. All rights reserved.

27 Drugs Used for Diuresis

Practice Quiz

CHAPTER

COMPLETION

Complete the following statements.

Two major diseases treated with diuretics are:
1.

2.

List four laboratory tests used to assess the state of hydration:

3.

4.

5.

6.

The normal range for the following electrolytes is:

7. Sodium (Na^+) = _____ mEq/L
8. Potassium (K^+)= _____ mEq/L
9. The most frequently used loop diuretic is
   _____.
10. _____ is known to occur when a loop diuretic is combined with an aminoglycoside or cisplatin.
11. Diabetic patients receiving a diuretic must be checked regularly for _____.
12. _____ occurs with diuretics that inhibit the excretion of uric acid.
13. _____ can occur with diuretic therapy due to reduction in total circulating fluid volume.

Name three loop diuretics.
14.

15.

16.

Name three thiazide diuretics.

17.

18.

19.

Name one potassium-sparing diuretic.

20.

ESSAY

21. Why is it important to know a patient's vital signs, mental status, and general appearance before administering a diuretic?
22. What action can diuretics have on uric acid in the body?
23. Which electrolytes are most commonly affected by diuretic therapy?
24. Why can the administration of a diuretic sometimes cause digoxin toxicity?
25. What antibiotics, given concurrently with diuretics, may cause ototoxicity?
26. What drug classification does each of the following diuretics belong to?
    a. furosemide = _____
    b. torsemide = _____
    c. hydrochlorothiazide = _____
    d. spironolactone = _____
27. Why are combination diuretic products used?
28. What side effects to report may occur when an angiotensin-converting enzyme inhibitor is given concurrently with spironolactone?

Copyright © 2004 Mosby Inc. All rights reserved.

END-OF-CHAPTER MATH REVIEW

1. Order: ethacrynic acid 50 mg, IV in 50 ml D$_5$W. Infuse the medication over 30 minutes. The patient has an IV pump running that is calibrated in ml/hr.
   Set the pump at _____ ml/hr to infuse the ethacrynic acid.

2. Order: furosemide 40 mg, PO, stat
   On hand: furosemide 20 mg tablets
   Give: _____ tablet(s)

CRITICAL THINKING QUESTIONS

1. The health care provider orders furosemide 80 mg, stat, IV push. The drug resource book states, "The rate of administration should not exceed 4 mg per minute." Based on this information, how long would it take to administer the furosemide? What other facts should be checked prior to initiating IV push of the drug?

2. A patient is being treated for hypertension with diuretic therapy. She calls the health care provider's office to report feeling weak, light-headed, and fatigued. What additional information would be useful prior to discussing her symptoms with the health care provider?

REVIEW QUESTIONS

_____ 1. Lasix (furosemide) is a commonly prescribed diuretic with an onset of action of _____ orally; and _____ after IV administration.
   a. 30 minutes; 5–15 minutes
   b. 1–2 hours; 5–10 minutes
   c. 3 hours; 25 minutes
   d. 4–6 hours; 5–10 minutes

_____ 2. Thiazide diuretics may cause:
   a. nephrotoxicity.
   b. ototoxicity.
   c. hyperuricemia.
   d. hypertension.

_____ 3. Nonsteroidal anti-inflammatory medications taken concurrently with certain diuretics (e.g., bumetanide, furosemide, and ethacrynic acid) can:
   a. increase diuresis.
   b. decrease diuresis.
   c. have no effect on diuresis.
   d. require a decreased dosage of the diuretic.

_____ 4. Potassium supplements and salt substitutes should not be given with which class of diuretic?
   a. thiazide
   b. loop
   c. potassium-sparing
   d. carbonic anhydrase inhibitors

Copyright © 2004 Mosby Inc. All rights reserved.

CHAPTER 28

Drugs Used to Treat Thromboembolic Disorders

Syllabus

CHAPTER CONTENT

Thromboembolic Diseases (p. 401)
Treatment of Thromboembolic Diseases (p. 402)
Drug Therapy for Thromboembolic Diseases (p. 402)
    Drug Class: Platelet Inhibitors (p. 404)
    Drug Class: Anticoagulants (p. 408)
    Drug Class: Fibrinolytic Agents (p. 414)

CHAPTER OBJECTIVES

1. State the primary purposes of anticoagulant therapy.
2. Analyze Figure 28-1 to identify the site of action of warfarin, heparin, and fibrinolytic medicine.
3. Identify the effects of anticoagulant therapy on existing blood clots.
4. Describe conditions that place an individual at risk for developing blood clots.
5. Identify specific nursing interventions that can prevent clot formation.
6. Explain laboratory data used to establish dosing of anticoagulant medications.
7. Describe specific monitoring procedures to detect hemorrhage in the anticoagulated patient.
8. Describe procedures used to ensure that the correct dose of an anticoagulant is prepared and administered.
9. Explain the specific procedures and techniques used to administer heparin subcutaneously, via intermittent administration through a heparin lock, and via intravenous infusion.
10. Identify the purpose, dosing determination, and scheduling factors associated with the use of protamine sulfate.
11. State the nursing assessments needed to monitor therapeutic response and the development of side effects to expect or report from anticoagulant therapy.
12. Develop objectives for patient education for patients receiving anticoagulant therapy.

KEY TERMS

thromboembolic diseases
thrombosis
thrombus
embolus
intrinsic clotting pathway
extrinsic clotting pathway
platelet inhibitors
anticoagulants
thrombolytic agents
fibrinolytic agents

ASSIGNMENTS

Read textbook, pp. 401-415.
Study Key Terms associated with chapter content.
Study Review Sheet for Chapter 28.
Complete Chapter 28 Practice Quiz.
Complete End-of-Chapter Math Review and Critical Thinking Questions.
Complete Chapter 28 Exam.

WEB RESEARCH ACTIVITIES

Access: www.dvt.org
Click on: VTE Education
Read: *Preventing Deep Vein Thrombosis and Pulmonary Embolism*
Activities:

1. Examine Table 1.3. "Percentage risks venous thrombosis." Read the section on clinical conditions linked with thromboembolism, then summarize the three approaches to address the problem of postoperative venous thrombosis.
2. Cite the advantages and disadvantages of heparin use. How long does it take for oral anticoagulants (e.g., warfarin) to reach a maximum level of anticoagulant effectiveness?
3. What prophylactic treatment is considered most effective for prophylaxis in hip surgery, knee surgery, and following major trauma?

Copyright © 2004 Mosby Inc. All rights reserved.

Drugs Used to Treat Thromboembolic Disorders

Review Sheet

The QUESTION column and the ANSWER column have been offset so you can cover the answer while reading the question, allowing you to assess your knowledge.

Question	Answer
1. Differentiate among thromboembolic disease, thrombosis, thrombus, and embolus.	
2. Explain factors that trigger blood clot formation.	1. See textbook, p. 401.
3. List factor(s) that trigger(s) the intrinsic blood clotting pathway.	2. See textbook, p. 401.
4. Identify factor(s) that trigger(s) the extrinsic pathway triggers.	3. Factor XII
5. What is the difference between red and white blood clots?	4. Factor VII to VIIa (factor VIIa can also activate factor X)
6. Describe appropriate nonpharmacologic patient education for prevention and treatment of thromboembolic disease.	5. Red embolus is a venous thrombus. White thrombi develop in arteries. See also textbook, pp. 401-402.
7. Differentiate among the drug actions of platelet inhibitors, anticoagulants, thrombolytic agents, and thromboembolic agents.	6. See textbook, p. 404.
8. Summarize the nursing actions that can help in the prevention of clot formation.	7. Thromboembolic agents either prevent platelet aggregation or inhibit a variety of steps in fibrin clot formation. Anticoagulants prevent new clot formation. Platelet inhibitors reduce arterial clot formation by inhibiting platelet aggregation. Thrombolytic agents dissolve thromboemboli already formed.
9. State hydration information that should be provided to an individual for whom an anticoagulant is prescribed.	8. See textbook, p. 403.
10. Identify laboratory tests used to evaluate anticoagulant therapy.	9. Adequate hydration to maintain fluidity of blood should be encouraged. Check to be certain the patient does not have coexisting disease that precludes forcing fluids.
11. Explain the desired therapeutic outcomes for platelet inhibitors.	10. Textbook, anticoagulant monographs. Prothrombin time (PT) is reported as international normalized ratio (INR) and is routinely used for warfarin therapy; APTT is most commonly used for heparin therapy.

Copyright © 2004 Mosby Inc. All rights reserved.

12. List premedication assessments that should be performed before administering aspirin as a platelet inhibitor.

13. Differentiate the between the actions of low molecular weight heparins (LMWHs) and heparin.

14. Name three commonly used LMWH drugs.

15. What laboratory studies are used to monitor for adverse effects of LMWHs?

16. What drug is used as an antidote in case of heparin overdose?

17. What is the normal therapeutic range for warfarin therapy?

18. What is the antidote for hemorrhage that occurs with warfarin therapy?

19. List six fibrinolytic agents.

20. When are fibrinolytic agents administered?

21. How long a time is required before clopidogrel (Plavix) achieves full antiplatelet activity level?

22. What is the primary use of ticlopidine (Ticlid)?

11. Reduce the frequency of transient ischemic attacks (TIAs), strokes, and myocardial infarction

12. Neurological assessment, gastrointestinal symptoms present, check for any concurrent anticoagulant therapy being taken; if on oral hypoglycemics, baseline serum glucose levels

13. Heparin acts at several specific points in the coagulation pathway. LMWHs act at fewer specific steps in the coagulation pathway (factors Xa and thrombin), reducing the potential for hemorrhage. LMWHs also have a longer duration of action. Dalteparin, enoxaparin, and tinzaparin have no antiplatelet activity and only minimal effect on PT and APTT.

14. Dalteparin (Fragmin), enoxaparin (Lovenox) and tinzaparin (Innohep)

15. Periodic CBC, daily platelet counts, and periodic checking of stools for occult blood are tests used to monitor for adverse effects of LMWHs.

16. Protamine sulfate; see textbook, p. 411, for details.

17. PT is used to monitor warfarin therapy. PT is expressed as the INR. The optimal dosage of warfarin is that which prolongs the PT and maintains the INR at 2–3. In some medical conditions the INR may be maintained at 2.5–3.5.

18. In most cases of hemorrhage, the dosage of warfarin is withheld until the INR returns to therapeutic levels. In rare cases, vitamin K is administered. In cases of severe hemorrhage, a transfusion with plasma or whole blood may be required.

19. Streptokinase, urokinase, anistreplase, alteplase, reteplase, and tenecteplase

20. Fibrinolytic agents are used to dissolve clots secondary to an MI, pulmonary or cerebral embolism, or deep vein thrombosis (DVT).

21. Three to seven days of continuous therapy is required.

22. To reduce risk of additional strokes in persons who have had a stroke or TIA.

Copyright © 2004 Mosby Inc. All rights reserved.

28 Drugs Used to Treat Thromboembolic Disorders

CHAPTER

Practice Quiz

COMPLETION

Complete the following statements.

A(n) 1. _____ is a circulating blood clot that may be trapped in a distal capillary causing an obstruction. A 2. _____ is a stationary blood clot.

A class of drugs used to prevent blood clot formation is 3. _____. The class of drugs used to dissolve recently formed thrombi is known as 4. _____.

The therapeutic effect of heparin is monitored by the use of the laboratory test known as 5. _____ time. The normal therapeutic range desired is 6. _____.

LMWHs (low molecular weight heparins) are monitored for adverse effects using the following laboratory tests: 7. _____, 8. _____, and 9. _____.

Side effects to be reported when heparin therapy is used include: 10. _____, 11. _____, 12. _____, and 13. _____.

The antidote for excessive bleeding during warfarin therapy is 14. _____.

MATCHING

Select the laboratory test(s) used to monitor the drug therapy listed.

_____ 15. warfarin
_____ 16. therapeutic effect of heparin
   a.   whole blood clotting time
   b.   PT or INR
   c.   APTT
   d.   bleeding time

CALCULATION

17. Order: 1000 ml D_5W with 10,000 U heparin added. Infuse at a rate of 80 U/hr IV. Set the infusion pump, calibrated in ml/hr, at _____ ml/hr.
18. Order: 1 liter D_5W/0.9% NaCl to infuse at 80 ml/hr. Using a microdrip administration set, at how many drops/minute should the infusion be set? _____

END-OF-CHAPTER MATH REVIEW

1.   Ordered: heparin 2000 U, SC, stat.
     On hand: heparin 10,000 U /ml is available.
     Give: _____ ml.
2.   Ordered: 100 ml D_5W with 30,000 U heparin. Infuse at a rate of 800 U/hr, IV. Set the infusion pump, calibrated in ml/hr, at _____ ml/hr. Three hours after the infusion is started, the physician changes the order to 1200 U/hr. How much heparin has already infused? _____ units What rate would the infusion pump be adjusted to?
     Set infusion pump at: _____ ml/ hr.
3.   Ordered: Persantine 75 mg, qid.
     How many 75 mg tablets should the patient be dismissed with in order to take the medication for the next 7 days?
     Give: _____ tablets

Copyright © 2004 Mosby Inc. All rights reserved.

CRITICAL THINKING QUESTIONS

1. A patient comes from surgery following a femoral bypass with a heparin drip running through a pump. What nursing assessments should be made to monitor this patient's postoperative progress? The operative record indicates she received a total of 50,000 U of heparin during the operative procedure. The postoperative orders do not state a specific rate of flow for the heparin drip that is currently running through the pump at 8 ml/hr. What actions should be taken by the nurse?

2. Review the procedure for administration of enoxaparin subcutaneously. What patient monitoring should be done during therapy with this drug?

REVIEW QUESTIONS

_____ 1. How long does the antiplatelet activity of fondaparinux (Arista) remain in a (non-renal compromised) patient after it is discontinued?
   a. unknown
   b. 2–4 days
   c. 4–6 days
   d. 7–12 days

_____ 2. The laboratory test used to monitor the dosage of warfarin is:
   a. INR and PT.
   b. INR and WBCT (whole blood clotting time).
   c. INR and ACT (activated coagulation time).
   d. PT and APTT.

_____ 3. The action of aspirin on clotting is to:
   a. prevent the clotting cascade.
   b. prevent thrombus formation.
   c. prevent platelet aggregation.
   d. decrease bleeding time.

_____ 4. Fibrinolytic agents have the action of:
   a. preventing the clotting cascade.
   b. preventing thrombus formation.
   c. preventing platelet aggregation.
   d. dissolving recently formed thrombi.

Copyright © 2004 Mosby Inc. All rights reserved.

CHAPTER 29

Drugs Used to Treat Upper Respiratory Disease

Syllabus

CHAPTER CONTENT

Upper Respiratory Tract Anatomy and Physiology (p. 416)
Common Upper Respiratory Diseases (p. 417)
Treatment of Upper Respiratory Diseases (p. 418)
Drug Therapy for Upper Respiratory Diseases (p. 419)
    Drug Class: Sympathomimetic Decongestants (p. 420)
    Drug Class: Antihistamines (p. 421)
    Drug Class: Respiratory Anti-inflammatory Agents (p. 422)

CHAPTER OBJECTIVES

1. State the causes of allergic rhinitis and nasal congestion.
2. Explain the major actions (effects) of sympathomimetic, antihistaminic, and corticosteroid decongestants and cromolyn.
3. Define *rhinitis medicamentosa* and describe the patient education needed to prevent it.
4. Review the procedure for administration of medications by nose drops, sprays, and inhalation.
5. Explain why all decongestant products should be used cautiously in persons with hypertension, hyperthyroidism, diabetes mellitus, cardiac disease, increased intraocular pressure, or prostatic disease.
6. State the premedication assessments and nursing assessments needed to monitor therapeutic response and side effects to expect or report from the use of decongestant drug therapy.
7. Identify essential components involved in planning patient education that will enhance compliance with the treatment regimen.

KEY TERMS

rhinitis
sinusitis
allergic rhinitis
antigen-antibody
histamine
rhinorrhea

decongestants
rhinitis medicamentosa
antihistamines
anti-inflammatory
    agents

ASSIGNMENTS

Read textbook, pp. 416-426.
Study Key Terms associated with chapter content.
Complete Collaborative Activity as assigned.
Study Review Sheet for Chapter 29.
Complete Chapter 29 Practice Quiz.
Complete End-of-Chapter Math Review and Critical Thinking Questions.
Complete Chapter 29 Exam.

WEB RESEARCH ACTIVITY

Access: www.aaaai.org
View Case Study 1: Rhinitis/Rhinosinusitis/Conjunctivitis/Recurrent Otitis Media. Answer review questions at the end of the case study.
View Case Study 5: General Diagnosis and Management of Allergic Disorders. Answer review questions at the end of the case study.

Copyright © 2004 Mosby Inc. All rights reserved.

COLLABORATIVE ACTIVITY

Complete the following as preparation for in-class discussion and group work that may be assigned by the instructor.

A 58-year-old patient comes to the physician's office with complaints of a large amount of cloudy nasal discharge, a cough, headache, and "aching all over" the body. He has a fever of 99.8° F.

The doctor prescribes phenylephrine (Neo-Synephrine) nasal spray 0.25%, two sprays in each nostril q 3–4 hours; ASA 650 mg q 4 h for temperature above 100° F and relief of discomfort.

What health education would you perform prior to the patient's leaving the doctor's office?

Copyright © 2004 Mosby Inc. All rights reserved.

Drugs Used to Treat Upper Respiratory Disease

Review Sheet

The QUESTION column and the ANSWER column have been offset so you can cover the answer while reading the question, allowing you to assess your knowledge.

Question	Answer
Question	**Answer**

1. What is allergic rhinitis?
2. What are the drugs of choice for treating allergic rhinitis?
3. What is the mechanism of action of decongestants?
4. What is a "rebound" effect associated with nasally administered decongestants?

5. Name two commonly used decongestants administered intranasally, and one administered orally.

6. Explain how to administer a nasal spray, nose drops, and medications by inhalation.

7. What response does histamine release have on the mucous membranes?
8. What is an antigen?
9. When is histamine released?

10. How do antihistamines act?

11. What side effects can be anticipated whenever an antihistamine is administered?

12. What actions should be initiated to offset the drying effects of antihistamines?
13. What patient education should accompany the use of antihistamines?

1. Inflamed nasal mucosa associated with an allergic reaction.
2. Antihistamines

3. Decongestants are alpha-adrenergic receptor stimulants that constrict blood vessels in the nasal passages, reducing swollen tissues and obstruction.
4. Excessive or prolonged use of nasal decongestants causes a rebound swelling in the nasal passages that requires further use of nasal decongestants to unblock nasal passages. It is difficult to break this cycle, so it is particularly important not to overuse nasal decongestants.
5. Pseudoephedrine (Sudafed)—oral tablets phenylephrine (NeoSynephrine)—nasal spray oxymetazoline (Afrin)—nasal spray xylometazoline (Otrivin)—nasal spray See Table 29-1, p. 420.
6. See Chapter 8, pp. 107-114.

7. Urticaria (itching), redness, and edema
8. A substance that elicits an immunologic response such as the production of a specific antibody against that substance.
9. In cases of tissue damage (trauma), allergic reactions, and infection.
10. Histamines block the H_1 receptor sites on the target cells; they do not affect the amount or the release of histamine.
11. Sedation and dryness of mucous membranes (anticholinergic effects)
12. Consume an adequate fluid intake of 8–12 8 oz glasses daily.

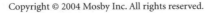

Copyright © 2004 Mosby Inc. All rights reserved.

14. What is the action of cromolyn sodium (Nasalcrom)?

15. What condition is treated with cromolyn sodium (Nasalcrom) that affects the upper respiratory tract?

16. What are the desired therapeutic outcomes from the use of respiratory anti-inflammatory agents?

17. When a drug monograph says that a drug produces anticholinergic effects, what does this mean?

13. Maintain adequate hydration. If the person knows he/she is going to be exposed to an allergen (e.g., pollen outdoors), take the dose 30–45 minutes prior to possible exposure to block receptors before histamine can attach. If exposure is unanticipated, take a dose immediately upon recognition of an allergic response (e.g., runny nose and burning, itchy eyes). Exercise caution when operating any power equipment or while driving because of the medicine's sedative effects.

14. Cromolyn prevents release of histamine from its storage sites, the mast cells.

15. Cromolyn is used with other medications to treat severe allergic rhinitis and prevent release of histamine that causes the symptoms of allergic rhinitis.

16. Reduction in rhinorrhea, rhinitis, itching, and sneezing

17. Blurred vision; constipation; urinary retention; dryness of mucosa of mouth, throat, and nose

Copyright © 2004 Mosby Inc. All rights reserved.

CHAPTER 29

Drugs Used to Treat Upper Respiratory Disease

Practice Quiz

COMPLETION

Complete the following statements.

1. Decongestants cause the blood vessels in the nasal mucosa to _____.
2. Rhinitis medicamentosa can be prevented by _____.
3. The drug class of choice to treat the symptoms of allergic rhinitis is _____.
4. Cromolyn sodium should be administered _____.
5. The desired therapeutic outcome from the use of respiratory anti-inflammatory agents (intranasal corticosteroids) is _____.

ESSAY

6. Explain the correct technique for administering nose drops and nasal spray.

END-OF-CHAPTER MATH REVIEW

Cetirizine hydrochloride (Zyrtec) is available in 5 and 10 mg tablets and a liquid 1 mg/ml for oral administration.
Order: cetirizine hydrochloride (Zyrtec), 2 teaspoonfuls daily at hs

1. Using the 1 mg/ml liquid form of cetirizine, give _____ total ml per dose.
   As the child grows, the mother asks to switch to an oral tablet. How many tablets would be administered to give the oral dose prescribed above?
2. Give: _____ tablets
3. Order: pseudoephedrine (Sudafed) 60 mg, q 6 h, PO
   On hand: pseudoephedrine (Sudafed) 30 mg/5 ml
   Give: _____ ml

CRITICAL THINKING QUESTIONS

1. A patient has been using phenylephrine nasal drops 2–3 times per day for the past 3 weeks. He comes to the physician's office complaining that his symptoms are worse than when he initiated treatment. What assessments should the nurse make?
2. A patient has been using chlorpheniramine maleate tablets three times per day and is now having considerable sedation. Her once productive cough has become nonproductive. What nursing actions should be considered?
3. A patient calls the office and asks the nurse how she can tell if her inhaler is almost empty. What would your response be?
4. Explain how to properly administer a medication by inhalation such as fluticasone, 2 sprays in each nostril once daily.
5. Perform health teaching for the proper administration of nose drops.

REVIEW QUESTIONS

_____ 1. The reason that intranasal corticosteroids are used for short periods to treat seasonal allergies is:
   a. bronchospasm/chronic cough may occur with prolonged therapy.
   b. to prevent elevated blood sugar.
   c. to minimize adrenal suppression.
   d. to prevent central nervous system depression.

Copyright © 2004 Mosby Inc. All rights reserved.

_____ 2. Premedication assessment for sympatho-mimetic decongestants (e.g. Afrin, Neo-Synephrine, Sudafed) includes checking the history for:

a. evidence of hypertension, hyperthyroidism, diabetes mellitus, glaucoma, or prostatic hyperplasia.

b. gastrointestinal symptoms that are present prior to initiation of therapy.

c. any diseases or disorders of the hepatobiliary system.

d. urinary retention, constipation, or blurred vision.

_____ 3. Prior to initiation of antihistamine medications the history should be checked for:

a. evidence of hypertension, hyperthyroidism, diabetes mellitus, glaucoma, or prostatic hyperplasia.

b. urinary retention, constipation, or blurred vision.

c. glaucoma, prostatic hyperplasia, asthma, and concurrent use of sedating drugs.

d. hypertension, hyperthyroidism, and concurrent use of nasal decongestants.

Copyright © 2004 Mosby Inc. All rights reserved.

CHAPTER 30

Drugs Used to Treat Lower Respiratory Disease

Syllabus

CHAPTER CONTENT

CHAPTER OBJECTIVES

1. Compare the physiologic responses of the respiratory system to emphysema, chronic bronchitis, and asthma.
2. Describe the physiology of respirations.
3. Identify components of blood gases.
4. Cite nursing assessments used to evaluate the respiratory status of a patient.
5. Implement patient education for patients receiving drug therapy for lower respiratory disease.
6. Distinguish the mechanisms of action of expectorants, antitussives, and mucolytic agents.
7. Review the procedures for administration of medication by inhalation.
8. State the nursing assessments needed to monitor therapeutic response and the development of side effects to expect or report from expectorant, antitussive, and mucolytic therapy.
9. State the nursing assessments needed to monitor therapeutic response and the development of side effects to expect or report from sympathomimetic bronchodilator therapy.
10. State the nursing assessments needed to monitor therapeutic response and the development of side effects to expect or report from anticholinergic bronchodilator therapy.
11. List side effects known to occur with the use of xanthine derivatives, and correlate these with the needed nursing assessments and interventions.
12. State the nursing assessments needed to monitor therapeutic response and the development of side effects to expect or report from corticosteroid inhalant therapy.

KEY TERMS

ventilation
perfusion
diffusion
goblet cells
obstructive airway
    diseases
bronchospasm
chronic obstructive
    pulmonary disease
chronic airflow
    limitation disease
restrictive airway
    diseases
arterial blood gases

oxygen saturation
spirometry
cough
asthma
bronchitis
emphysema
bronchodilation
expectorants
antitussives
mucolytic agents
bronchodilators
anti-inflammatory
    agents
immunomodulator

Copyright © 2004 Mosby Inc. All rights reserved.

ASSIGNMENTS

Read textbook, pp. 426-451.
Study Key Terms associated with chapter content.
Complete Collaborative Activity as assigned.
Study Review Sheet for Chapter 30.
Complete Chapter 30 Practice Quiz.
Complete End-of-Chapter Math Review and Critical
    Thinking Questions.
Complete Chapter 30 Exam.

WEB RESEARCH ACTIVITY

Access: www.aaaai.org
Click on Professional.
Access NAEPP Guidelines Update
Answer the following question:
Does chronic use of inhaled corticosteroids im-
prove long-term outcomes for children with mild or
moderate persistent asthma, in comparison to the
following treatments?
  • "As-needed" beta$_2$ agonists?
  • Long-acting beta$_2$ agonists?
  • Theophylline?
  • Cromolyn/nedocromil?
  • Combinations of above drugs?

COLLABORATIVE ACTIVITY

*Complete the following as preparation for in-class
discussion and group work that may be assigned by the
instructor.*

Research the effects of smoking on the respiratory
tract. Include current statistics on the incidence of
smoking in young people. Discuss cigarettes as ad-
dictive drugs and as entry drugs leading to marijuana and cocaine use.

Copyright © 2004 Mosby Inc. All rights reserved.

Drugs Used to Treat Lower Respiratory Disease

Review Sheet

The QUESTION column and the ANSWER column have been offset so that you can cover the answers while reading the questions, allowing you to assess your knowledge.

Question	Answer
1. Define *ventilation, perfusion,* and *diffusion.*	
2. What are the differences between obstructive and restrictive respiratory diseases?	1. Ventilation is the movement of air in and out of the lungs; perfusion is blood flow through the pulmonary arteries to the capillaries surrounding the alveoli to the pulmonary veins; and diffusion is the process by which oxygen passes across the alveolar membrane to the blood in the capillaries and carbon dioxide passes from the blood to the alveolar sacs.
3. Why are pulmonary function tests performed?	2. Obstructive disease is associated with narrowed air passages and increasing resistance to air flow (e.g., asthma, acute bronchitis). Restrictive airway disease is characterized by restricted alveolar expansion due to loss of elasticity of tissue or physical deformity of the chest itself.
4. Why is the SaO_2 ratio valuable in an assessment of respiratory function?	3. To assess ventilation and diffusion capacity of the lungs and to determine whether medicines are having a therapeutic effect.
5. What is asthma?	4. It reflects the percent of oxygen bound to the hemoglobin compared with the maximum amount of oxygen that could be attached.
6. What is bronchitis?	5. Asthma is a chronic inflammatory disease of bronchi and bronchioles.
7. What is emphysema?	6. Bronchitis is inflammation and edema with excessive mucus secretions leading to airflow obstruction.
8. What are the goals of therapy for asthma?	7. Emphysema is a disease of alveolar destruction without fibrosis.
9. What is the action of expectorants?	8. Goals are: maintain normal activity levels, maintain near-normal pulmonary function rates, prevent chronic and troublesome symptoms, prevent recurrent exacerbations, and avoid adverse effects from asthma medications.
10. What is the action of an antitussive agent?	9. Expectorants liquefy mucus by stimulating natural lubricant fluids.

Copyright © 2004 Mosby Inc. All rights reserved.

11. What is the action of a mucolytic agent?

12. What is the purpose of administering a bronchodilator?

13. What types of drugs are known as anti-inflammatory agents?

14. What data should be collected as part of a respiratory assessment?

15. Explain desirable peak expiratory flow (PEF) used to assess the severity of asthma symptoms.

16. What dietary considerations should be made for a person with a respiratory disease?

17. How should persons with known respiratory disease prevent infection?

18. What medication administration considerations should be made for the delivery of aerosol therapy to a child or elderly person?

19. Cite important aspects of patient education and health promotion for individuals with a lower respiratory disease.

20. What posture does a dyspneic patient assume?

21. Describe appropriate health teaching for patients requiring respiratory therapy.

22. What is the primary action of an expectorant?

23. What precautions must be used when administering an iodine product?

24. When should SSKI not be administered?

25. What types of respiratory diseases may be treated with mucolytic agents [e.g., acetylcysteine (Mucomyst)]?

26. The patient receiving medication by inhalation should be placed in what position?

27. The patient should be instructed to exhale through _____ lips.

28. What patient teaching should be performed for a patient taking an expectorant?

10. Antitussives suppress the cough center in the brain.

11. Mucolytic agents reduce stickiness and viscosity of pulmonary secretions by acting directly on the mucus plug to cause dissolution.

12. It causes a widening of the opening of the bronchioles and alveolar ducts and a decrease in resistance to airflow into the alveolar sacs.

13. Corticosteroids are the most effective anti-inflammatory agents. Other agents are leukotriene modifiers, cromolyn, and nedocromil.

14. See textbook, p. 433.

15. See textbook, pp. 430-431; p. 434.

16. Well-balanced diet to maintain near-normal weight. With dyspnea, eat small servings throughout day, take small bites, and eat slowly. Administer oxygen during meals as needed.

17. Good hygiene; influenza and pneumococcal vaccinations. Seek medical attention at earliest signs of suspected infection.

18. See textbook, p. 435.

19. See textbook, p. 436.

20. Sits upright and leans forward from the waist, resting the elbows on the knees. When hospitalized, will be placed in a high-Fowler's position.

21. See pp. 435-436, Patient Education and Health Promotion.

22. Expectorants enhance the output of respiratory tract fluids.

23. Dilute in water or fruit juice. Use a straw placed well back on the tongue to administer iodine products; this prevents permanent staining of the teeth.

24. Do *not* give to a patient allergic to iodine or one who has hyperthyroidism, hyperkalemia, or experiences a skin eruption after taking the medication.

25. Emphysema, bronchitis, pneumonia, cystic fibrosis

26. Sitting

27. Pursed

Copyright © 2004 Mosby Inc. All rights reserved.

29. What is the desired action for giving saline solution by nebulizer?

30. What classes of antitussive agents are available?
31. What are the major drawbacks to using an opiate antitussive?
32. In what type of patient must great caution be exercised if an opiate antitussive is to be administered?

33. Give one example of an antitussive agent.

34. What premedication assessments should be made prior to administering an antitussive agent, mucolytic agent, expectorant, anticholinergic bronchodilating agent, xanthine derivative bronchodilating agent, respiratory anti-inflammatory agent, antileukotriene agents, and immunomodulators?
35. What are the four components of asthma therapy?

36. Review the premedication assessments associated with acetylcysteine therapy.

37. What types of patients benefit from beta-adrenergic bronchodilator therapy?
38. What two classes of drugs are prescribed as bronchodilators?
39. What is the drug ipratropium bromide (Atrovent) primarily used to treat?
40. How do sympathomimetic (adrenergic) agents act?

41. Which drugs are classified as xanthine derivatives?

28. Teach the patient the difference between a productive and nonproductive cough, as well as measures to combat nonproductive coughs.
29. Hydration of viscous mucus
30. Opiate and nonopiate cough suppressants

31. Codeine may cause dependence (rarely), respiratory depression, bronchial constriction, central nervous system (CNS) depression, and constipation.
32. Patients with preexisting pulmonary distress; persons already taking sedative/hypnotics, CNS depressants, or psychotropic agents; persons using alcohol.
33. Codeine

34. Antitussive agent, p. 439; mucolytic agents, p. 440; expecorants, p. 438; anticholinergic bronchodilating agents, p. 442; xanthine derivative bronchodilating agents, p. 443 respiratory anti-inflammatory agents, p. 444 antileukotriene agents, p. 445; immunomodulators, p. 448
35. Patient education, environmental control, comprehensive pharmacologic therapy, and objective monitoring via regular use of a peak flow meter
36. See textbook, p. 440.

37. Patients with diseases that cause constriction of the tracheobronchial tree, obstructing the airways.
38. Sympathomimetics and xanthine derivatives

39. Ipratropium bromide (Atrovent) is used as a bronchodilator for long-term treatment of reversible bronchospasm associated with chronic obstructive pulmonary disease (COPD).
40. Adrenergic agents stimulate beta$_2$ receptors, causing bronchodilation. Many of the drugs also stimulate beta$_1$ receptors in the heart. Always monitor patients taking adrenergic agents for changes in cardiac function (e.g., hypertension, tachycardia), CNS stimulation (exhibited as insomnia, nervousness, anxiety, tremors), and gastrointestinal (GI) disturbances.

Copyright © 2004 Mosby Inc. All rights reserved.

42. How do xanthines work?

43. What pharmacologic effects do xanthines cause?

44. How can dosages of theophylline be measured?

45. Describe the clinical uses of montelukast (Singulair), zafirlukast (Accolate), and zileuton (Zyflo).

46. Describe premedication assessments for omalizumab (Zolair).

41. Aminophylline, theophylline, dyphylline, oxtriphylline (*Note:* all xanthine derivatives except caffeine end in "-phylline.")

42. They cause an increase in cyclic adenosine monophosphate (cAMP), a substance that is associated with bronchodilation and smooth muscle relaxation.

43. They stimulate the CNS, cause diuresis, increase gastric secretions, and stimulate the heart to beat rapidly. Always monitor patients for nausea, changes in cardiac function, and CNS stimulation.

44. Theophylline levels can be monitored by a blood test.
Adult: 10–20 mcg/ml; Newborn: 6–11 mcg/ml.

45. See textbook, pp. 445-446.

46. See textbook, p. 449.

Copyright © 2004 Mosby Inc. All rights reserved.

CHAPTER 30

Drugs Used to Treat Lower Respiratory Disease

Practice Quiz

DEFINITIONS

Define the following terms.
1. Perfusion:
2. Ventilation:
3. Bronchitis:
4. Emphysema:
5. Expectorants (action):
6. Antitussives (action):
7. Mucolytics (action):

COMPLETION

Complete the following statements.
8. The _____ measures the ratio of actual oxygen content of hemoglobin compared with the hemoglobin's oxygen-carrying capacity.
9. _____ is an inflammatory disease of the bronchi and bronchioles. There are intermittent periods of acute, reversible airflow obstruction (bronchoconstriction) caused by bronchiolar inflammation and overresponsiveness to a variety of stimuli.
10. A _____ is an instrument used to measure volumes of air during inhalation and exhalation.
11. Guaifenesin (Robitussin) is a drug known as a(n) _____.
12. This drug may produce a goiter when used over an extended length of time in children such as those with cystic fibrosis: _____.
13. _____ is a medicine that acts by dissolving mucus by disrupting the chemical bonds.
14. The side effects of sympathomimetic bronchodilator therapy, _____ and _____ _____, should be reported to the health care provider.

15. _____ (drug class) therapy requires a period of up to 4 weeks of therapy for maximum benefits on obstructive lung disease.
16. _____ agents must NOT be considered as the primary treatment for an acute episode of asthma.

END-OF-CHAPTER MATH REVIEW

1. Ordered: diphenhydramine (Benylin) 25 mg, q 4 h
   On hand: diphenhydramine (Benylin) 13.3 mg/5 ml
   Give: _____ ml or _____ tsp.
2. Ordered: terbutaline (Brethine) 0.25 mg, SC
   On hand: terbutaline 1 mg/ml
   Give: _____ ml.
3. Ordered: theophylline elixir 9 mg/kg/24 hrs in 4 divided doses
   The patient weighs 86 lbs.
   Give: _____ mg per individual dose
4. On hand: theophylline elixir 50 mg/5 ml
   Give: _____ml per individual dose

CRITICAL THINKING QUESTIONS

1. Explain why the action of a beta-adrenergic blocking agent may interfere with the therapeutic effects of bronchodilating agents [e.g., albuterol (Proventil)].
2. Differentiate among the actions of acetylcysteine, guaifenesin, and potassium iodide on mucus in the respiratory tract.

Copyright © 2004 Mosby Inc. All rights reserved.

Student Name_____

REVIEW QUESTIONS

_____ 1. The action of antileukotriene agents (e.g., zileuton [Zyflo], zafirlukast [Accolate]) is to:
   a. dilate the bronchi.
   b. inhibit release of histamine.
   c. reduce release of leukotrienes.
   d. dissolve chemical bonds of mucus.

_____ 2. Prior to the administration of xanthine-derivative bronchodilators (e.g., aminophylline and theophylline) the nurse should assess for:
   a. concurrent use of antihistamines or nasal decongestants.
   b. prior history of angina pectoris, peptic ulcer, glaucoma, or diabetes mellitus.
   c. liver function test results.
   d. history of angle-closure glaucoma.

_____ 3. An antitussive agent acts to:
   a. dissolve mucus.
   b. suppress cough reflex response in the brain.
   c. stimulate increased bronchial gland secretions.
   d. reduce the release of leukotrienes.

_____ 4. Guaifenesin (Robitussin) is classified as a(n):
   a. antitussive.
   b. expectorant.
   c. mucolytic.
   d. beta-adrenergic bronchodilator.

_____ 5. Whenever administering a beta-adrenergic bronchodilator, preassessment data should include checking for:
   a. liver function tests.
   b. history of glaucoma, diabetes mellitus, or peptic ulcer disease.
   c. palpitations, arrhythmias, and baseline mental status data.
   d. history of concurrent use of antihistamines or nasal decongestants.

Copyright © 2004 Mosby Inc. All rights reserved.

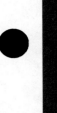

Drugs Used to Treat Oral Disorders

Syllabus

CHAPTER CONTENT

Mouth Disorders (p. 452)
Drug Therapy of Mouth Disorders (p. 453)
    Drug Class: Dentifrices (p. 456)
    Drug Class: Mouthwashes (p. 456)

CHAPTER OBJECTIVES

1. Cite the treatment alternatives and associated nursing assessments to monitor response to drug therapy for common mouth disorders.
2. Identify baseline data the nurse should collect on a continuous basis for comparison and evaluation of drug effectiveness.
3. Identify important nursing assessments and interventions associated with the drug therapy and treatment of diseases of the mouth.

KEY TERMS

xerostomia	dental caries
cold sores	tartar
fever blisters	gingivitis
canker sores	halitosis
candidiasis	dentifrice
stomatitis	mouthwashes
plaque	

ASSIGNMENTS

Read textbook, pp. 452-457.
Study Key Terms associated with chapter content.
Study Review Sheet for Chapter 31.
Complete Chapter 31 Practice Quiz.
Complete End-of-Chapter Critical Thinking Question.
Complete Chapter 31 Exam.

WEB RESEARCH ACTIVITY

Access: www.ada.org
Select: Gum Disease—Preventing Periodontal Disease
    What are the warning signs of periodontal disease and how can periodontal disease be prevented?

Copyright © 2004 Mosby Inc. All rights reserved.

Drugs Used to Treat Oral Disorders

Review Sheet

The QUESTION column and the ANSWER column have been offset so that you can cover the answers while reading the questions, allowing you to assess your knowledge.

Question	Answer

Question

1. Cite the major goals of treatment and drug therapy used for cold sores, canker sores, stomatitis, plaque, halitosis, and xerostomia.

2. Explain how to perform an assessment of the oral cavity.

3. Cite basic nursing interventions used for cold sores, canker sores, stomatitis, plaque, halitosis, xerostomia, and denture wearers.

4. What is the only FDA-approved over-the-counter medicine for the enhancement of healing of cold sores?

5. What types of mouthwashes should be recommended for use to:
   a. reduce plaque accumulation and gingivitis?
   b. treat oral stomatitis?
   c. decrease bleeding or irritation?

6. When lidocaine, a local anesthetic, is used as an oral spray or as a viscous solution, what precautions should be taught to the patient?

7. Describe the stomatitis scale.

Answer

1. See textbook, pp. 453-454.

2. See textbook, pp. 454-455.

3. See textbook, pp. 455-456.

4. Docosanol (Abreva)

5. a. Medicinal mouthwashes (e.g., Listerine)
   b. Chlorhexidine (Peridex)
   c. Mouthwashes containing zinc chloride

6. Do not smoke, eat, or drink for at least 30 minutes after use. Test ability to swallow before taking oral foods or drink. These products decrease normal sensations in the mouth, test temperature of foods or drinks before ingesting to prevent accidental burning of the oral mucosa.

7. See textbook, Box 31-1, p. 453.

Copyright © 2004 Mosby Inc. All rights reserved.

Drugs Used to Treat Oral Disorders

Practice Quiz

DEFINITIONS

Define the following terms.

1. Fever blisters:

2. Candidiasis:

3. Halitosis:

4. Xerostomia:

List five medicines that may be used to treat stomatitis.

5.

6.

7.

8.

9.

CRITICAL THINKING QUESTION

Compare oral hygiene measures appropriate in a person with a healthy mouth versus those measures needed in a person with a moderate to severe mouth disorder.

REVIEW QUESTIONS

_____ 1. When painful oral lesions are present, the best approach to oral hygiene is to:
   a. wait until the lesions are healed.
   b. use commercial mouthwashes for rinsing after meals and at bedtime.
   c. use normal saline, baking soda, or half-strength hydrogen peroxide rinses.
   d. give prescribed oral analgesic medications.

_____ 2. Mouthwashes given for the purpose of debriding and cleansing minor oral lesions will contain:
   a. lidocaine.
   b. chlorhexidine (Peridex).
   c. hydrogen peroxide.
   d. lidocaine (Xylocaine).

Copyright © 2004 Mosby Inc. All rights reserved.

Drugs Used to Treat Gastroesophagel Reflux and Peptic Ulcer Disease

Syllabus

CHAPTER CONTENT

Physiology of the Stomach (p. 458)
    Common Stomach Disorders (p. 458)
        Treatment of Gastroesophageal Reflux and
            Peptic Ulcer Disease (p. 459)
        Drug Therapy for Gastroesophageal Reflux
            and Peptic Ulcer Disease (p. 459)
        Drug Class: Antacids (p. 461)
        Drug Class: Histamine (H_2)-Receptor
            Antagonists (p. 463)
        Drug Class: Gastrointestinal
            Prostaglandin (p. 465)
        Drug Class: Gastric Acid Pump
            Inhibitors (p. 466)
        Drug Class: Coating Agent (p. 467)
        Drug Class: Prokinetic Agents (p. 467)
        Drug Class: Antispasmodic Agents
            (p. 469)

CHAPTER OBJECTIVES

1. Cite common stomach disorders that require drug therapy.
2. Identify factors that prevent breakdown of the body's normal defense barriers resulting in ulcer formation.
3. State the drug classifications and actions used to treat stomach disorders.
4. Develop health teaching for an individual with stomach disorders that incorporates pharmacologic and nonpharmacologic treatment modalities.

KEY TERMS

parietal cells
hydrochloric acid
gastroesophageal reflux
   disease (GERD)
heartburn
peptic ulcer disease
   (PUD)
Helicobacter pylori

ASSIGNMENTS

Read textbook, pp. 458-471.
Study Key Terms associated with chapter content.
Complete Collaborative Activities as assigned.
Study Review Sheet for Chapter 32.
Complete Chapter 32 Practice Quiz.
Complete End-of-Chapter Math Review and Critical
   Thinking Questions.
Complete Chapter 32 Exam.

WEB RESEARCH ACTIVITIES

Access: http://gerdonline.itgo.com
Research the Bard EndoCinch procedure and the Stretta procedure used for treatment of GERD.
1. How are each of these procedures performed?
2. What are the advantages of each procedure?
3. How long after the Stretta procedure are dietary restrictions required and GERD medications continued?

Copyright © 2004 Mosby Inc. All rights reserved.

COLLABORATIVE ACTIVITIES

Complete the following as preparation for in-class discussion and group work that may be assigned by the instructor.

A patient develops diarrhea after taking a prescribed antacid for 5 days.

1. What type of antacids may initiate diarrhea?
2. What nursing diagnosis should be initiated on the patient's care plan?

3. The patient is also taking digoxin 0.25 mg daily and levodopa 1 gm qid. Using the MAR record that follows or one distributed by the instructor, develop a time schedule for the administration of the drugs ordered.
4. When levodopa, digoxin, and an antacid are prescribed together, what nursing assessments should be performed?

MEDICATION ADMINISTRATION RECORD

NAME: RM-BD: Init   Signature   Title
  ID NO.:   AGE:
  DIAGNOSIS: SEX:

PHYSICIAN: Ht: Wt:

SCHEDULED MEDICATIONS

DATE	MEDICATION-STRENGTH-FORM-ROUTE	0030-0729	0730-1529	1530-0029

** PRN MEDICATIONS**

Copyright © 2004 Mosby Inc. All rights reserved.

Drugs Used to Treat Gastroesophagel Reflux and Peptic Ulcer Disease

Review Sheet

The QUESTION column and the ANSWER column have been offset so that you can cover the answers while reading the questions, allowing you to assess your knowledge.

Question	Answer
1. What types of conditions are treated with antacids?	
2. What is the difference between GERD and PUD?	1. Antacids decrease hyperacidity associated with PUD, GERD, gastritis, and hiatal hernia.
3. What are the major treatment goals for GERD and PUD?	2. See textbook, pp. 458-459.
4. What premedication assessments should be made prior to beginning antacid therapy?	3. See textbook, p. 459.
5. What effect does the administration of an antacid have on the pH of the gastric secretions?	4. Prior to antacid therapy, check for any abnormal renal function. If present, avoid magnesium-containing products. Check bowel pattern for diarrhea or constipation. Record any gastric pain or symptoms present. If patient is pregnant or has edema, heart failure, hypertension, or salt restrictions, ensure that a low-sodium antacid is prescribed. Check scheduling of antacids in relation to other prescribed medications to avoid interactions.
6. Are antacids alkaline or acidic?	5. Antacids buffer the hydrogen ion concentration, reducing the acidity of the gastric secretions and raising the pH of the gastric contents to neutralize gastric secretions.
7. Describe effect(s) of the following active ingredients of antacids: simethicone aluminum hydroxide magnesium oxide or hydroxide magnesium trisilicate calcium carbonate	6. Mildly alkaline
8. What ingredients in an antacid may produce constipation?	7. Simethicone is an antiflatulent. Aluminum hydroxide, magnesium oxide and hydroxide, magnesium trisilicate, and calcium carbonate all buffer gastric acidity.

Copyright © 2004 Mosby Inc. All rights reserved.

9. What ingredients in antacids may cause diarrhea?
10. What ingredient(s) in antacids should not be administered to patients with renal disease?
11. Define *acid rebound*.

12. Should antacids be given on an empty stomach or with food in the stomach?

13. What types of products can produce a systemic alkaline effect?

14. Patients with chronic renal failure who have hyperphosphatemia can benefit from taking which type of antacid and why?
15. What class of antibiotics, when given with antacids (Mg, Ca, or Al types), interact to result in a decrease in the absorption of the antibiotic?
16. Because antacids alter the absorption rate of digoxin and iron compounds, what dosing schedule should be used to administer antacids when these medicines are also ordered?
17. In order to obtain the most rapid onset of action, should an antacid be administered in a liquid or a tablet form?
18. Are antacid tablets recommended for the treatment of PUD?
19. Compare the actions of antihistamines and H_2 antagonists.
20. What premedication assessments should be performed for H_2 antagonists?

21. When should the H_2 antagonist agents cimetidine (Tagamet), famotidine (Pepcid), nizatidine (Axid), or ranitidine (Zantac) be administered in relation to food intake?

8. Calcium and aluminum products may cause constipation.
9. Magnesium

10. Magnesium should not be administered to patients with renal failure because they are unable to excrete it.
11. Acid rebound is found with calcium compounds and sodium bicarbonate; acid is neutralized followed by hypersecretion of gastric acid.
12. Given on an empty stomach, the neutralizing effects of antacids last only approximately 30 minutes. With food in the stomach, the neutralizing action is extended to 2–4 hours.
13. Sodium bicarbonate (baking soda)

14. Aluminum hydroxide and aluminum carbonate gel, because the aluminum ion binds the phosphate in the gastrointestinal tract
15. Tetracyclines

16. Administer 1 hour before or 2 hours after the antacid.

17. Liquid form

18. Tablets do not contain enough antacid to be effective for treatment of peptic ulcers.
19. Antihistamines block the receptor sites on target cells (e.g., arterioles, capillaries, glands) so that the histamine cannot attach there. This prevents the symptoms of an allergic reaction such as rhinorrhea and lacrimation. To be effective, antihistamines need to be taken 30–40 minutes before exposure to allergens such as pollen or as soon as symptoms first appear. Antihistamines do not have a direct effect on gastric acid secretion. H_2 antagonists (e.g., cimetidine, famotidine, nizatidine, ranitidine) block the action of histamine on the gastric acid-secreting cells (parietal cells) in the stomach.
20. See textbook, p. 464. Assess patient's mental status to detect CNS alterations, particularly with cimetidine therapy.

Copyright © 2004 Mosby Inc. All rights reserved.

22. Compare the dosage and scheduling of the H_2 antagonists.

23. If antacid therapy is continued concurrently with the use of cimetidine (Tagamet), what scheduling for the antacid should be used?

24. What advantages does famotidine (Pepcid) have when compared to cimetidine (Tagamet)?

25. How does the coating agent sucralfate (Carafate) differ from histamine H_2 antagonists?

26. List the actions of gastrointestinal prostaglandins.

27. What premedication assessments should be performed before misoprostol therapy?

28. Cite the most common side effect of misoprostol therapy.

29. How can diarrhea associated with misoprostol therapy be minimized?

30. Should misoprostol be taken during pregnancy?

31. What drugs can have altered absorption as a result of a reduction in gastric acid secretions?

32. What is the more common name for the substituted benzimidazoles?

33. What is the action of the gastric acid pump inhibitors?

34. What are gastric acid pump inhibitors used to treat?

35. What is the ending on the generic name of all gastric acid pump inhibitors?

21. Cimetidine, famotidine, and ranitidine are administered with food. Nizatidine may be administered with or without food.

22. Cimetidine (Tagamet) 300 mg, 4 times per day with meals and at bedtime; famotidine (Pepcid) 40 mg once daily at bedtime or 20 mg twice daily; ranitidine (Zantac) 150 mg, twice daily or 300 mg at bedtime. Nizatidine (Axid) 300 mg, PO, once daily at bedtime or 150 mg two times daily.

23. Antacids should be administered 1 hour before or 2 hours after the H_2 antagonist.

24. Famotidine is taken once daily, does not produce gynecomastia, and has fewer significant drug interactions reported with its use.

25. Coating agents do not affect the amount of hydrochloric acid secreted; they adhere to the crater of the ulcer.

26. Gastrointestinal prostaglandins stimulate GI motility, gastric acid and pepsin secretion, and protect the stomach and duodenal lining against ulceration.

27. Determine if the patient is pregnant. This drug is a uterine stimulant and may induce a miscarriage. Check pattern of bowel elimination. Misoprostol may induce diarrhea.

28. Diarrhea

29. Take misoprostol with meals and at bedtime; avoid antacids containing magnesium (e.g., Maalox, Mylanta).

30. Discontinue if that patient is pregnant.

31. Digoxin, ketoconazole, ampicillin, and iron

32. Substituted benzimidazoles are more commonly known as *gastric acid pump inhibitors*.

33. Gastric acid pump inhibitors inhibit gastric acid secretion.

34. Gastric acid pump inhibitors are used to treat severe esophagitis, GERD, gastric and duodenal ulcers, and hypersecretory disorders, such as Zollinger-Ellison syndrome. They may also be used in combination with antibiotics (e.g., ampicillin, amoxicillin, clarithromycin) to eradicate *Helicobacter pylori*, a common cause of PUD.

Copyright © 2004 Mosby Inc. All rights reserved.

36. What is the action of metoclopramide (Reglan)?

35. All generic names of gastric acid pump inhibitors end in "-prazole."

36. Metoclopramide is a gastric stimulant thought to block dopamine in the chemoreceptor trigger zone. It increases stomach contractions, relaxes the pyloric valve, and increases peristalsis in GI tract resulting in increased rate of gastric emptying and intestinal transit.

Copyright © 2004 Mosby Inc. All rights reserved.

Drugs Used to Treat Gastroesophagel Reflux and Peptic Ulcer Disease

Practice Quiz

TRUE OR FALSE

Mark each statement "T" for true and "F" for false. <u>*Correct all false statements.*</u>

_____ 1. Antacid tablets are effective in treating PUD.

_____ 2. Patients with renal failure may develop hypermagnesemia if magnesium-containing antacids are taken.

_____ 3. The pH of the stomach decreases when the hydrochloric acid content is reduced.

_____ 4. Smoking causes an increase in hydrochloric acid secretion.

_____ 5. Premedication assessments needed with misoprostol (Cytotec) include checking to see if the individual is pregnant and checking the normal pattern of bowel elimination.

_____ 6. The desired therapeutic outcome with omeprazole (Prilosec) is a reduction in heartburn and discomfort and healing of irritated gastrointestinal mucosa.

_____ 7. Sucralfate (Carafate) decreases gastric secretions.

_____ 8. Metoclopramide (Reglan) should be prescribed for nausea and vomiting associated with chemotherapy because it decreases peristalsis.

_____ 9. Antacids containing magnesium may be dangerous to patients with renal disease.

COMPLETION

Complete the following statements.

10. _____ coats the ulcer crater to protect it from gastric acid secretions.

11. Patients with renal failure should not take antacids containing _____.

12. The action of antacids is longest when given _____ food in the stomach.

13. Cimetidine (Tagamet) and famotidine (Pepcid) are examples of drugs that belong to which class of drugs? _____

14. Hypersecretion of gastric acid after taking calcium compounds and sodium bicarbonate is called _____.

ESSAY

15. Name two antispasmodic agents.

16. Compare the daily dosages and side effects of cimetidine, ranitidine, and famotidine.

CALCULATIONS

17. Ordered: famotidine (Pepcid) 20 mg, PO, bid
On hand: famotidine (Pepcid) suspension 40 mg/5 ml
Give: _____ ml.

18. Ordered: propantheline (Pro-Banthine) 15 mg, ac and 30 mg at hs
On hand: propantheline (Pro-Banthine) 15 mg tablets
The ac dose will require _____ tablets and the hs dose will require _____ tablets.

Copyright © 2004 Mosby Inc. All rights reserved.

END-OF-CHAPTER MATH REVIEW

1. Ordered: ranitidine (Zantac) 50 mg in 100 ml D_5W IV over 20 minutes.
   Using an infusion pump, calibrated in ml/hr, at what rate would the infusion pump be set?
   _____ ml/hr

2. Ordered: Pepcid 35 mg, PO, stat
   On hand: Pepcid 40 mg/ml oral suspension.
   Give _____ ml

CRITICAL THINKING QUESTIONS

1. A 45-year-old patient has PUD and seems unaware that lifestyle changes are needed to treat the disorder. The patient has an H_2 antagonist ordered. What teaching approaches would be appropriate for her?

2. A patient is complaining of intermittent diarrhea. No physical basis for the diarrhea has been identified. She also complains of heartburn. Explore self-treatments available with over-the-counter medicines that could cause the diarrhea.

REVIEW QUESTIONS

_____ 1. Antacid therapy requires a premedication assessment of:
   a. renal function studies and/or renal disease present.
   b. mental status data.
   c. serum electrolyte studies.
   d. closed-angle glaucoma.

_____ 2. Metoclopramide therapy has possible major reportable side effects of:
   a. irregular heartbeat.
   b. persistent vesicular rash.
   c. extrapyramidal symptoms.
   d. hepatotoxicity.

_____ 3. Drugs whose generic names all end in "-dine" belong to a class of drugs known as:
   a. prokinetic agents.
   b. coating agents.
   c. gastric acid pump inhibitors.
   d. histamine (H_2)-receptor antagonists.

_____ 4. Which classification of drugs has the side effects of blurred vision; constipation; urinary retention; and dryness of mucosa of the mouth, nose, and throat?
   a. anticholinergics
   b. gastric acid pump inhibitors
   c. histamine (H_2)-receptor antagonists
   d. prokinetic agents

Copyright © 2004 Mosby Inc. All rights reserved.

Drugs Used to Treat Nausea and Vomiting

Syllabus

CHAPTER CONTENT

Nausea and Vomiting (p. 472)
Common Causes of Nausea and Vomiting (p. 472)
Drug Therapy for Selected Causes of Nausea and
   Vomiting (p. 474)
   Drug Class: Dopamine Antagonists (p. 476)
   Drug Class: Serotonin Antagonists (p. 477)
   Drug Class: Anticholinergic Agents (p. 477)
   Drug Class: Corticosteroids (p. 482)
   Drug Class: Benzodiazepines (p. 483)
   Drug Class: Cannabinoids (p. 483)

CHAPTER OBJECTIVES

1. Compare the purposes of using antiemetic
   products.
2. State the therapeutic classes of antiemetics.
3. Discuss scheduling of antiemetics for maximum
   benefit.

KEY TERMS

nausea
vomiting
emesis
retching
postoperative nausea
   and vomiting
   (PONV)
hyperemesis
   gravidarum

psychogenic vomiting
chemotherapy-induced
   emesis (CIE)
anticipatory nausea
   and vomiting
delayed emesis

ASSIGNMENTS

Read textbook, pp. 472-484.
Study Key Terms associated with chapter content.
Complete Collaborative Activities as assigned.
Study Review Sheet for Chapter 33.
Complete Chapter 33 Practice Quiz.
Complete End-of-Chapter Math Review and Critical
   Thinking Questions.
Complete Chapter 33 Exam.

WEB RESEARCH ACTIVITY

Access: www.umm.edu/ency/article/003117.htm
Research treatment of nausea and vomiting.
Describe the home care of nausea and vomiting and
cite instances when a health care provider should be
contacted for further treatment options.

COLLABORATIVE ACTIVITIES

*Complete the following as preparation for in-class
discussion and group work that may be assigned by the
instructor.*
1. What is the usual dosage scheduling of serotonin antagonists in relation to a prescribed
   dose of chemotherapy?
2. What premedication assessments should be
   completed and recorded prior to administering
   a serotonin antagonist?

Copyright © 2004 Mosby Inc. All rights reserved.

CHAPTER 33

Drugs Used to Treat Nausea and Vomiting

Review Sheet

The QUESTION column and the ANSWER column have been offset so that you can cover the answers while reading the questions, allowing you to assess your knowledge.

Question	Answer
1. What is an antiemetic?	
2. What six classes of drugs are used to treat nausea and vomiting?	1. A medication used to prevent nausea and vomiting.
3. What is the mechanism of action for the six drug classes used to treat nausea and vomiting?	2. Dopamine antagonists, serotonin antagonists, anticholinergic agents, corticosteroids, benzodiazepines, and cannabinoids
	3. See sections labeled "Action" for each drug class.
4. Name the most widely used antiemetic in the phenothiazine class used to treat nausea and vomiting associated with surgery, radiation, and cancer chemotherapy.	
5. What is the action of metoclopramide (Reglan) on the gastrointestinal tract that makes it useful as an antiemetic?	4. Prochlorperazine (Compazine)
6. When is ondansetron (Zofran) administered in relation to chemotherapy?	5. Metoclopramide is thought to work as an antiemetic by blocking dopamine in the chemoreceptor trigger zone. It has also been suggested that it inhibits serotonin when administered in higher doses.
	6. Ondansetron (Zofran) is administered 30 minutes before chemotherapy and at 4-hour intervals after chemotherapy for 2 doses.
7. What drugs are recommended for nausea and vomiting associated with pregnancy?	7. Administration of meclizine, cyclizine, or dimenhydrinate is recommended first for nausea and vomiting associated with pregnancy.
8. What herbal medicine is used by some cultures to treat pregnancy-induced nausea and vomiting?	8. Ginger
9. What are the usual nursing implementations used for an adult and for an infant experiencing nausea and vomiting?	
10. What are the usual premedication assessments performed for any antiemetic?	9. See textbook, pp. 475-476.
11. Define *hyperemesis gravidarum, psychogenic vomiting, anticipatory vomiting*, and *chemotherapy-induced vomiting*.	10. See textbook, p. 477.
	11. See textbook, pp. 472-474.

Copyright © 2004 Mosby Inc. All rights reserved.

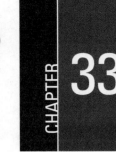

CHAPTER 33

Drugs Used to Treat Nausea and Vomiting

Practice Quiz

DEFINITIONS

Define the following terms.

1. Hyperemesis gravidarum:

2. Psychogenic vomiting:

COMPLETION

Complete the following statements.

3. CIE is an abbreviation for _____.

Antiemetics act by:

4.

5.

6. Dopamine antagonists act by:

7. Ondansetron (Zofran) or granisetron (Kytril) are generally prescribed for _____ and _____-type vomiting.

8. Anticholinergic agents such as Dramamine are generally prescribed for _____-type vomiting.

ESSAY

9. When should an antiemetic be administered to a patient having postoperative nausea?

10. What is the cause of motion sickness?

11. How long after administration of chemotherapy can it take for delayed emesis to occur?

12. What six classes of drugs are used to treat nausea and vomiting?

13. What information should be included in a nursing assessment performed on a patient having nausea and vomiting?

14. Compare the premedication assessments listed for each of the six drug classes used in the treatment of nausea and vomiting.

END-OF-CHAPTER MATH REVIEW

1. Ordered: ondansetron (Zofran) 0.15 mg/kg, IV in 50 ml D_5W over 20 minutes before chemotherapy. The client's weight today is 135 lbs.
   Weight is: _____ kg
   The total amount of ondansetron to administer is _____.
   When administering this order using an infusion pump calibrated in ml/hr, set the pump at _____ml/hr.

2. Ordered: dexamethasone 6 mg by IM injection stat.
   On hand: dexamethasone 4 mg/ml.
   Give: _____ ml

CRITICAL THINKING QUESTIONS

1. A 65-year-old patient has been vomiting intermittently for 3 days with the "flu." He is a resident on your unit in the nursing home. What data should be collected and reported to the physician for further evaluation and action?

2. A patient has been vomiting repeatedly following administration of chemotherapy and received metoclopramide an hour ago. What is the action of this drug and what further actions by the nurse are appropriate?

Copyright © 2004 Mosby Inc. All rights reserved.

REVIEW QUESTIONS

_____ 1. A patient scheduled to receive ondansetron (Zofran) as a prechemotherapy medication has a weight loss recorded of 4 pounds since yesterday when the orders were written. The nurse should:
   a. recheck the accuracy of the weight.
   b. give the prescribed dosage of medication.
   c. notify the health care provider of the weight.
   d. recheck weight and notify the health care provider if appropriate.

_____ 2. A neighbor is going on a deep-sea fishing trip and tells you she plans on using transdermal patches of scopolamine. How far in advance should the patches be applied?
   a. 30 minutes
   b. 60 minutes
   c. 2 hours
   d. 4 hours

_____ 3. You are told that two children, ages 6 and 8, will accompany your neighbor on the deep-sea fishing trip. You should:
   a. ask what specific medication she plans to give the children, if any.
   b. encourage her not to premedicate the children.
   c. have her consult the family health care provider for specific orders.
   d. tell her to wait and see if the children develop seasickness before medicating them.

_____ 4. People using dronabinol (THC) (Marinol) for nausea and vomiting should be taught to report:
   a. headache, diarrhea, constipation, and sedation.
   b. sedative effects.
   c. depression, paranoia, or hallucinations.
   d. blurred vision, constipation, or urinary retention.

Copyright © 2004 Mosby Inc. All rights reserved.

34 Drugs Used to Treat Constipation and Diarrhea

Syllabus

CHAPTER CONTENT

Constipation (p. 485)
Diarrhea (p. 485)
    Drug Therapy for Constipation and Diarrhea
        (p. 486)
        Drug Class: Laxatives (p. 488)
        Drug Class: Antidiarrheal Agents (p. 489)

CHAPTER OBJECTIVES

1. State the underlying causes of constipation.
2. Explain the meaning of "normal" bowel habits.
3. Identify the indications for use, method of action, and onset of action for contact or stimulant laxatives, saline laxatives, lubricant or emollient laxatives, bulk-forming laxatives, and fecal softeners.
4. Describe medical conditions in which laxatives should not be used.
5. List nine causes of diarrhea.
6. State the differences between locally acting and systemically acting antidiarrheal agents.
7. Identify electrolytes that should be monitored whenever prolonged or severe diarrhea is present.
8. Describe nursing assessments needed to evaluate the state of hydration in patients suffering from either constipation or dehydration.
9. Cite conditions that generally respond favorably to antidiarrheal agents.
10. Prepare a list of medications that may cause diarrhea.

KEY TERMS

constipation
diarrhea
laxative

ASSIGNMENTS

Read textbook, pp. 485-492.
Study Key Terms associated with chapter content.
Complete Collaborative Activity as assigned.
Study Review Sheet for Chapter 34.
Complete Chapter 34 Practice Quiz.
Complete End-of-Chapter Critical Thinking
    Questions.
Complete Chapter 34 Exam.

WEB RESEARCH ACTIVITIES

Access: www.acg.gi.org
Select Patient Information
1. What medications can contribute to constipation in a patient?
2. What tips are given for constipation and fecal incontinence?

COLLABORATIVE ACTIVITY

Complete the following as preparation for in-class discussion and group work that may be assigned by the instructor.
Explain the health teaching needed for an elderly patient who consistently takes one or more laxatives daily.

Copyright © 2004 Mosby Inc. All rights reserved.

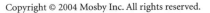

Drugs Used to Treat Constipation and Diarrhea

Review Sheet

The QUESTION column and the ANSWER column have been offset so that you can cover the answers while reading the questions, allowing you to assess your knowledge.

Question	Answer

Question

1. What is the mechanism of action of:
   a. contact or stimulant laxatives?
   b. saline laxatives?
   c. lubricant or emollient laxatives?
   d. bulk-forming laxatives?
   e. fecal softeners?
2. What is the onset of action for:
   a. contact or stimulant laxatives?
   b. saline laxatives?
   c. lubricant or emollient laxatives?
   d. bulk-forming laxatives?
   e. fecal softeners?

3. When administering fecal softeners, what factors must be considered to promote the action of these laxative agents?

4. Differentiate between the action of systemic and local antidiarrheal agents.
5. What premedication assessments should be performed before administration of an antidiarrheal agent?

6. Examine Table 34-1 to identify the names and types of laxatives commonly prescribed and Table 34-2 for antidiarrheals prescribed.

Answer

1. a. Promote peristalsis by irritation.
   b. Attract water into intestines from surrounding tissues, promote peristalsis.
   c. Lubricate intestinal wall and soften the stool; peristalsis does not appear to be increased.
   d. Cause water to be retained in stool, thus increasing bulk that stimulates peristalsis.
   e. Draw water into stool causing it to soften. No stimulation of peristalsis.
2. a. 6–10 hours orally; 60–90 minutes rectally
   b. 1–3 hours
   c. 6–8 hours
   d. 12–24 hours, up to 72 hours
   e. up to 72 hours
3. Adequate fluid intake is essential.

4. Systemic: Decrease peristalsis and GI mobility via the autonomic nervous system, allowing the mucosal lining to absorb nutrients, water, and electrolytes and leaving a formed stool from the residue remaining in the colon. Local: Adsorb excess water to cause a formed stool and to adsorb irritants or bacteria that cause diarrhea.
5. Take medication history and examine for drugs that may be contributing to the diarrhea; review for precipitating factors.
6. See textbook, pp. 489-490.

Copyright © 2004 Mosby Inc. All rights reserved.

Student Name_____

CHAPTER 34

Drugs Used to Treat Constipation and Diarrhea

Practice Quiz

COMPLETION

Complete the following statements.

1. Describe the mechanism of action of the following:

   a. Bulk-forming laxatives:

   b. Lubricant or emollient laxatives:

   c. Locally acting antidiarrheal agents:

   d. Systemically acting antidiarrheal agents:

2. What are the most common causes of intestinal infections?

3. What type of diet should be used to treat constipation?

4. What ingredient in antacid products is known to cause diarrhea?

5. What type of laxative is the drug of choice for treatment of persons requiring regular use of laxatives?

CRITICAL THINKING QUESTIONS

1. The physician asks a nurse to instruct the mother of a 6-month-old infant on the procedure to insert a glycerin suppository. What information would you give?

2. An 80-year-old resident asks for a laxative daily. What health teaching should be done? Would you give the prn laxative daily?

REVIEW QUESTIONS

_____ 1. All systemic antidiarrheal agents act by:
   a. softening the stool.
   b. inhibiting peristalsis.
   c. adsorbent action.
   d. increasing bulk.

_____ 2. Kaopectate, a common OTC medication for diarrhea, acts by:
   a. softening the stool.
   b. inhibiting peristalsis.
   c. adsorbent action.
   d. increasing bulk.

_____ 3. Stimulant laxatives increase peristalsis within _____ hour(s) when given orally.
   a. 0.5
   b. 1–3
   c. 6–8
   d. 12–24

_____ 4. Bulk-forming laxatives have an onset of action of _____ hour(s).
   a. 0.5
   b. 1–3
   c. 6–10
   d. 12–24

Copyright © 2004 Mosby Inc. All rights reserved.

Drugs Used to Treat Diabetes Mellitus

Syllabus

CHAPTER CONTENT

Diabetes Mellitus (p. 493)
Treatment of Diabetes Mellitus (p. 494)
Drug Therapy (p. 495)
Drug Therapy for Diabetes Mellitus (p. 503)
    Drug Class: Insulins (p. 503)
    Drug Class: Biguanide Oral Hypoglycemic
        Agents (p. 507)
    Drug Class: Sulfonylurea Oral Hypoglycemic
        Agents (p. 508)
    Drug Class: Meglitinide Oral Hypoglycemic
        Agent (p. 510)
    Drug Class: Thiazolidinedione Oral
        Hypoglycemic Agents (p. 511)
    Drug Class: Antihyperglycemic Agents (p. 512)
    Drug Class: Antihypoglycemic Agent (p. 514)

CHAPTER OBJECTIVES

1. State the current definition of diabetes mellitus.
2. Identify the incidence of the disease in the United States.
3. Describe the current classification system for diabetes mellitus.
4. Differentiate between the symptoms of type 1 (formerly IDDM) and type 2 (formerly NIDDM) diabetes mellitus.
5. Identify the objectives of dietary control of diabetes mellitus.
6. Discuss the action and use of insulin as opposed to oral hypoglycemic and antihyperglycemic agents to control diabetes mellitus.
7. Identify the major nursing considerations associated with the management of diabetes (such as nutritional evaluation, dietary prescription, activity and exercise, and psychologic considerations).

8. Differentiate between the signs, symptoms, and management of hypoglycemia and hyperglycemia.
9. Discuss the contributing factors of, nursing assessments for, and nursing interventions for patients exhibiting complications associated with diabetes mellitus.
10. Develop a health teaching plan for persons taking any type of insulin or oral hypoglycemic agent.

KEY TERMS

diabetes mellitus
type 1 diabetes mellitus
type 2 diabetes mellitus
neuropathies
paresthesia
gestational diabetes
   mellitus

impaired glucose
   tolerance (IGT)
impaired fasting
   glucose (IFG)
hypoglycemia
hyperglycemia

ASSIGNMENTS

Read textbook, pp. 493-515.
Study Key Terms associated with chapter content.
Complete Collaborative Activities as assigned.
Study Review Sheet for Chapter 35.
Complete Chapter 35 Practice Quiz.
Complete End-of-Chapter Math Review and Critical
   Thinking Questions.
Complete Chapter 35 Exam.

WEB RESEARCH ACTIVITIES

Access: http://www.joslin.org
Research High Protein Diets and Diabetes.
1. What are the benefits of the Adkins diet?
2. How do you increase whole grains in the diet?

Copyright © 2004 Mosby Inc. All rights reserved.

COLLABORATIVE ACTIVITIES

Complete the following as preparation for in-class discussion and group work that may be assigned by the instructor.

1. Practice mixing short- and intermediate-acting insulin in the same syringe using the technique taught in your educational setting.
2. Explain the treatment(s) of hypoglycemia in response to excessive insulin intake.

Copyright © 2004 Mosby Inc. All rights reserved.

Drugs Used to Treat Diabetes Mellitus

Review Sheet

The QUESTION column and the ANSWER column have been offset so that you can cover the answers while reading the questions, allowing you to assess your knowledge.

Question	**Answer**
1. Diabetes mellitus is a disease that causes abnormal metabolism of _____.	
2. "Insulin-dependent diabetes" (formerly IDDM) is now known as _____.	1. Fats, proteins, and carbohydrates
3. "Type 2 diabetes" was formerly known as _____.	2. Type 1 diabetes mellitus
4. "Gestational diabetes" (GDM) is _____.	3. Noninsulin-dependent diabetes mellitus (NIDDM)
5. "Hypoglycemia" is _____.	4. The development of an abnormal glucose tolerance in pregnant women
6. "Hyperglycemia" is _____.	5. Low blood sugar
7. "Polydipsia" is _____.	6. High blood sugar
8. "Polyuria" is _____.	7. Increased thirst
9. What are the symptoms of neuropathies?	8. Increased frequency of urination
10. What is the immediate goal for treatment of diabetes mellitus?	9. Numbness and tingling of extremities (paresthesia), loss of sensations, postural hypotension, impotence, and difficulty controlling urination.
11. What does the treatment of type 2 diabetes mellitus require?	10. Prevent ketoacidosis and symptoms resulting from hyperglycemia.
12. What does the treatment of type 1 diabetes mellitus require?	11. Adequate weight reduction, dietary control, and possibly the use of oral hypoglycemic or antihyperglycemic agents.
13. What laboratory values of the fasting plasma glucose (FPG) are considered normal, impaired, or result in a provisional diagnosis of diabetes mellitus?	12. Adequate weight reduction, dietary control, and use of exogenous insulin.
14. What are the recommended guidelines for glucose levels while exercising?	13. FPG less than 110 mg/dl = normal fasting glucose FPG at 110 mg/dl or greater but less than 126 mg/dl = impaired fasting glucose (IFG) FPG at 126 mg/dl or greater = provisional diagnosis of diabetes mellitus
15. What are the usual causes of hypoglycemia?	14. Individuals should not exercise with glucose level above 250 mg/dl or less than 100 mg/dl.

Copyright © 2004 Mosby Inc. All rights reserved.

16. When should ketone testing of the urine be performed?

17. What is the difference between the glycosylated hemoglobin and fructosamine tests to measure glucose?

18. What signs and symptoms result from peripheral vascular disease?

19. What types of visual complications are persons with diabetes mellitus more susceptible to?

20. How often should persons with diabetes mellitus have an eye exam?

21. How can complications of diabetes affecting the kidneys be identified?

22. What is the source of endogenous insulin? What are the primary animal sources of exogenous insulins?

23. What methods are used to produce human exogenous insulin?

24. Is insulin required for glucose transport into the brain or liver tissue?

25. Why can't insulin be administered orally?

26. Differentiate among *onset, peak,* and *duration* in relation to insulin therapy.

27. What are the most rapid-acting forms of insulin manufactured today?

15. Too much insulin, insufficient food intake to cover insulin taken, imbalances from diarrhea and vomiting, or excessive exercise without additional carbohydrate intake are common causes of hypoglycemia.

16. When serum glucose is 240 mg/dl or above, test for the presence of ketones.

17. The glycosylated hemoglobin measures glucose control over the previous 8–10 weeks, while the fructosamine test measures the amount of glucose bonded to the protein fructosamine over the previous 1–3 weeks. Each has a benefit in measuring glucose control.

18. Cyanosis or reddish-blue discoloration in the hands, feet, and legs. Pallor and coolness in the feet and legs. Ulcerations may develop. When any circulatory impairment is found, pedal and radial pulses should be checked at least every 4 hours.

19. Blurred vision may occur with hyperglycemia. With advanced diabetes mellitus, there are changes in small blood vessels in the eyes (microangiopathies). Retinal hemorrhages, degeneration of retinal vascular tissue, cataracts, and blindness may also occur.

20. Regular eye exams to detect changes in the eye should be performed at least annually and more often as deemed appropriate by the HCP.

21. Presence of proteinuria, elevated serum creatinine, and blood urea nitrogen. Persons with diabetes mellitus are more likely to have urinary tract infections.

22. Endogenous insulin is produced by the beta cells of the pancreas. Synthetic insulin is the primary source of insulin for recently diagnosed diabetics. Beef and pork pancreases are the primary animal sources of exogenous insulin, but fish and sheep pancreases have been used as well.

23. Most common source of human insulin production is with recombinant DNA.

24. No

25. Insulin is destroyed by the proteolytic enzymes in the gastrointestinal tract.

26. Onset is the time required for the initial effect of insulin to occur. Peak is the time of the maximum effect of insulin. Duration is the length of time insulin remains active.

Copyright © 2004 Mosby Inc. All rights reserved.

28. Do short-acting, intermediate-acting, and long-acting insulins differ in terms of onset, peak, and duration of action?

29. How far in advance of a meal should a rapid-acting insulin be administered?

30. How far in advance of a meal should a short-acting insulin be administered?

31. Examine Table 35-3, textbook p. 506, and identify compatibility of insulin combinations.

32. What is the major advantage of the new glargine, biosynthetic long-acting insulin?

33. Why should insulin stored at room temperature be discarded after 1 month of use?

34. What does "U-100" mean?

35. What kind of syringe is used to measure U-100 insulin?

36. What is the only type of insulin used intravenously?

37. Why is it important to teach the patient to rotate insulin sites within one area before proceeding to the next area on a rotation schedule?

38. What effect does the long-term use of one injection site have on insulin absorption?

39. With increased activity and exercise, what adjustment may be required in the insulin dose?

40. When are patients who are receiving rapid-acting, short-acting, intermediate-acting, or long-acting insulin most likely to develop hypoglycemia if the dose is excessive or meals are not taken as planned?

27. Insulin analog injection lispro (Humalog) onset: 0.2–0.33 hr; peak: 0.1–2 hrs; duration: 3–5 hrs. Insulin analog injection aspart (Novolog) onset: 0.2–0.33 hr; peak: 0.1–2 hr.; duration: 3–5 hrs.

28. Yes. See Table 35-2, p. 505.

29. Rapid-acting (aspart and lispro) are given 10–15 minutes before a meal.

30. Short-acting (Humulin R, Novolin R, Regular Iletin I, Regular Iletin II, and Velosulin BR) are given 30 minutes before a meal.

31. See Table 35-3, textbook p. 506.

32. Glargine insulin is absorbed more uniformly, thereby reducing the possibility of hypoglycemic reactions.

33. After 1 month at room temperature insulin starts loosing potency.

34. U-100 means 100 units of insulin are contained in 1 ml of solution.

35. An insulin syringe calibrated in 100 units has been available for years; however, because U-100 = 100 units in 1 ml, a tuberculin syringe could also be used to accurately measure the dosage.

36. Regular insulin

37. To prevent hypertrophy or atrophy of subcutaneous tissue.

38. Absorption is prolonged and control of glucose may require an increase in the insulin dose. If switching from an injection site that has been used repeatedly to one used infrequently, the dose of insulin may need to be decreased to prevent hypoglycemia. Each patient is somewhat variable, but patients may become hypoglycemic. A snack may be required to cover the action of the insulin, or the insulin dose could be reduced if the increased activity can be anticipated.

39. Because of risk of hypoglycemia, the insulin dose could be reduced if increased activity can be anticipated.

Copyright © 2004 Mosby Inc. All rights reserved.

41. When are blood or urine tests for glucose performed in relation to meals and insulin administration?

42. Differentiate between the symptoms of hypoglycemia and hyperglycemia.

43. What are the treatments for hypoglycemia and hyperglycemia?

44. If uncertain whether a patient is hypoglycemic or hyperglycemic, what action should be taken?

45. Why do allergic reactions to insulins occur?
46. What complications are associated with diabetes mellitus?

47. Describe the procedure for mixing two insulins in the same syringe.

48. What effect does the administration of beta-adrenergic blocking agents concurrent with insulin have on symptoms of hypoglycemia?

40. If the patient injects insulin at 7 AM, rapid-acting insulin may induce hypoglycemia within 1–3 hrs; short-acting insulin: occurs before lunch; intermediate-acting insulin: between 3 PM and supper; and long-acting insulin: between 2 AM and breakfast.
41. 1/2 hour ac and hs

42. Hypoglycemia: rapid onset, nervousness, tremors, headache, apprehension, sweating, hunger, double or blurred vision, lack of coordination, unconsciousness
hyperglycemia: gradual onset, increased thirst, headache, nausea and vomiting, rapid pulse, shallow respirations, acetone odor on breath, unconsciousness
43. Hypoglycemia: If conscious and able to swallow: 2–4 oz fruit juice with 2 teaspoons sugar or honey added, or 1 cup skim milk, 4 oz nondiet soft drink, or piece of candy (not chocolate), or frosting added. If unable to swallow: 20–50 ml glucose 50% IV. Hyperglycemia: Hospitalize patient, identify the cause, hydrate the patient and give insulin IV; stabilize electrolytes, especially potassium.
    See also drug monograph for glucagon.

44. Treat for hypoglycemia.
45. Allergy may be caused by a protein from the animal source of insulin (e.g., pork, beef) or from the protein modifiers used to extend the duration of insulin (e.g., isophane). An acute reaction with a rash over the entire body is a rare, but possible, symptom of an anaphylactic reaction that must be treated with antihistamines, epinephrine, and steroids. Allergic reactions can be minimized by changing to an insulin without protein modifiers or to insulins derived from biosynthetic (nonanimal) sources; by using unscented alcohol swabs. Local irritation can be minimized by using disposable syringes and needles and by checking the patient's injection technique.
46. Peripheral vascular disease, renal vascular disease, increased frequency of infections, progressive blindness, neuropathies
47. When mixing rapid- or short-acting insulin with intermediate- or long-acting insulin, the clear rapid- or short-acting insulin should be drawn into the syringe first (ADA Guidelines 2003).
See Ch. 10, textbook, Fig. 10-26, p. 146.

Copyright © 2004 Mosby Inc. All rights reserved.

49. What drug class does the drug metformin (Glucophage) belong to and what is its mechanism of action compared to oral sulfonylureas?
50. How do oral hypoglycemic agents differ from insulin?

51. Which type of diabetes mellitus requires treatment with insulin and which type may be treated with oral hypoglycemic agents?

52. For what type of allergy should you check the chart and the patient before initiating therapy with an oral sulfonylurea hypoglycemic agent?

53. What is the effect of sulfonylurea hypoglycemic agents combined with ethanol on blood glucose levels?
54. When should a diabetic patient perform urine testing for ketones?

55. What are the therapeutic outcomes expected from a biguanide oral hypoglycemic agent, sulfonylurea oral hypoglycemic agents, meglitinide oral hypoglycemic agents, thiazolidinedione oral hypoglycemic agents, and antihyperglycemic agents?

48. Beta-adrenergic blocking agents mask the signs of hypoglycemia.

49. Biguanide oral hypoglycemic agents—mechanism of action unknown. It does not stimulate release of insulin from the pancreas like the sulfonylureas.

50. For sulfonylurea oral hypoglycemic agents (e.g., chlorpropamide [Diabinese], tolazamide [Tolinase], and others), and meglitinide oral hypoglycemic agents (repaglinide and nateglinide) to be effective, the diabetic patient must still have beta cells in the pancreas that are capable of producing insulin. These agents act by stimulating the release of insulin from the beta cells. Oral hypoglycemic agents are not an oral form of insulin. The biguanide oral hypoglycemic [e.g., metformin (Glucophage)], does not stimulate release of insulin from the pancreas; the mechanism of its action is unknown. For thiazolidinedione (TZDs) oral hypoglycemic agents, (pioglitazone [Actos] and rosiglitazone [Avandia]), the blood glucose is lowered by increasing the sensitivity of muscle and fat issue to insulin, allowing more glucose to enter the cells in the presence of insulin metabolism. The antihyperglycemic agents (acarbose [Precose] and miglitol [Glyset]) inhibit the pancreatic alpha-amylase and gastrointestinal alpha-glycoside hydrolase enzymes used in the digestion of sugars resulting in delayed glucose absorption and lowering of postprandial hyperglycemia.

51. Type 1 diabetes mellitus uses insulin; type 2 diabetes mellitus may be treated with diet and oral hypoglycemic agents. In certain cases, type 2 diabetes mellitus may also be treated with low doses of insulin.

52. Sulfonamides. The patient who is allergic to sulfonamides may also be allergic to sulfonylureas.

53. Hypoglycemia. Also may result in an Antabuse-like reaction manifested by facial flushing, pounding headache, breathlessness, and nausea.

54. Perform urine testing for ketones whenever the blood glucose is 240 mg/dl or above and whenever under stress or having an infection. Perform at least four times daily under these circumstances.

Copyright © 2004 Mosby Inc. All rights reserved.

56. What side effects can be expected with acarbose (Precose) and miglitol (Glyset)?

57. What affect can acarbose and miglitol have on digoxin absorption?
58. What is the action of glucagon?

55. More appropriate control of FPG and glycosylated hemoglobin concentration with fewer long-term complications from poorly controlled type 2 diabetes
56. Abdominal cramps, diarrhea, flatulence. Resolves with continued use of acarbose or miglitol.
57. These drugs may inhibit digoxin absorption.
58. Glucagon breaks down stored glycogen to glucose to be used as an energy source.

Copyright © 2004 Mosby Inc. All rights reserved.

CHAPTER 35

Drugs Used to Treat Diabetes Mellitus

Practice Quiz

COMPLETION

Complete the following statements.

1. Treatment of hypoglycemia in a conscious patient includes:

2. Treatment of hyperglycemia includes:

3. Insulin is required to transport glucose into skeletal and heart muscle and fat. It is not required for glucose transport into _____.

4. _____ type insulin may be given intravenously and subcutaneously.

5. Long-acting, suspension form of insulin is _____.

6. Insulin should be stored _____.

7. Lispro (Humalog) _____ be administered IV because it is a clear form of insulin.

8. When examining a diabetic patient the nurse detects a "fruity-smelling breath." This would likely indicate the patient is _____.

9. The nurse should administer aspart insulin _____ minutes before a meal.

10. After giving an intermediate-acting insulin at 7 AM, the nurse should assess the patient for hypoglycemia at what time? _____

11. (Hyperglycemic, Hypoglycemic) reactions require treatment with IV insulin, hydration, and stabilization of electrolytes.

12. _____ of the skin can be prevented by rotating the insulin injection sites.

13. U-100 = _____ units of insulin in 1 ml.

14. A provisional diagnosis of diabetes mellitus is made when the FBG = _____.

15. The _____ test measures the amount of glucose bonded to a protein in the blood over the previous 8–10-week period.

16. Blurred vision may be a symptom of _____.

17. The development of an abnormal glucose tolerance test in a pregnant woman is an indication of _____.

18. Short-acting (Regular) insulins (Humulin R and Novolin R) have a _____ hour duration of action.

19. Ultralente (Humulin U) is an example of a(n) _____ type insulin.

20. Type _____ diabetes mellitus is treated with insulin, and type _____ diabetes mellitus may be treated with oral hypoglycemic agents, antihyperglycemic agents, and/or insulin.

21. If the glucose level is less than _____ mg/dl or above_____ mg/dl, the diabetic patient should not exercise.

22. Numbness and tingling of the extremities is known as _____.

23. Endogenous insulin is produced by what type of cells _____ in what organ?

_____

24. Short-acting insulin, regular Iletin II, has an onset of action of _____.

END-OF-CHAPTER MATH REVIEW

1. Ordered: 22 U NPH (human) insulin to be administered 30 minutes before breakfast.
   Available: U-100 NPH (human) insulin
   Volume of insulin to be administered: _____ ml

2. Ordered: 27 U NPH (human) insulin + 7 U Regular (human) insulin to be administered before breakfast.
   Available: U-100 NPH (human) insulin
   U-100 Regular (human) insulin
   a. Volume of NPH insulin to be drawn up: _____ ml
   b. Volume of Regular insulin to be drawn up: _____ ml
   c. Total volume to be injected: _____ ml

Copyright © 2004 Mosby Inc. All rights reserved.

CRITICAL THINKING QUESTIONS

An 18-year-old patient was recently diagnosed with type 1 diabetes mellitus. After several days of treatment with adjustment of diet, exercise, and regular insulin, the patient was placed on U-100 NPH (human) insulin, 20 U 30 minutes before breakfast and 10 U before the evening meal.

1. What are the nursing interventions to be considered when administering the NPH insulin?
2. The patient is having trouble injecting himself. In a moment of frustration, he asks, "Why can't I take insulin pills like my grandfather?" What is your response?

Five days later, the health care provider adds 5 U of Regular (human) insulin to the morning dose to be administered with the NPH insulin.

3. Describe how you would teach the patient to mix the morning insulin dose for a single administration.
4. While continuing with the patient's education, he asks again for the difference between the symptoms of hypoglycemia and hyperglycemia. What is your response?

REVIEW QUESTIONS

_____ 1. The most rapid-acting type of insulins available are:
   a. Lispro and Aspart.
   b. Humulin R.
   c. Regular Iletin I.
   d. Humulin N.

_____ 2. After injection, regular insulin takes _____ minutes to start acting and its peak action is in _____ hours.
   a. 10; 1–2
   b. 20; 2–4
   c. 30; 2.5–5
   d. 50; 4–6

_____ 3. Hypoglycemia can occur as a result of:
   a. increased carbohydrate intake; usual daily insulin dose.
   b. increased protein intake with decreased physical activity.
   c. intake of diuretic agents with insulin.
   d. insulin overdose; decreased carbohydrate intake.

_____ 4. Which classification of commonly prescribed drugs may mask the symptoms of hypoglycemia when taken concurrently with insulin?
   a. glucagons
   b. oral contraceptives
   c. corticosteroids
   d. beta-adrenergic blocking agents

_____ 5. The action of thiazolidinediones (TZDs) lower blood glucose by:
   a. stimulating release of insulin from beta cells in the pancreas.
   b. an unknown mechanism of action.
   c. increasing muscle and fat tissue sensitivity to allow more glucose to enter the cell in presence of insulin.
   d. affects certain enzymes used in digestion of sugars that results in delayed glucose absorption.

Copyright © 2004 Mosby Inc. All rights reserved.

CHAPTER 36

Drugs Used to Treat Thyroid Disease

Syllabus

CHAPTER CONTENT

Thyroid Gland (p. 516)
Thyroid Diseases (p. 516)
Treatment of Thyroid Diseases (p. 517)
Drug Therapy for Thyroid Diseases (p. 517)
    Drug Class: Thyroid Replacement Hormones
      (p. 519)
    Drug Class: Antithyroid Medicines (p. 522)

CHAPTER OBJECTIVES

1. Describe the signs, symptoms, treatment, and nursing interventions associated with hypothyroidism and hyperthyroidism.
2. Identify the two classes of drugs used to treat thyroid disease.
3. Name the drug of choice for hypothyroidism.
4. Explain the effects of hyperthyroidism on dosages of warfarin and digitalis glycosides and on persons taking oral hypoglycemic agents.
5. Discuss the actions of antithyroid medications on the formation and release of the hormones produced by the thyroid gland.
6. State the three types of treatment for hyperthyroidism.
7. Explain the nutritional requirements and activity restrictions needed for individuals with hyperthyroidism.
8. Identify the types of conditions that respond favorably to the use of radioactive iodine 131 (^{131}I).
9. Explain the action of propylthiouracil on the synthesis of T_3 and T_4.

KEY TERMS

thyroid stimulating
    hormone
triiodothyronine (T_3)
thyroxine (T_4)
hypothyroidism

myxedema
cretinism
hyperthyroidism
thyrotoxicosis

ASSIGNMENTS

Read textbook, pp. 516-525.
Study Key Terms associated with chapter content.
Complete Collaborative Activities as assigned.
Study Review Sheet for Chapter 36.
Complete Chapter 36 Practice Quiz.
Complete End-of-Chapter Math Review and Critical Thinking Questions.
Complete Chapter 36 Exam.

WEB RESEARCH ACTIVITY

Access: www.thyroidfoundation.org/
Select: Thyroid Disease: Effects of Thyroxine as Compared with Thyroxine plus Triiodothyronine in Patients with Hypothyroidism
    Compare the effects of thyroxine alone with those of thyroxine plus triiodothyronine (liothyronine) on the treatment of hypothyroidism.

COLLABORATIVE ACTIVITIES

Complete the following as preparation for in-class discussion and group work that may be assigned by the instructor.

1. Research the hospital policy for management of radioactive spills.
2. Research the hospital guidelines/policy for handling patient excreta following the administration of ^{131}I.

Copyright © 2004 Mosby Inc. All rights reserved.

Drugs Used to Treat Thyroid Disease

Review Sheet

The QUESTION column and the ANSWER column have been offset so that you can cover the answers while reading the questions, allowing you to assess your knowledge.

Question	Answer
1. What glands regulate the function of the thyroid gland?	
2. What body functions are regulated by the thyroid gland?	1. Hypothalamus and anterior pituitary gland
3. What is another name for myxedema?	2. Growth and maturation; carbohydrate, protein, and lipid metabolism; thermal regulation; cardiovascular function; lactation; and reproduction are all processes affected by thyroid function.
	3. Hypothyroidism in adult patients
4. Excessive thyroid secretion results in what conditions?	4. Hyperthyroidism, also known as thyrotoxicosis
5. What is a normal thyroid state called?	5. Euthyroid state
6. Thyroid replacement hormones are used to replace what hormones secreted by the thyroid gland?	
7. What focused assessment should be performed by the nurse when a patient has hypothyroid or hyperthyroid disorders?	6. Liothyronine (T_3) and levothyroxine (T_4)
8. If a patient has hypothyroidism, what change in his or her weight over the past few months could be anticipated?	7. See textbook, pp. 517-519.
9. A patient with hyperthyroidism may require what dietary changes?	8. Weight gain
10. What type of environment does a patient with hypothyroidism or hyperthyroidism need?	9. Increase in calories to meet metabolic needs—as much as 4000 to 5000 calories daily.
11. List the thyroid hormone replacement products' brand names and ingredients.	10. Hypothyroidism = warm environment; hyperthyroidism = cool environment
12. Of the thyroid products available, which has the most rapid onset of action?	11. Levothyroxine (T_4)—(Synthroid, Levoxyl) liothyronine (T_3)—(Cytomel) liotrix (T_3, T_4)—(Thyrolar) thyroid USP
	12. Liothyronine (T_3) (Cytomel)
13. Are thyroid replacement hormones given to a patient with hypothyroidism or hyperthyroidism?	
14. List the signs and symptoms of hypothyroidism and hyperthyroidism.	13. Hypothyroidism

Copyright © 2004 Mosby Inc. All rights reserved.

15. What are the three products available to treat hyperthyroidism?
16. State the action of propylthiouracil and methimazole.
17. Describe the desired therapeutic outcome(s) for antithyroid medications.

18. What are the side effects to assess when propylthiouracil or methimazole are administered?

19. What laboratory studies should be performed at periodic intervals for people taking propylthiouracil?
20. Would a patient with hyperthyroidism be more likely to require a smaller or larger dose of a digitalis glycoside?

14. See textbook, pp. 516-517.

15. Radioactive iodine (^{131}I), propylthiouracil (PTU, Propacil), and methimazole (Tapazole)
16. Propylthiouracil (PTU) and methimazole block the synthesis of T_3 and T_4 in the thyroid gland; the drugs do not destroy T_3 and T_4 already produced.
17. The primary therapeutic outcome expected from propylthiouracil or methimazole is a gradual return to normal thyroid metabolic function.
18. Skin eruptions, pruritus, headaches, salivary or lymph node enlargement, sore throat, purpura, jaundice, and progressive weakness
19. RBC, WBC, and differential counts

20. A larger dose

Copyright © 2004 Mosby Inc. All rights reserved.

CHAPTER 36

Drugs Used to Treat Thyroid Disease

Practice Quiz

TRUE OR FALSE

Mark "T" for true and "F" for false. <u>Correct all false statements.</u>

_____ 1. Hyperthyroidism is a condition caused by excessive production of thyroid hormone.

_____ 2. Thyroid replacement hormones block the release of T_3 and T_4 in the body, thereby making the hormones available for metabolic functioning.

_____ 3. Baseline premedication assessments prior to initiation of thyroid replacement hormones are vital signs, weight, bowel elimination pattern, and laboratory studies to identify thyroid hormone levels.

_____ 4. The hypothyroid patient will be hyperactive.

_____ 5. The resting pulse rate of a hyperthyroid patient upon awakening will be low.

_____ 6. A patient with hypothyroidism would show dramatic weight loss as one of their symptoms.

_____ 7. Drugs used as thyroid replacement include iodine, propylthiouracil (PTU), and methimazole (Tapazole).

ESSAY

8. List the signs and symptoms of hypothyroidism and hyperthyroidism. When thyroid replacement hormones are administered, how should these signs and symptoms be monitored?

9. After initiating therapy with propylthiouracil, what regularly scheduled observations should be made of the patient?

10. When ^{131}I is administered, what type of precautions must be used when handling excreta or linens on which excreta has been spilled?

END-OF-CHAPTER MATH REVIEW

1. Ordered: levothyroxine (Synthroid) 0.1 mg, PO, daily
    On hand: levothyroxine (Synthroid) 0.05 mg tablets
    Give: _____ tablets.

2. Ordered: levothyroxine (Synthroid) 200 mcg
    Convert 200 mcg to mg.
    _____ mg

CRITICAL THINKING QUESTIONS

A patient's baseline vital signs are BP 140/60, pulse 104, respirations 24. He has been receiving levothyroxine (Synthroid) 0.1 mg, PO, daily for the past 6 weeks for treatment of hypothyroidism.

The patient reports that his resting pulse on awakening has been 90–112 over the past week.

1. Should these findings be reported to the health care provider?

2. If so, what additional data should be assembled before initiating health care provider contact?

A patient is taking propylthiouracil 50 mg, PO, tid.

3. What patient education should be provided regarding side effects to expect and side effects to report?

Copyright © 2004 Mosby Inc. All rights reserved.

REVIEW QUESTIONS

_____ 1. A patient receiving levothyroxine should be monitored for which signs and symptoms of overdose?
  a. bradycardia, weight gain
  b. cold intolerance, bradycardia
  c. palpitations, tachycardia, heat intolerance
  d. sluggish, slow speech; increasing confusion

_____ 2. Patients with hyperthyroidism would require a _____ dose of digoxin.
  a. normal
  b. decreased
  c. increased
  d. staggered

_____ 3. Propylthiouracil acts by:
  a. converting iodine to active iodine.
  b. blocking synthesis of T_3 and T_4 in the thyroid gland.
  c. destroying T_3 and T_4.
  d. being a synthetic form of thyroid.

Copyright © 2004 Mosby Inc. All rights reserved.

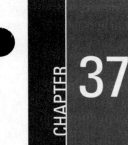

CHAPTER 37

Corticosteroids

Syllabus

CHAPTER CONTENT

Corticosteroids (p. 526)
Drug Therapy with Corticosteroids (p. 529)
    Drug Class: Mineralocorticoids (p. 529)
    Drug Class: Glucocorticoids (p. 530)

CHAPTER OBJECTIVES

1. Review the functions of the adrenal gland.
2. State the normal actions of mineralocorticoids and glucocorticoids in the body.
3. Cite the disease states caused by hypersecretion or hyposecretion of the adrenal gland.
4. Identify the baseline assessments needed for a patient receiving corticosteroids.
5. Prepare a list of the clinical uses of mineralocorticoids and glucocorticoids.
6. Discuss the potential side effects associated with the use of corticosteroids and give examples of specific patient education needed for patients taking these agents.
7. Develop measurable objectives for patient education for persons taking corticosteroids.

KEY TERMS

corticosteroids
mineralocorticoids
glucocorticoids
cortisol

ASSIGNMENTS

Read textbook, pp. 526-533.
Study Key Terms associated with chapter content.
Complete Collaborative Activity as assigned.
Study Review Sheet for Chapter 37.
Complete Chapter 37 Practice Quiz.
Complete End-of-Chapter Math Review and Critical Thinking Questions.
Complete Chapter 37 Exam.

WEB RESEARCH ACTIVITY

Access: http://www.corticosteroid.com
How do topical steroids work and what factors affect their absorption?

COLLABORATIVE ACTIVITY

Complete the following as preparation for in-class discussion and group work that may be assigned by the instructor.

Develop a patient education plan for an individual with a glucocorticoid prescribed for treatment of rheumatoid arthritis. (Use drug monograph and other resources.)

Copyright © 2004 Mosby Inc. All rights reserved.

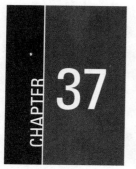

CHAPTER 37

Corticosteroids

Review Sheet

The QUESTION column and the ANSWER column have been offset so that you can cover the answers while reading the questions, allowing you to assess your knowledge.

Question

1. Define *corticosteroids*.
2. For what types of illnesses are glucocorticoids frequently prescribed?
3. What endogenous hormone is known as a glucocorticoid?
4. Do exogenous corticosteroids cure disease?
5. What side effects may be observed with the administration of glucocorticoids?

6. What time of day is best to administer glucocorticoids?

7. Why do corticosteroids and diuretics produce or enhance hypokalemia when given simultaneously?
8. Why must patients taking corticosteroids be cautioned to avoid contact with persons with infections?

Answer

1. Hormones secreted by the adrenal cortex of the adrenal gland
2. To treat diseases or disorders that are inflammatory or allergic in nature
3. Cortisol
4. Exogenous corticosteroids do not cure disease unless the adrenal glands have been surgically removed and corticosteroids are used for replacement therapy. Usually, steroids provide relief of symptoms without treating the underlying disease.
5. Hyperglycemia, glycosuria (corticosteroids stimulate formation of glucose while decreasing use of glucose by the body); electrolyte imbalances and fluid accumulation due to mineralocorticoid effects that cause sodium and water retention and potassium and hydrogen excretion; increased susceptibility to infection; peptic ulcer formation by decreasing the protective secretions of the gastric mucosa; delayed wound healing because of protein breakdown; visual changes, cataracts; osteoporosis—inhibits bone formation and growth; see textbook, pp. 530-532.
6. Between 6 AM and 9 AM to minimize suppression of normal adrenal function
7. Diuretics (except potassium-sparing diuretics) and corticosteroids cause the loss of potassium.

Copyright © 2004 Mosby Inc. All rights reserved.

9. What instructions should be given to a patient taking corticosteroids?

10. What baseline assessments should be completed for patients taking any type of corticosteroids?
11. Review the signs and symptoms of Addison's disease and Cushing's disease and contrast these with the signs and symptoms of adrenocortical excess and deficiency.

12. What effect do glucocorticoids have on blood glucose levels?
13. What type of health teaching should be done for a client receiving steroid therapy?
14. What is the major glucocorticoid secreted by the adrenal cortex?

15. Why is an alternate day schedule for administration of corticosteroids used?
16. What effect do corticosteroids have on potassium balance?

8. Corticosteroids diminish the production of antibodies, resulting in a suppressed immune system, making the patient susceptible to infection. The anti-inflammatory properties of these drugs also mask the presence of infection. Even the slightest signs and symptoms of an infection may indicate the presence of a major infection.
9. See textbook, pp. 527-532.

10. Daily weight; blood pressure in supine and sitting position; intake and output for hospitalized patients; electrolyte studies, especially sodium and potassium; check mental status; blood glucose; signs and symptoms of infection; signs and symptoms of ulcers
11. See a general medical/surgical nursing text.

12. Hyperglycemia

13. Identification bracelet, *do not* suddenly discontinue drug therapy. See textbook for specific drug therapy prescribed by reviewing the drug monograph.
14. Cortisol

15. Alternate day schedule, between 6 AM and 9 AM, minimizes suppression of normal adrenal function. Also administer with meals to minimize gastric irritation.
16. Enhance loss of potassium. Be especially alert when diuretics such as furosemide, thiazides, bumetanide, and other non-potassium–sparing diuretics are prescribed concurrently.

Copyright © 2004 Mosby Inc. All rights reserved.

Corticosteroids

CHAPTER **37**

Practice Quiz

TRUE OR FALSE

Mark "T" for true and "F" for false. <u>Correct all false statements.</u>

_____ 1. Corticosteroids are secreted from the adrenal medulla.

_____ 2. Psychotic behavior may be seen during corticosteroid therapy.

_____ 3. Individuals receiving glucocorticoid therapy should be monitored for hyperglycemia if they are diabetic or prediabetic.

_____ 4. Glucocorticoids taken for long-term therapy may produce cataracts.

_____ 5. Corticosteroid therapy does not mask the signs and symptoms of infection.

_____ 6. To minimize suppression of normal adrenal function, corticosteroids may be administered on alternate days.

_____ 7. Corticosteroids should not be discontinued abruptly.

_____ 8. Glucocorticoids should be administered between 6 PM and 9 PM to maintain normal adrenal function.

_____ 9. The major glucocorticoid secreted by the adrenal cortex is cortisol.

END-OF-CHAPTER MATH REVIEW

1. The package insert accompanying prednisone states that the physiologic replacement (pediatric) is 0.1–0.15 mg/kg/day, PO, in equal divided doses q 12 h. The child's weight is 22 lbs.
   22 lbs = _____ kg.

2. Using the dosage parameters described above, calculate the minimum and maximum dose per day for this child's weight.
   _____ mg minimum
   _____ mg maximum

CRITICAL THINKING QUESTIONS

1. A 75-year-old patient receiving prednisone for treatment of hypercalcemia associated with cancer tells you, with great excitement, that young grandchildren are coming to stay at his home for the next several months. What precautions should be taught to the patient and immediate family members regarding exposure to the grandchildren, especially when the children receive pediatric immunizations?

2. What data would indicate a positive clinical response following the administration of adrenal cortical hormones prescribed for the treatment of Addison's disease?

REVIEW QUESTIONS

_____ 1. Patients receiving a corticosteroid should be questioned regarding any history of:
   a. ulcers.
   b. blood dyscrasias.
   c. heart disease.
   d. respiratory disease.

_____ 2. Fludrocortisone (Florinef) is used for:
   a. inflammatory processes.
   b. allergic reactions.
   c. severe itching and hives.
   d. mineralocorticoid replacement.

_____ 3. The use of alternate-day administration of corticosteroids is to:
   a. minimize the suppression of normal adrenal activity.
   b. maximize the effects on the electrolytes.
   c. reduce likelihood of hypokalemia.
   d. reduce potential for cataract development.

Copyright © 2004 Mosby Inc. All rights reserved.

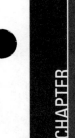

CHAPTER 38

Gonadal Hormones

Syllabus

CHAPTER CONTENT

The Gonads and Gonadal Hormones (p. 534)
Drug Therapy with Gonadal Hormones (p. 535)
    Drug Class: Estrogens (p. 535)
    Drug Class: Progestins (p. 537)
    Drug Class: Androgens (p. 537)

CHAPTER OBJECTIVES

1. Describe the body changes that can be anticipated with the administration of androgens,
   estrogens, or progesterone.
2. State the uses of estrogens and progestins.
3. Compare the side effects of estrogen hormones
   with those of a combination of estrogen and
   progesterone.
4. Differentiate between the side effects to expect
   and those requiring consultation with the health
   care provider that occur with the administration
   of estrogen or progesterone.
5. Identify the rationale for administering androgens to women who have certain types of breast
   cancer.

KEY TERMS

gonads
testosterone
androgens
ovaries
estrogen
progesterone

ASSIGNMENTS

Read textbook, pp. 534-540.
Study Key Terms associated with chapter content.
Complete Collaborative Activity as assigned.
Study Review Sheet for Chapter 38.
Complete Chapter 38 Practice Quiz.
Complete End-of-Chapter Math Review and Critical
    Thinking Question.
Complete Chapter 38 Exam.

WEB RESEARCH ACTIVITY

Access: www.nida.nih.gov/pdf/monographs/102.pdf
    Research the effects of use of anabolic steroids
on bone growth of boys at puberty.
    What long-term effect does anabolic steroid use
have on bone growth during puberty?

COLLABORATIVE ACTIVITY

*Complete the following as preparation for in-class
discussion and group work that may be assigned by the
instructor.*

Explain the rationale for administering androgens to
women with certain types of breast cancer.

Copyright © 2004 Mosby Inc. All rights reserved.

Gonadal Hormones

Review Sheet

The QUESTION column and the ANSWER column have been offset so that you can cover the answers while reading the questions, allowing you to assess your knowledge.

Question

1. What is another name for the male sex hormones?
2. What male characteristics are attributed to androgens?
3. When androgens are given to females, what effects can be anticipated?

4. Describe the effect of the administration of testosterone to boys before completion of bone growth.

5. When would androgens be prescribed for females?
6. Why is testosterone derived naturally from animal testes not administered orally?
7. What type of testosterone can be administered orally?
8. Review the uses and effects of estrogens on the body systems.
9. What are the side effects to expect and those to report for persons taking estrogen products?
10. What are progestins used to treat?

11. What happens to the progesterone level if fertilization does not take place?

12. What premedication assessments should be performed prior to therapy with estrogens, progestins, and androgens?

Answer

1. Androgens; testosterone is the primary hormone.
2. Normal growth and development of male sex organs and secondary sex characteristics (e.g., growth and maturation of prostate, seminal vesicles, penis, and scrotum; development and distribution of male hair on the body; deepening of the voice)
3. Masculinization, if given in sufficient doses (e.g., deepening voice, hirsutism, acne, menstrual irregularity); electrolyte imbalance of Na^+, K^+, Cl^-, and Ca^{++}; gastric irritation
4. May cause premature closure of the epiphyseal line, inhibiting normal bone growth.
5. In some types of breast cancer
6. It is rapidly inactivated by the liver.
7. Synthetic forms (e.g., methyltestosterone, fluoxymesterone)
8. See textbook, pp. 535-537.
9. Expect: weight gain, edema, breast tenderness, nausea; report: hypertension, hyperglycemia, thrombophlebitis, breakthrough vaginal bleeding
10. Secondary amenorrhea, breakthrough bleeding, endometriosis, and when combined with estrogen, used as an oral contraceptive
11. Progesterone production drops and menstruation occurs.

Copyright © 2004 Mosby Inc. All rights reserved.

13. What effect can androgen therapy have on calcium in patients being treated for breast cancer?
14. Identify common estrogen, progestin, and androgen medications.

12. See textbook: estrogens, p. 536; progestins, p. 537; androgens, p. 538.
13. Hypercalcemia

14. Examine Tables 38-1, 38-2, and 38-3.

Copyright © 2004 Mosby Inc. All rights reserved.

Gonadal Hormones

Student Name_____

Practice Quiz

COMPLETION

Complete the following statements.
The gonads are called:
1. _____ in males.
2. _____ in females.

Progesterone's major body functions include:
3.
4.
5.
Premedication assessment before initiation of estrogen therapy should include:
6.
7.
8.
9. and any history of:
Progestins prevent:
10.
11.
12. Androgen therapy in females produces
    _____.
13. Levonorgestrel (Norplant system) is an example of a(n) _____.
14. Fluoxymesterone (Halotestin) is an example of a(n) _____.
15. Estropipate (Ogen) is an example of a(n)
    _____.

END-OF-CHAPTER MATH REVIEW

1. Ordered: hydroxyprogesterone 375 mg, IM.
    On hand: hydroxyprogesterone 250 mg/ml
    Give: _____ ml.
2. Ordered: progesterone 10 mg, IM, daily times 6 days.
    On hand: progesterone 50 mg/ml
    Give: _____ ml daily

CRITICAL THINKING QUESTION

A 62-year-old patient is receiving methyltestosterone 200 mg, PO, daily for palliation of breast cancer. She asks you why she is taking this particular medication and expresses concern that this, like other medications she has taken for treatment of the cancer, will make her feel ill. What should you tell her?

REVIEW QUESTIONS

_____ 1. Androgens, when given to an immobilized patient or a patient with breast cancer, may result in development of:
    a. hypertension.
    b. fluid loss and dehydration.
    c. feminization.
    d. hypercalcemia.
_____ 2. Androgens given to male children may result in:
    a. hypercalcemia.
    b. premature closure of epiphyseal line.
    c. delayed closure of epiphyseal line.
    d. developmental delay.
_____ 3. Conjugated estrogens (Premarin) is prescribed during menopause for:
    a. amenorrhea.
    b. breast cancer.
    c. hot flashes.
    d. breakthrough uterine bleeding.
_____ 4. An action of progestin is to:
    a. inhibit ovulation.
    b. promote ovulation.
    c. promote growth of secondary sex characteristics.
    d. treat prostatic cancer.

Copyright © 2004 Mosby Inc. All rights reserved.

39 Drugs Used in Obstetrics

Syllabus

CHAPTER CONTENT

Obstetrics (p. 541)
Drug Therapy with Pregnancy (p. 549)
    Drug Class: Uterine Stimulants (p. 549)
    Drug Class: Uterine Relaxants (p. 554)
    Drug Class: Other Agents (p. 556)
Neonatal Ophthalmic Solutions (p. 559)

CHAPTER OBJECTIVES

1. Describe nursing assessments and nursing interventions needed for the pregnant patient during the first, second, and third trimesters of pregnancy.

2. Identify appropriate nursing assessments, nursing interventions, and treatment options used for the following obstetric complications: infection, hyperemesis gravidarum, miscarriage, abortion, preterm labor, premature rupture of membranes, gestational diabetes, and pregnancy-induced hypertension (PIH).
3. State the methods and time parameters of each approach to the termination of a pregnancy.
4. Summarize the care needs of the pregnant woman during labor and delivery and the immediate postpartum period, including the patient education needed before discharge to promote safe self-care and care of the newborn.
5. State the purpose of administering glucocorticoids to certain women in preterm labor.
6. State the actions, primary uses, nursing assessments, and monitoring parameters for uterine stimulants, uterine relaxants, clomiphene citrate, magnesium sulfate, and $Rh_O(D)$ immune globulin (RhoGAM).
7. Compare the effects of uterine stimulants and uterine relaxants on the pregnant woman's uterus.

8. Describe specific nursing concerns and appropriate nursing actions when uterine stimulants are administered for induction of labor, augmentation of labor, and postpartum atony and hemorrhage.
9. Cite the effects of adrenergic agents on $beta_1$ and $beta_2$ receptors, then identify the relationship of these actions to the side effects to report when adrenergic agents are used to inhibit preterm labor.
10. Describe specific assessments needed before and during the use of terbutaline or magnesium sulfate.
11. Identify emergency supplies that should be available in the immediate vicinity during magnesium sulfate therapy.
12. Identify the action, specific dosage, administration precautions, and proper timing of the administration of RhoGAM and rubella vaccine in relation to pregnancy.
13. Summarize the immediate nursing care needs of the newborn infant following delivery.

KEY TERMS

pregnancy-induced hypertension (PIH)
lochia
precipitous labor and delivery
augmentation
dysfunctional labor

ASSIGNMENTS

Read textbook pp. 541-561.
Study Key Terms associated with chapter content.
Complete Collaborative Activities as assigned.
Study Review Sheet for Chapter 39.
Complete Chapter 39 Practice Quiz.

Copyright © 2004 Mosby Inc. All rights reserved.

Complete End-of-Chapter Math Review and Critical
   Thinking Questions.
Complete Chapter 39 Exam.

WEB RESEARCH ACTIVITIES

Access: www.obgyn.net/newsheadlines/womens_
health-Pre_eclampsia_20030731-65.asp
Select: Low-Dose Aspirin During Pregnancy May
Lower Risk of Preeclampsia

1. What type of obstetrical patient may benefit
    from low-dose aspirin therapy during pregnan-
    cy?
2. What other benefits, in addition to a reduction
    in the frequency of preeclampsia, were found
    with the administration of low-dose aspirin
    therapy during pregnancy?

COLLABORATIVE ACTIVITIES

*Complete the following as preparation for in-class
discussion and group work that may be assigned by the
instructor.*

1. Research the hospital policy for administration
    of oxytocin.
2. Prepare a detailed listing of nursing interven-
    tions needed during IV infusion of oxytocin.

Copyright © 2004 Mosby Inc. All rights reserved.

CHAPTER 39

Drugs Used in Obstetrics

Review Sheet

The QUESTION column and the ANSWER column have been offset so that you can cover the answers while reading the questions, allowing you to assess your knowledge.

Question	Answer
1. Identify the factors that need to be assessed during prenatal management of a pregnant woman and during and following normal labor and delivery.	
2. Describe nursing assessments and interventions needed for the pregnant patient experiencing potential obstetrical complications (e.g., infection; hyperemesis gravidarum; miscarriage; abortion; pregnancy-induced hypertension (PIH); hemolysis, elevated liver enzymes, low platelet syndrome (HELLP); and bleeding disorders).	1. See textbook, pp. 541-544.
3. State the methods and time parameters of each approach to the termination of a pregnancy.	2. See text (p. 542) for details of the following categories: miscarriage, placental separation and abortion, PIH, HELLP, etc.
4. Cite the recommended times of administration for RhoGAM (human) and rubella vaccine in relation to pregnancy.	3. Before 12 weeks gestation: dilatation and evacuation (D&E); 12–20 weeks gestation: saline or prostaglandin administered intra-amniotically, intramuscularly, or by vaginal suppository; intrauterine fetal death after 20 weeks gestation: prostaglandin suppositories with or without oxytocin augmentation.
5. Describe the nursing assessments and interventions used for PIH.	4. *Previous immunization.* Although there is no need to administer RhoGAM to a woman who is already sensitized to the Rh factor, the risk is no more than that when given to a woman who is not sensitized. When in doubt, administer RhoGAM.
	Before administration:
	1. *Never* administer the IGIM full dose or microdose products intravenously. (The IGIV full dose product may be administered intramuscularly or intravenously).
	2. *Never* administer to a neonate.

Copyright © 2004 Mosby Inc. All rights reserved.

3. *Never* administer to an Rh-negative patient who has been previously sensitized to the Rh antigen.
4. *Confirm* that the mother is Rh negative.

Pregnancy. Postpartum prophylaxis—one standard dose vial of IGIM intramuscularly or one standard dose vial of IGIV intramuscularly or intravenously. Additional vials may be necessary if there was unusually large fetal-maternal hemorrhage.

Antepartum prophylaxis—one standard dose vial IM at about 28 weeks gestational age. This must be followed by another vial administered within 72 hours of delivery. After amniocentesis, miscarriage, abortion, or ectopic pregnancy—less than 13 weeks of gestation: one microdose vial IM within 72 hours; 13 or more weeks of gestation: one standard dose vial IM within 72 hours.

Transfusion accident. Rh-negative, premenopausal women who receive Rh-positive red cells by transfusion: one standard dose vial IM for each 15 ml of transfused packed red cells.

Idiopathic thrombocytopenic purpura:
Before administration:
1. *Confirm* that the mother is Rh positive.
2. *Follow* manufacturer's instructions on dilution and administration of Rh_o[D] IGIV.
    IV—Initial dose: 250 U/kg as a single injection. Additional doses are dependent upon response.
Rubella vaccine should be given to a patient whose rubella titer is low, immediately after pregnancy. She should be counseled to use birth control for at least the next 3 months.

6. State the purpose of administering glucocorticoids to certain women in preterm labor.

5. Take vital signs at regularly scheduled intervals and compare with baseline readings. Report elevations of systolic pressure of 30 mm Hg or more above the previous readings, or systolic blood pressure of 140 mm Hg or more, or diastolic pressure of 90 mm Hg or more. Edema may be present: monitor I & O and check state of hydration. Intake of 1000 ml more than the output over the preceding 24 hours is generally allowed. Perform assessment of edema: daily weights, report a weight gain of 2 or more

Copyright © 2004 Mosby Inc. All rights reserved.

7. Summarize the care needs of the pregnant woman during normal labor and delivery.

8. Identify the name, dosage, route of administration, and correct time for administering oxytocic agents.
9. Describe the normal sequence of changes in the appearance of lochia during the postpartum period.
10. Summarize the immediate nursing care needs of the newborn infant following delivery.
11. Discuss the rationale for inspection of the placenta and cord following delivery of the newborn.
12. Summarize the Centers for Disease Control recommendations for prophylaxis of ophthalmia neonatorum.

13. Identify assessment data essential in detecting postpartum hemorrhage.

14. State the drug actions and nursing assessments needed to monitor therapeutic response and development of side effects to expect or report from uterine stimulants, uterine relaxants, clomiphene citrate, magnesium sulfate, RhoGAM, and erythromycin or tetracycline ophthalmic ointment.
15. List premedication assessments needed prior to an oxytocin infusion.
16. What are signs and symptoms of fetal distress?

pounds in any 1-week period. Discourage the heavy use of salt. Monitor urine for the presence of protein. Electrolyte studies should be done at regular intervals. Hematocrit will become elevated as the patient becomes dehydrated. Information from the serum estriols and L/S ratio give indications of fetal maturity. Seizure precautions: monitor for drowsiness, hyperreflexia, visual disturbances, or severe pain. Report any of these symptoms immediately. Give prescribed medications (e.g., sedatives, antihypertensives, anticonvulsants). Observe for complications (e.g., started labor, pulmonary edema, heart failure).

6. Glucocorticoids are administered IM to the woman in preterm labor to accelerate fetal lung maturation and to minimize hyaline membrane disease.
7. See textbook, pp. 546-549, for summary of normal labor and delivery needs.

8. See textbook, pp. 553-554, for a discussion of oxytocic agents.

9. Blood red immediately after delivery, progressing to a more watery or pinkish color
10. See text discussion: Immediate Neonatal Care, pp. 546-547.

11. Verify presence of one vein and two arteries in the cord and inspect the placenta to be certain it is intact and no fragments or pieces have been retained.
12. See textbook, p. 547, for acceptable agents that prevent gonococcal ophthalmia neonatorum and chlamydial ophthalmia neonatorum.
13. Fundus height and firmness, lochia color and amount, vital signs

14. See individual drug monographs for details.

15. Maternal vital signs, especially blood pressure and pulse rate; mother's hydration status including urine output and I & O. (This will form baseline data for subsequent monitoring during drug therapy.) Monitor characteristics of uter-

Copyright © 2004 Mosby Inc. All rights reserved.

ine contractions (e.g., frequency, rate, duration, and intensity); report duration over 90 seconds. Monitor fetal heart rate and rhythm. Perform reflex testing as specified in drug monograph. Check amount and characteristics of vaginal discharge.

17. If fetal distress occurs during oxytocin therapy, what actions should be taken immediately?

18. State the primary clinical indications for use of uterine stimulants.

19. Describe specific nursing concerns and appropriate nursing actions when uterine stimulants are administered for induction of labor, augmentation of labor, and postpartum atony and hemorrhage.

20. Explain the limitations of the use of oxytocin for the purpose of initiating a therapeutic abortion.

16. Normal fetal heart rate (120–160 beats/min); report bradycardia (below 120) or tachycardia (over 160)

17. Slow oxytocin infusion to lowest rate in accordance with hospital policy. Turn mother to left lateral position, administer O_2 by mask or cannula, call the health care provider immediately.

18. Four primary clinical uses: (1) induction or augmentation of labor; (2) control of postpartum atony and hemorrhage; (3) control of postsurgical hemorrhage (e.g., C-section); and (4) induction of therapeutic abortion.

19. Induction of labor: check vital signs q 15 minutes, use an infusion pump, monitor contractions (e.g., frequency, duration, and intensity), and fetal heart tones. Monitor for fetal distress (fetal heart rate of 160 bpm followed by bradycardia below 120 bpm). If fetal distress occurs, reduce oxytocin infusion to the slowest rate, turn mother to left lateral position, and administer oxygen. Monitor I & O of all patients receiving oxytocin and report accumulation of water by the body, known as "water intoxication."

21. Review the procedure for insertion of vaginal suppositories.

22. Differentiate among the uses and actions on the uterus of dinoprostone, ergonovine maleate, methylergonovine maleate, and oxytocin.

23. Identify specific nursing assessments, interventions, and evaluation criteria used during the administration of uterine stimulants.

20. Uterine smooth muscle is not very responsive to oxytocin stimulation until late in the third trimester.

21. See Administration of Vaginal Medications (pp. 114-116).

22. Dinoprostone: uterine smooth muscle stimulant. Used during pregnancy to increase the frequency and strength of uterine contractions and produce cervical softening and dilatation. Used to expel uterine contents in cases of intrauterine fetal death, benign hydatidiform mole, missed spontaneous miscarriage, and second trimester abortion.

Ergonovine maleate, methylergonovine maleate: both stimulate contractions of the uterus. Cannot be used for induction of labor because they cause sudden, intense uterine activity. Used in postpartum patients to control bleeding and maintain uterine firmness.

Copyright © 2004 Mosby Inc. All rights reserved.

24. Compare the effects of methylergonovine maleate and ergonovine maleate on lactation.
25. Identify specific actions, dosage and administration, and nursing assessments needed during the use of oxytocin therapy.
26. What is the effect of oxytocin on fluid balance?

27. Compare the effects of uterine stimulants and uterine relaxants on the pregnant uterus.

28. Review the effects of adrenergic agents on beta$_1$ and beta$_2$ receptors and identify the relationship of these actions to the side effects to report when adrenergic agents are used to inhibit preterm labor.
29. What are the effects of adrenergic agents on serum glucose and electrolyte balance?

30. Describe specific assessments needed before and during the use of terbutaline.

31. What are the baseline laboratory studies needed before the initiation of terbutaline therapy?

32. Describe the potential effects of terbutaline on the neonate.

33. For what clinical condition is clomiphene citrate used?

Oxytocin: stimulates smooth muscle of the uterus, blood vessels, and mammary glands. Can be used during the third trimester to initiate labor. Drug of choice to induce labor at term or to augment uterine contractions during first and second stages of labor.
23. See number 19 above.

24. Do not use ergonovine in patients who wish to breastfeed. Methylergonovine may be used.

25. Observe the rate of infusion of oxytocin and the fetal monitor for measurement of contractions. Assess for nausea, vomiting, fetal distress, hypertension or hypotension, seizure activity, and water intoxication.
26. Oxytocin can alter fluid balance by stimulating antidiuretic hormone, causing the body to accumulate water. Signs and symptoms include drowsiness, listlessness, headache, confusion, oliguria, edema, and in extreme cases, seizures.
27. Uterine stimulants increase uterine activity. Uterine relaxants are used to delay or prevent labor and delivery in selected patients.

28. Adrenergic or sympathetic control
Beta$_1$: increase rate and force of heart contractions. Beta$_2$: relaxation of smooth muscles in bronchi, uterus, gastrointestinal tract, and peripheral vascular area. Monitor for tachycardia and hypotension.
29. May cause hyperglycemia because of stimulation of the sympathetic system, resulting in an increase in glycogenolysis. Continuous, long-term infusions of terbutaline may also cause hypokalemia. Monitor serum electrolytes periodically.
30. Obtain baseline vital signs and weight. Monitor maternal and fetal heart rates. Perform baseline mental status assessment (e.g., alertness, orientation, anxiety level, muscle strength, tremors). Monitor diabetic patients for hyperglycemia.
31. Serum glucose, chloride, sodium, potassium, hematocrit, and carbon dioxide before initiation of therapy.
32. Neonatal adverse effects include hyperglycemia followed by hypoglycemia, hypotension, hypocalcemia, and paralytic ileus.

Copyright © 2004 Mosby Inc. All rights reserved.

34. Identify the preliminary screening needed before initiation of clomiphene citrate therapy.

35. What safety precautions are needed in the event that visual disturbances occur with the use of clomiphene citrate?

36. At what specific time during the menstrual cycle can ovulation be anticipated with the use of clomiphene citrate?

37. What is the action of magnesium sulfate on the central nervous system?

38. What is the normal range of blood levels of magnesium sulfate when it is used as an anticonvulsant?

39. Prepare a list of assessments that should be implemented during the administration of magnesium sulfate to detect toxicity.

40. Explain the rationale for monitoring urine output during magnesium sulfate therapy.

41. What methods are used to assess deep tendon reflexes and what specific findings would require notification of the physician?

42. Identify treatment for magnesium sulfate toxicity.

43. Describe specific procedures and precautions needed during the intravenous administration of magnesium sulfate.

44. What nursing assessments are needed to monitor infants born to mothers receiving magnesium sulfate?

45. What emergency supplies should be available in the immediate vicinity during magnesium sulfate therapy?

46. What are the action and purpose of administration of RhoGAM?

33. It is used to induce ovulation in women who are not ovulating because of reduced circulating estrogen levels.

34. A complete physical exam must rule out other pathologic causes for lack of ovulation.

35. See a health care provider for an eye exam. Avoid tasks requiring visual acuity (e.g., driving or operating power machinery). Visual disturbances usually subside in a few days to weeks following discontinuation of the medication.

36. Usually 6–10 days after the last dose of medication

37. It depresses the central nervous system (CNS) and blocks peripheral nerve transmission, causing muscle relaxation.

38. 4–8 mEq/L

39. Deep tendon reflexes: Patellar reflex qh (IV), or before every dose (IM). Hourly urine output: report output of less than 30 ml/hour or less than 100 ml/4 hours. Vital signs: take q 15–30 minutes. Respirations must be at least 16/minute before further doses are administered. If blood pressure drops, do not administer another dose. Fetal distress: do not administer. Mental status: check orientation and alertness before initiating therapy.

40. With reduced urine output, toxicity is more likely to occur.

41. See text on Deep Tendon Reflex, pp. 557-558.

42. Administer calcium gluconate 10%. Stop magnesium infusion.

43. Use an infusion pump. Periodic neurologic exam, I & O, fetal assessment, vital signs.

44. Monitor for hyporeflexia and respiratory depression. May also be hypotensive.

45. Calcium gluconate 10% solution ready for IV administration. Ambu bag, in case of respiratory depression. Discontinue the IV infusion.

Copyright © 2004 Mosby Inc. All rights reserved.

47. Identify the specific dosage, administration precautions, and proper timing of the administration of RhoGAM.

48. State the appropriate treatment of fever, arthralgia, and generalized aches and pains that can be anticipated following RhoGAM administration.

49. What is the purpose of erythromycin ophthalmic ointment?

50. Describe the specific procedures used to instill erythromycin ophthalmic ointment.

51. What is the causative organism of ophthalmia neonatorum?

52. Explain the rationale for administering phytonadione to the neonate.

53. What is the preferred site for intramuscular administration of vitamin K to a neonate?

54. Review the anatomical structures associated with the administration of intramuscular medications in an infant.

55. What side effects to report are associated with phytonadione therapy?

46. It is used to prevent Rh immunization of the Rh− patient exposed to Rh+ blood as a result of a transfusion accident, during termination of pregnancy, or as a result of a delivery of an Rh+ infant. Action: prevents Rh hemolytic disease in subsequent delivery. Also used in the treatment of idiopathic thrombocytopenic purpura.

47. See drug monograph, p. 559.

48. Use acetaminophen, not aspirin or other anti-inflammatory agents.

49. Used prophylactically to prevent ophthalmia neonatorum caused by *Neisseria gonorrhoeae* or *Chlamydia trachomatis*

50. See Therapeutic Outcome, textbook pp. 559-560.

51. *Neisseria gonorrhoeae* or *Chlamydia trachomatis*

52. Newborns are often deficient in bacteria to produce vitamin K. They are also deficient in clotting factors and are more susceptible to hemorrhagic disease.

53. Lateral aspect of the thigh

54. See Parenteral Medications and Administration: Intradermal, Subcutaneous, and Intramuscular Administration (pp. 153-157).

55. Bruising, hemorrhage, petechiae, bleeding from any site or orifice

Copyright © 2004 Mosby Inc. All rights reserved.

CHAPTER 39

Drugs Used in Obstetrics

Practice Quiz

COMPLETION

Complete the following statements.

1. _____ are given to a woman to accelerate fetal lung development and to minimize hyaline membrane disease.
2. RhoGAM is given to an Rh-_____ mother.
3. The hematocrit will be _____ in a dehydrated patient.
4. When inspecting the umbilical cord following delivery, it should have _____vein(s) and _____ artery(ies).
5. Name two ophthalmic agents used in the prevention of ophthalmia neonatorum: _____ and _____.
6. Fetal distress would be indicated by _____ or _____.
7. Oxytocin does not induce contractions in the pregnant uterus until _____.
8. Dinoprostone is a uterine smooth muscle _____.
9. _____ and _____ are two drugs used in postpartum patients to control uterine bleeding and maintain uterine firmness.
10. An adverse effect of _____ is water intoxication.
11. Beta$_1$ adrenergic agents cause an (increase, decrease) in the rate and an (increase, decrease) in the force of heart contractions.
12. _____ is a drug that may produce hyperglycemia followed by hypoglycemia, hypotension, and hypocalcemia in the neonate.
13. Magnesium sulfate blood levels should be maintained between _____ mEq/L when used as an anticonvulsant.
14. Urine output is monitored during administration of magnesium sulfate because reduced urine output may induce _____.
15. _____ is the emergency drug used to treat magnesium sulfate toxicity.
16. _____ is the preferred site for administration of vitamin K to a neonate.

END-OF-CHAPTER MATH REVIEW

1. Ordered: methylergonovine maleate (Methergine) 0.2 mg, IM, immediately after delivery of the placenta.
   On hand: Check the drug monograph in the textbook to determine the availability of the drug.
   Give: _____ ml.
2. Ordered: magnesium sulfate 1 g/hr by continuous infusion.
   On hand: magnesium sulfate 4 g added to 250 ml D$_5$W
   Set the infusion pump at: _____ ml/hr.

CRITICAL THINKING QUESTIONS

1. After delivery of a newborn, an Rh– mother asks why she must receive RhoGAM. Give an explanation of the rationale that a lay person would understand.
2. Why is it necessary to prehydrate the mother before administration of terbutaline IV?
3. During administration of terbutaline IV, the woman's pulse elevates to l50 beats per minute and the fetal heart rate is 200 beats/minute. What actions would you take?

Copyright © 2004 Mosby Inc. All rights reserved.

Student Name _____

REVIEW QUESTIONS

_____ 1. Oxytocin (Pitocin) is administered:
   a. subcutaneously.
   b. intramuscularly.
   c. intravenously using an infusion pump.
   d. in fractional doses every hour.

_____ 2. During terbutaline (Brethine) administration, the patient's pulse rate is 150 and blood pressure is 170/100 mm Hg. The nurse should:
   a. increase the infusion rate and retake vitals in 20 minutes.
   b. administer antihypertensive PRN.
   c. check fetal heart rate and report all findings to the health care provider.
   d. report findings to the health care provider.

_____ 3. During the administration of magnesium sulfate the nurse should have _____ available.
   a. calcium carbonate
   b. calcium gluconate
   c. calcium citrate
   d. calcium chloride

_____ 4. Phytonadione (AquaMEPHYTON) is given to the newborn to:
   a. prevent intestinal flora from developing.
   b. increase water-soluble vitamin supply.
   c. prevent production of prothrombin (factor II).
   d. prevent hemorrhagic disease.

40 Drugs Used in Men's and Women's Health

Syllabus

CHAPTER CONTENT

CHAPTER OBJECTIVES

1. Identify common organisms known to cause leukorrhea.
2. Cite the generic and brand names of products used to treat *Candida albicans, Trichomonas vaginalis,* and *Gardnerella vaginalis.*
3. Review specific techniques for administering vaginal medications.
4. Develop a plan for teaching self-care to women and men with sexually transmitted diseases. Include personal hygiene measures, medication administration, methods of pain relief, and prevention of spread of infection or reinfection.
5. Discuss specific interviewing techniques that can be used to obtain a patient's history of sexual activity.
6. Compare the active ingredients in the two types of oral contraceptive agents.
7. Differentiate between the actions and the benefits of the combination pill and the minipill.

8. Describe the major adverse effects of and contraindications to the use of oral contraceptive agents.
9. Develop specific patient education plans to be used to teach a patient to initiate oral contraceptive therapy with the combination pill and the minipill.
10. Identify the patient teaching necessary with the administration of the transdermal contraceptive and the intravaginal hormone contraceptive.
11. Describe pharmacologic treatments of benign prostatic hyperplasia.
12. Describe the pharmacologic treatment of erectile dysfunction.

KEY TERMS

leukorrhea
dysmenorrhea
sexually transmitted diseases

ASSIGNMENTS

Read textbook, pp. 562-579.
Study Key Terms associated with chapter content.
Complete the Collaborative Activity as assigned.
Study Review Sheet for Chapter 40.
Complete Chapter 40 Practice Quiz.
Complete End-of-Chapter Math Review and Critical Thinking Questions.
Complete Chapter 40 Exam.

WEB RESEARCH ACTIVITY

Access: www.cdc.gov/STD/treatment
Search: Healthy People 2010
Identify the trends in sexually transmitted diseases (STDs) and significant biological, social, and behavioral factors that are having an impact on the spread and treatment of STDs.

Copyright © 2004 Mosby Inc. All rights reserved.

COLLABORATIVE ACTIVITY

Complete the following as preparation for in-class discussion and group work that may be assigned by the instructor.

Develop a health teaching plan for a woman with a vaginal infection.

Copyright © 2004 Mosby Inc. All rights reserved.

40 Drugs Used in Men's and Women's Health

Review Sheet

The QUESTION column and the ANSWER column have been offset so that you can cover the answers while read-ing the questions, allowing you to assess your knowledge.

Question	Answer
1. Define *leukorrhea*.	1. Leukorrhea is an abnormal, usually whitish, vaginal discharge.
2. What types of infection are known to develop in the mouth, gastrointestinal tract, or vagina with the use of broad-spectrum antibiotics?	2. *C. albicans* and others listed in Table 40-2
3. List the diseases collectively known as sexually transmitted diseases (STDs).	3. See Table 40-3, p. 565.
4. Identify the components of a female and/or male reproductive history.	4. See textbook, pp. 562-563.
5. What history of drug use would be of signifi-cance in a medication history and should be reported to the health care provider?	5. Steroids, antibiotics, illegal drugs, allergies, and previous drug treatment of the same condition
6. List laboratory studies used to detect infection in the male or female reproductive system.	6. See textbook, p. 565.
7. Identify basic hygiene measures that should be taught to men and women.	7. See textbook, pp. 565-567.
8. Explain in detail the proper method of applying vaginal medications topically or intravaginally and discuss medication regimens used for both partners in a sexual relationship.	
9. How is a psychosocial assessment that focuses on obtaining data related to STDs completed?	8. Patient Education and Health Promotion, Medications. Textbook, pp. 566-567.
10. Compare the active ingredients of combination and progestin-only oral contraceptive agents.	9. See textbook, pp. 564-565.
11. Differentiate between the actions and the bene-fits of the combination pill and the minipill oral contraceptives.	10. See textbook, pp. 567-569.
12. Describe the major adverse effects of and con-traindications for the use of oral contraceptives.	11. The combination pill prevents conception by inhibiting ovulation, making the cervical mucus thick and inhibiting sperm migration, and im-pairing implantation of the fertilized ovum. The minipill prevents conception through progestin activity on cervical mucus, uterine and fallopian transport, and implantation. Other mechanisms also contribute to preventing implantation.

Copyright © 2004 Mosby Inc. All rights reserved.

13. Develop a specific education plan for teaching patients about oral contraceptives.

14. What medications, when combined with oral contraceptive therapy, require the use of an alternate form of contraceptive therapy?
15. What herbal product may reduce the effectiveness of oral contraceptives?
16. Explain how the transdermal contraceptive, ethinyl estradiol/norelgestromin (Ortho-Evra) is applied and the patient teaching that should be done regarding its use.
17. What drugs are contained in the vaginal ring (NuvaRing)?
18. Describe the procedure for insertion of the NuvaRing.

19. Explain the health teaching that should be initiated when the NuvaRing is prescribed.
20. What side effects need to be reported with the use of the NuvaRing?
21. Differentiate between the symptoms of obstructive and irritative benign prostatic hypertrophy.

22. Compare the actions of alpha$_1$-adrenergic blocking agents and antiandrogen agents on the prostatic gland.
23. What is androgenetic alopecia?

24. What premedication assessments should be made prior to administering alpha$_1$ adrenergic blocking agents and antiandrogen agents?
25. Define *erectile dysfunction* and differentiate between vascular, neurologic, and psychologic causative factors.
26. Why is it important to check for a history of cardiovascular disease before initiating sildenafil (Viagra) therapy?

12. Diseases that may be aggravated by oral contraceptive therapy include hypertension, gallbladder disease, diabetes mellitus, severe varicose veins, seizure disorders, oligomenorrhea or amenorrhea, and rheumatic heart disease. Side effects common with oral contraceptive therapy are nausea, headache, weight gain, spotting, depression, fatigue, chloasma, yeast infections, vaginal itching or discharge, and changes in libido.
13. See textbook, Oral Contraceptive Therapy: Administration, pp. 569-571.

14. See textbook, p. 571.

15. St. John's wort

16. See textbook, p. 572.

17. Ethinyl estradiol (an estrogen) and norelestromin (a progestin) are contained in the NuvaRing.
18. See textbook, pp. 573-574.

19. See textbook, pp. 573-574.

20. Vaginal discharge, breakthrough bleeding, yeast infection, blurred vision, severe headaches, dizziness, leg pain, chest pain, shortness of breath, or acute abdominal pain
21. See Table 40-7, p. 574.

22. Alpha$_1$-adrenergic blocking agents relax the smooth muscles of the bladder and prostate, whereas antiandrogen agents block androgens at the prostate cellular level and cause the prostate gland to shrink.
23. Male pattern baldness. Elevated dihydrotestosterone (DHT) induces androgenetic alopecia.

24. See textbook, pp. 575-576.

25. See textbook, p. 576.

Copyright © 2004 Mosby Inc. All rights reserved.

27. What is the time of onset and duration of action of sildenafil?

26. Sildenafil can cause fatal interactions with nitroglycerin or isosorbide. Always check with the physician if a patient has any history of cardiovascular disease before initiating therapy.

27. Take 30 minutes to 4 hours before sexual activity; erectile function lasts for an hour or more but is highly variable and dependent on a number of factors.

Copyright © 2004 Mosby Inc. All rights reserved.

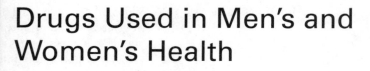

CHAPTER 40

Drugs Used in Men's and Women's Health

Practice Quiz

COMPLETION

Complete the following statements.

The combination pill contains 1. _____ and _____ hormones. These hormones are taken for 2. _____ days per month.

The progestin-only oral contraceptive is taken 3. _____ day of the month. This type of oral contraceptive is nicknamed the 4. _____.

List five common side effects associated with oral contraceptive therapy:

5.

6.

7.

8.

9.

10. Estrogen stimulates what action on the reproductive cycle?

11. The transdermal patch is applied weekly for _____ weeks.

12. What contraceptive hormones are the active ingredients in the Nuva-Ring?

END-OF-CHAPTER MATH REVIEW

1. Ordered: acyclovir (Zovirax) 200 mg, PO, q 4 h while awake for a total of five capsules per day. The total daily dose would be _____ mg. A prescription that is to last for 2 weeks until the patient is seen in the clinic again would need to include a total of _____ capsules.

2. Ordered: doxycycline (Doryx) 100 mg, q 12 h, PO for the first day; followed by 100 mg/day, PO, for a total of 10 days. When the prescription comes from the pharmacy, how many capsules should be in the bottle (the product is available in 100 mg capsules)? _____ capsules

CRITICAL THINKING QUESTIONS

1. A patient is being started on a combination oral contraceptive. You start the initial health teaching regarding the prescription. What would you explain?

2. A 22-year-old patient comes to the clinic for an annual physical and renewal of her oral contraceptives. She tests positive for Chlamydia and becomes very upset when informed of this. How would you address this situation?

3. A neighbor tells you he is obtaining Viagra through the "black market." What should you do in view of your knowledge of this drug and its action and potential interactions?

REVIEW QUESTIONS

_____ 1. When combination oral contraceptive products are administered, the action of the _____ is on the release of FSH (follicle stimulating hormone) and the action of _____ is on LH (luteinizing hormone).
   a. enzyme 5-alpha reductase; alpha-1 blocking agent
   b. progestins; estrogens
   c. estrogens; progestins
   d. sympathetic agents; alpha-adrenergic blocking agents

Copyright © 2004 Mosby Inc. All rights reserved.

_____ 2. Sildenafil (Viagra) requires a premedication assessment for:
a. sexually transmitted diseases (STDs).
b. diabetes mellitus.
c. gastritis or peptic ulcer disease.
d. cardiovascular disease.

_____ 3. A transdermal contraceptive is applied:
a. for 28 consecutive days.
b. for 1 week on, 1 week off.
c. for 21 days on, 7 days off.
d. for 14 days on, 14 days off.

_____ 4. If the NuvaRing has been out of the
vagina longer than 3 hours, the patient
should be instructed:
a. that no backup contraceptive is necessary.
b. to reinsert the ring and use a non-
hormonal contraceptive for 7 consecutive days.
c. to reinsert the ring and use the minipill for 7 consecutive days.
d. to reinsert the ring and use a combination contraceptive for 7 consecutive days.

Copyright © 2004 Mosby Inc. All rights reserved.

Drugs Used to Treat Disorders of the Urinary System

Syllabus

CHAPTER CONTENT

Urinary Tract Infections (p. 580)
Drug Therapy for Urinary Tract Infections (p. 584)
    Drug Class: The Fosfomycins (p. 584)
    Drug Class: The Quinolones (p. 584)
    Drug Class: Bladder-Active Drugs (p. 587)

CHAPTER OBJECTIVES

1. Explain the major action and effects of drugs used to treat disorders of the urinary tract.
2. Identify baseline data the nurse should collect on a continuous basis for comparison and evaluation of drug effectiveness.
3. Identify important nursing assessments and interventions associated with the drug therapy and treatment of diseases of the urinary system.
4. Identify essential components involved in planning patient education that will enhance compliance with the treatment regimen.
5. Analyze Table 41-1 and identify specific portions of a urinalysis report that would indicate proteinuria, dehydration, infection, or renal disease.
6. Prepare a chart of antimicrobial agents used to treat urinary tract infections. Give the drug names, the organisms treated, and special considerations (such as the need for acidic urine, changes in urine color, and effect on urine tests).
7. Develop a health teaching plan for an individual who has repeated urinary tract infections.

KEY TERMS

pyelonephritis
cystitis
prostatitis
urethritis
acidification
antispasmodic agent

ASSIGNMENTS

Read textbook, pp. 580-590.
Study Key Terms associated with chapter content.
Complete the Collaborative Activity as assigned.
Study Review Sheet for Chapter 41.
Complete Chapter 41 Practice Quiz.
Complete End-of-Chapter Math Review and Critical Thinking Questions.
Complete Chapter 41 Exam.

WEB RESEARCH ACTIVITY

Access: www.kidney.org
Select: Professional
A-Z Category
Treatment
Analgesic
What effect can the long-term or prolonged use of analgesics such as aspirin, acetaminophen, ibuprofen, ketoprofen, and naproxen sodium have on kidney function?

COLLABORATIVE ACTIVITY

Complete the following as preparation for in-class discussion and group work that may be assigned by the instructor.
Compare the premedication assessments needed for fosfomycins, quinolones, and bladder-active agents.

Copyright © 2004 Mosby Inc. All rights reserved.

Drugs Used to Treat Disorders of the Urinary System

Review Sheet

The QUESTION column and the ANSWER column have been offset so that you can cover the answers while reading the questions, allowing you to assess your knowledge.

Question	Answer
1. Differentiate among pyelonephritis, cystitis, prostatitis, and urethritis.	
2. Identify the components of an assessment of the urinary tract.	1. Pyelonephritis is kidney infection, cystitis is bladder infection, prostatitis is prostate gland infection, and urethritis is infection of the urethra.
3. Why is the use of strict aseptic technique needed with indwelling catheters?	2. See textbook, pp. 580-581.
4. In the elderly, what is a common sign of a urinary tract infection (UTI)?	3. Prevent UTIs
5. Study Table 41-1 to identify details found on a routine urinalysis report.	4. Confusion
6. What measures should be taught to prevent UTIs?	5. See Table 41-1, textbook p. 582.
7. Should a urine specimen for bacterial culture and sensitivity be collected before or after starting antimicrobial therapy?	6. Personal hygiene measures—wiping front to back in female, keeping perineal area clean, avoiding nylon underwear and constrictive clothing in perineal area, avoiding scented bubble bath products and colored toilet paper, washing the perineal area immediately before and after intercourse, and urinating after intercourse
8. What health teaching should be completed when a patient has a UTI?	7. Before giving the first dose of an antimicrobial agent
9. What is the action of a urinary antimicrobial agent?	8. Force fluids, 2000 ml or more per day. Continue medication for the entire course of treatment, even if symptoms have subsided fairly rapidly. Return for urine culture when scheduled. Have patient report perineal itching, vaginal discharge, or breakdown of tissue. Teach the patient ways to prevent future infections.
10. What criteria are used to select a urinary antimicrobial agent?	9. It is an antimicrobial agent that, if sufficiently concentrated in the urine, has an antiseptic effect on the urine and the urinary tract.
11. What is the mechanism of action of fosfomycin (Monurol)?	10. Identification of the specific pathogen by gram stain or urine culture and sensitivity

Copyright © 2004 Mosby Inc. All rights reserved.

12. What are the desired therapeutic outcomes of therapy with quinolone-type drugs?

13. Why are some urinary antimicrobial agents prescribed to be taken after the urine culture is sterile?

14. What drug class is newly approved for one-dose treatment of UTIs?

15. Identify premedication assessments used for quinolone therapy.

16. How is fosfomycin (Monurol) administered?

17. What are the major advantages of norfloxacin over other quinolones for the treatment of UTIs?

18. What type of anemia precludes the use of quinolone antibiotics?

19. Why must the urine be acidic during the administration of methenamine mandelate (Mandelamine)?

20. Urine pH should be maintained below what value for optimal results from methenamine mandelate therapy?

21. How is urinary tract acidification accomplished?

22. What drugs cause alkalinization of the urine?

23. What color change in the urine may occur with nitrofurantoin therapy?

24. Which urinary antimicrobial agent is more likely to cause photosensitivity?

25. Name two medicines that may be used in non-obstructive urinary retention (e.g., postoperatively, during postpartum period).

26. What drug should be readily available for treatment of serious adverse effects of bethanechol?

27. What is oxybutynin chloride (Ditropan) used to treat?

28. Name a urinary analgesic and describe its action.

29. What changes in urine color can often occur following the administration of phenazopyridine?

11. Inhibits bacterial cell wall synthesis and reduces adherence of bacteria to epithelial cells of urinary tract

12. Resolution of the urinary tract infection

13. To prevent recurrence of a urinary tract infection

14. Fosfomycin antibiotics (Fosfomycin, Monurol)

15. See textbook, p. 585.

16. Empty entire contents of single-dose packet into 3–4 oz of water (not hot), stir to dissolve, and ingest immediately.

17. It is broad-spectrum with activity against gram-positive and -negative microorganisms. It also can be administered orally to patients.

18. Glucose-6-phosphate dehydrogenase deficiency

19. For methenamine mandelate (Mandelamine) to be effective it must be converted to formaldehyde to suppress the growth of bacteria. The urine has to be acidic for this reaction to occur. Therefore, the patient may have vitamin C prescribed simultaneously for this purpose.

20. When the pH is above 5.5, methenamine is less likely to be converted to formaldehyde. Therefore, it needs to be maintained at 5.5 or below.

21. Vitamin C

22. Acetazolamide and sodium bicarbonate

23. Urine may become tinted yellow to rust-brown.

24. Nalidixic acid (NegGram)

25. Bethanechol chloride (Urecholine) and neostigmine (Prostigmin)

26. Atropine sulfate

27. Ditropan is a bladder antispasmodic.

28. Phenazopyridine hydrochloride (Pyridium) acts as a local anesthetic on the mucosa of the ureters and bladder, reducing spasm.

29. Reddish-orange urine. Inform the patient not to be alarmed.

Copyright © 2004 Mosby Inc. All rights reserved.

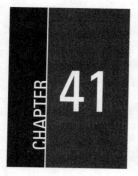

Student Name_____

CHAPTER 41

Drugs Used to Treat Disorders of the Urinary System

Practice Quiz

COMPLETION

Complete the following statements.

1. In the presence of acidic urine, methenamine mandelate (Mandelamine) forms

    _____.

2. Nitrofurantoin is an effective antibiotic for systemic infections. (<u>True or False</u>)

3. The urine color that may occur with nitrofurantoin therapy is _____.

4. Bethanechol and neostigmine are used to treat what urinary disorder? _____

5. The class of antibiotic used for single-dose treatment of a urinary tract infection is

    _____.

6. In order for methenamine mandelate (Mandelamine) to be active the urine must be at a pH of _____ or below.

7. The medication used to acidify urine is

    _____.

8. What laboratory tests should be completed before starting a urinary antimicrobial agent?

9. The action of _____ occurs as a result of altering the ability of bacteria to synthesize a cell wall and to adhere to the urinary tract epithelial cells.

10. A quinolone antibiotic should not be administered to a patient with _____.

11. Oxybutynin chloride (Ditropan) is used to treat

    _____.

12. The onset of action for phenazopyridine hydrochloride (Pyridium) is _____ after oral administration.

13. Tolterodine is used to _____.

END-OF-CHAPTER MATH REVIEW

1. Ordered: bethanechol chloride (Urecholine) 2.5 mg, SC, stat
    On hand: bethanechol chloride 5 mg/ml
    Give: _____ ml

2. Ordered: methenamine mandelate (Mandelamine) 750 mg, PO
    On hand: methenamine mandelate 0.5 g/5 ml suspension
    Give: _____ ml

CRITICAL THINKING QUESTIONS

A 64-year-old resident of Longmeadow nursing home has developed her third UTI in the past 4 months.

1. What assessments should be made?

2. Discuss appropriate nursing actions during the treatment of the current UTI and measures to prevent another episode.

REVIEW QUESTIONS

_____ 1. A patient receiving methenamine mandelate (Mandelamine) has a urine pH of 5.2. The nurse knows that the _____ given has _____ the urine sufficiently for the medication to be active.
   a. probenecid (Benemid); acidified
   b. ascorbic acid; acidified
   c. ascorbic acid; alkalinized
   d. probenecid (Benemid); alkalinized

_____ 2. Fosfomycin (Monurol) is given:
   a. once.
   b. bid.
   c. tid.
   d. qid.

Copyright © 2004 Mosby Inc. All rights reserved.

_____ 3. The use of _____ reduces the urinary excretion of cinoxacin and norfloxacin.
a. formaldehyde in a medication
b. probenecid (Benemid)
c. nitrofurantoin (Furadantin, Macrodantin)
d. bethanechol chloride (Urecholine)

_____ 4. _____ causes the urine to become reddish-orange in color.
a. Probenecid (Benemid)
b. Nitrofurantoin (Furadantin, Macrodantin)
c. Bethanechol chloride (Urecholine)
d. Phenazopyridine hydrochloride (Pyridium)

Copyright © 2004 Mosby Inc. All rights reserved.

Drugs Used to Treat Glaucoma and Other Eye Disorders

Syllabus

CHAPTER CONTENT

Anatomy and Physiology of the Eye (p. 591)
Glaucoma (p. 592)
Drug Therapy for Glaucoma (p 593)
    Drug Class: Osmotic Agents (p. 595)
    Drug Class: Carbonic Anhydrase Inhibitors
      (p. 598)
    Drug Class: Cholinergic Agents (p. 599)
    Drug Class: Cholinesterase Inhibitors
      (p. 599)
    Drug Class: Adrenergic Agents (p. 601)
    Drug Class: Beta-Adrenergic Blocking
      Agents (p. 602)
    Drug Class: Prostaglandin Agonist (p. 602)
Other Ophthalmic Drugs (p. 604)
    Drug Class: Anticholinergic Agents (p. 604)
    Drug Class: Antifungal Agents (p. 605)
    Drug Class: Antiviral Agents (p. 605)
    Drug Class: Antibacterial Agents (p. 606)
    Drug Class: Corticosteroids (p. 606)
    Drug Class: Anti-Inflammatory Agents
      (p. 606)
    Drug Class: Antihistamines (p. 607)
    Drug Class: Antiallergic Agents (p. 607)
    Drug Class: Sodium Fluorescein (p. 607)
    Drug Class: Artificial Tear Solutions (p. 607)
    Drug Class: Ophthalmic Irrigants (p. 608)

CHAPTER OBJECTIVES

1. Describe the normal flow of aqueous humor in
   the eye.
2. Identify the changes in normal flow of aqueous
   humor caused by open-angle and closed-angle
   glaucoma.
3. Explain baseline data that should be gathered
   when an eye disorder exists.

4. Review the correct procedure for instilling eye
   drops or eye ointments.
5. Develop teaching plans for a person with an eye
   infection and one receiving glaucoma medication.

KEY TERMS

cornea	near point
sclera	zonular fibers
iris	cycloplegia
sphincter muscle	lacrimal canaliculi
miosis	intraocular pressure
dilator muscle	closed-angle glaucoma
mydriasis	open-angle glaucoma
lens	

ASSIGNMENTS

Read textbook, pp. 591-608.
Study Key Terms associated with chapter content.
Complete Collaborative Activities as assigned.
Study Review Sheet for Chapter 42.
Complete Chapter 42 Practice Quiz.
Complete End-of-Chapter Math Review and Critical
    Thinking Questions.
Complete Chapter 42 Exam.

WEB RESEARCH ACTIVITY

Access: www.eyesearch.com/eye.medications.htm
Select: Eye Medication Questions
What are common questions asked by patients of
the health care provider regarding eye medications?

Copyright © 2004 Mosby Inc. All rights reserved.

COLLABORATIVE ACTIVITIES

Complete the following as preparation for in-class discussion and group work that may be assigned by the instructor.

A 55-year-old patient was found to have an elevated intraocular pressure (IOP) in both eyes on routine examination. Further examination revealed cupping of the optic discs and a nerve fiber bundle defect consistent with glaucoma. Gonioscopy indicated that the anterior chamber angles were open in both eyes. Upon questioning, the patient reveals a family history of glaucoma. The patient's diagnosis is primary open-angle glaucoma of genetic origin. A prescription order was written to start treatment:

Timolol 0.25% 1 drop in each eye twice daily

1. What is the action of the medicine prescribed?
2. Explain the procedure the nurse would use to teach the patient to administer this medication.
3. What additional patient education should be performed?

Copyright © 2004 Mosby Inc. All rights reserved.

Drugs Used to Treat Glaucoma and Other Eye Disorders

Review Sheet

The QUESTION column and the ANSWER column have been offset so that you can cover the answers while reading the questions, allowing you to assess your knowledge.

Question	Answer
1. Identify the major structures of the eye (e.g., cornea, pupil, iris, canal of Schlemm).	
2. Define: *miosis, mydriasis, cycloplegia, intraocular pressure,* and *glaucoma.*	1. Refer to textbook for a review of the basic structure and function of the eye. In particular, examine the location of the canal of Schlemm, Fig. 42-3. Note that dilation of the iris could result in a blockage of the canal of Schlemm.
3. Explain the normal drainage system of the eye.	2. Miosis: contraction of the iris sphincter muscle causing narrowing of the pupil of the eye. Mydriasis: contraction of the dilator muscle and relaxation of the sphincter muscle causing dilation of the pupil of the eye. Cycloplegia: paralysis of the ciliary muscles. IOP results from the excessive production of the aqueous humor or from decreased fluid outflow. Glaucoma: an eye disorder characterized by an increase in the IOP.
4. What are the symptoms of acute closed-angle glaucoma?	3. Aqueous humor flows between the lens and the iris into the anterior chamber of the eye. It drains through channels located near the junction of the cornea and the sclera through meshwork into the canal of Schlemm and then into the venous system of the eye.
5. What is the principal treatment of open-angle glaucoma?	4. Gradual onset of intermittent symptoms, especially when the pupil is dilated. Symptoms include blurred vision, halos around white lights, frontal headache, and eye pain.
6. Identify the normal intraocular pressure (IOP) reading when taken with a tonometer.	5. Historically, miotic agents (e.g., pilocarpine) were commonly used to increase outflow of aqueous humor; recently beta-adrenergic blocking agents (e.g., timolol maleate) are the initial drugs of choice. Other agents used are sympathomimetic agents (e.g., epinephrine), the carbonic anhydrase inhibitors (e.g., acetazolamide), and the cholinesterase inhibitors (e.g., echothiophate iodide).

Copyright © 2004 Mosby Inc. All rights reserved.

7. Compare the mechanisms of action of drugs used to lower IOP.

8. Describe the actions of drugs known as mydriatic agents and miotic agents.

6. 10–21 mm Hg

7. Osmotic agents: elevate osmotic pressure of the plasma, causing fluid from the extravascular spaces to be drawn into the blood, thereby reducing IOP.
   Carbonic anhydrase inhibitors: inhibit the enzyme carbonic anhydrase resulting in a decrease of aqueous humor production, thereby lowering IOP.
   Cholinergic agents: produce contraction of the iris (miosis) and ciliary body musculature (accommodation), thereby permitting outflow of aqueous humor by widening the filtration angle, thus decreasing IOP.
   Cholinesterase inhibitors: prevent destruction of acetylcholine, the cholinergic neurotransmitter within the eye. This results in increased cholinergic activity, and because of miosis the IOP is reduced.
   Adrenergic agents: have several uses in ophthalmology. These agents cause pupil dilation, increased outflow of aqueous humor, vasoconstriction, relaxation of ciliary muscle, and decreased formation of aqueous humor.
   Beta-adrenergic blocking agents: thought to reduce production of aqueous humor.
   Prostaglandin agonists: increase outflow of aqueous humor.

9. What should the nurse look for when performing an assessment of the pupil?

10. What action does an osmotic diuretic have on the IOP?

11. What are side effects from osmotic agents that can be anticipated?

12. Osmotic agents may produce fluid overload or heart failure. What are the signs and symptoms of this?

13 Describe the nursing assessments needed during the administration of osmotic agents.

8. Mydriatic agents dilate the pupil and miotic agents constrict the pupil.

9. Pupil size, shape, and accommodation when exposed to light.

10. Osmotic agents reduce the volume of intraocular fluid present.

11. Thirst, nausea, dehydration, electrolyte imbalance (potassium, sodium, and chloride), headache, and circulatory overload.

12. Fluid overload/pulmonary edema; apprehension; cyanosis; diaphoresis; rapid pulse; dyspnea; and moist, gurgling-type respirations. Patients may also develop a productive cough with frothy, pink-tinged sputum.

14. Explain the administration techniques involved with osmotic agents.

13. Check urinary output frequently and record the amount accurately. An indwelling catheter is usually inserted, depending on the circumstances. Assess the intravenous site q 15 min, and take vital signs q 15 min, or more frequently, as ordered. Check the rate of infusion at least q 30 minutes.

Copyright © 2004 Mosby Inc. All rights reserved.

15. Before administering a carbonic anhydrase inhibitor, the nurse should check the patient's chart for _____.
16. Cholinergic agents cause the pupil to _____.

17. List common side effects of cholinergic agents.

18. Explain how the systemic effects of cholinergic agents can be minimized.
19. Cholinesterase inhibitors block the destruction of what neurotransmitter, causing prolonged cholinergic activity and resulting in miosis and decreased IOP?
20. An overdose of a cholinesterase inhibitor will cause what symptoms?
21. What actions should be taken when cholinesterase inhibitors are used by farmers handling insecticides and pesticides?

22. Adrenergic agents cause pupil _____, and a _____ in formation of _____.

23. Adrenergic-blocking agents _____ IOP.
24. What premedication assessments should be made with adrenergic agents?
25. What types of patients should not receive beta-adrenergic blocking agents?
26. What are beta-adrenergic blocking agents used to treat?

27. What are some advantages of using beta-adrenergic blocking agents to reduce IOP?

28. When should beta-adrenergic blocking agents be withheld?

29. What is the action of a prostaglandin agonist on the eye?

14. See textbook, p. 587.

15. A history of allergy to sulfonamides, whether the patient is pregnant; contact lenses are removed (before dorzolamide drops); gastric symptoms, and IOP value.
16. Constrict; this increases or widens the filtration angle near the canal of Schlemm, permitting outflow of the aqueous humor.
17. Reduced visual acuity, conjunctival irritation, headache, pain, and discomfort.
18. To reduce systemic absorption from the highly vascular nasal tissues, block the inner canthus of the eye for 1–2 minutes immediately after instilling the eye drop(s).
19. Acetylcholine

20. Systemic toxicity manifested by sweating, salivation, vomiting, abdominal cramping, urinary incontinence, diarrhea, bronchospasms, arrhythmias, and bradycardia
21. Added absorption of insecticides and pesticides may occur through the skin and respiratory tract. Respiratory masks and frequent washing and clothing changes are advisable.
22. Dilation; decrease; aqueous humor
23. Reduce IOP; also may reduce production of aqueous humor
24. Vital signs including blood pressure, visual acuity, and IOP
25. Patients with a respiratory condition (e.g., bronchitis, emphysema, and asthma) because beta blockers may produce severe bronchoconstriction. Use in patients with heart failure should be limited to those persons whose disease is under control because hypotension, bradycardia, and/or heart failure may develop with use of these agents.
26. In ophthalmology beta-adrenergic blockers are used to reduce elevated IOP in chronic open-angle glaucoma or ocular hypertension.
27. Beta-adrenergic blocking agents do not blur the vision and have little or no effect on pupil size or visual acuity.
28. Withhold the beta-adrenergic blocking agent and notify the health care provider if bradycardia, hypertension, or respiratory disorders are present.

Copyright © 2004 Mosby Inc. All rights reserved.

30. Explain the precautions for instilling ophthalmic prostaglandin agonist medications to a person who wears contacts.
31. The class of drugs that produces both mydriasis and cycloplegia is _____.
32. What effect does the use of an anticholinergic agent have on IOP?
33. When mydriatic agents are administered, what patient reaction to bright lights is observed?
34. What specific medication is used to treat an ophthalmic fungal infection?
35. Antiviral agents may produce what adverse effects?
36. What is the major use of corticosteroid therapy in the eye?
37. What eye complications can occur with the long-term use of corticosteroids?

38. What is the desired action of an antihistamine on eye disorders?

39. Review the procedures and abbreviations used for administering eye medications.

40. The drug sodium fluorescein is used for what purpose?

41. When are artificial tears used?

29. Decrease IOP and increase outflow of aqueous humor

30. Remove contact lenses, instill medication, and wait 15 minutes to reinsert the contact lenses
31. Anticholinergic agents

32. Increase IOP

33. Squinting because of excessive dilation; reduced visual acuity
34. Natamycin (Natacyn)

35. Sensitivity to bright lights, visual haze, lacrimation, redness, and burning
36. For allergic reactions of the eye and other acute, noninfectious inflammatory conditions of the eye
37. Increased IOP, glaucoma, and cataracts. Do not use with bacterial, fungal, or viral infections of the eye because corticosteroids decrease defense mechanisms and reduce resistance to pathologic organisms.
38. Antihistamines relieve signs and symptoms and prevent itching associated with allergic conjunctivitis.
39. os = left eye
    od = right eye
    ou = both eyes (See textbook, pp. 108-109.)
40. Fitting hard contact lenses and as diagnostic aid to identify foreign bodies in the eye or corneal abrasions
41. Artificial tear solutions are products made to mimic natural secretions of the eye. They provide lubrication for dry eyes and for artificial eyes. They are also used to prevent drying when a person has lost the blink reflex such as during surgery or when comatose.

Copyright © 2004 Mosby Inc. All rights reserved.

CHAPTER 42

Drugs Used to Treat Glaucoma and Other Eye Disorders

Practice Quiz

COMPLETION

Complete the following statements.

The abbreviation 1. _____ means left eye, 2. _____ means right eye, and 3. _____ means both eyes.

When administering eye medications, it is important to 4. _____ for 5. _____ minutes immediately after instilling the eye drops to minimize systemic effects.

Cholinesterase inhibitors destroy cholinesterase, an enzyme that destroys the neurotransmitter 6. _____. The prolonged action of the neurotransmitter lowers IOP and causes 7. _____ of the pupil.

Adrenergic agents cause 8. _____ of the pupil.

The action of osmotic agents on glaucoma is to 9. _____.

The mechanism of action of carbonic anhydrase inhibitors used to treat glaucoma is 10. _____.

Antiviral agents may cause what side effects? (List minimum of four.)
11.

Corticosteroids are used in the eye to treat 12. _____.

When carbonic anhydrase inhibitors are administered, IOP is reduced by 13._____.

Beta-adrenergic blocking agents should not be administered to patients with 14._____.

Before administering any beta-adrenergic blocking agent, the nurse should check and record the 15._____.

Carbonic anhydrase inhibitors should not be administered to a patient who is allergic to 16._____.

END-OF-CHAPTER MATH REVIEW

1. Ordered: 1.5 g/kg mannitol 15% solution IV over 30 minutes.
    The patient weighs 156 lbs. What is the weight in kg? _____
    The total g of mannitol to administer is: _____.

CRITICAL THINKING QUESTIONS

1. While working in the eye clinic, the nurse observes that several of the patients being treated for glaucoma complain that the medications cause pain and headache and that reading ability is diminished. How would you respond to these statements?
2. Develop a teaching plan for a patient who is to self-administer Betoptic, one drop twice daily.

REVIEW QUESTIONS

_____ 1. Osmotic agents act by:
   a. pulling fluid from the extravascular spaces into the blood.
   b. shifting fluid from the blood into the extravascular spaces.
   c. inhibiting enzymes from producing aqueous humor.
   d. causing pupil dilation and increased outflow of aqueous humor.

Copyright © 2004 Mosby Inc. All rights reserved.

Student Name_____

_____ 2. The therapeutic outcome when instilling an adrenergic agent in the eyes is to:
a. produce miosis.
b. produce mydriasis.
c. act as an irritant.
d. prevent production of aqueous humor.

_____ 3. Sodium fluorescein is used to:
a. inhibit the release of histamine.
b. treat an infection.
c. stain the eye for examination.
d. prevent production of aqueous humor.

_____ 4. Before administering a beta-adrenergic blocking agent for reduction of IOP, the nurse should check to see if the patient has a history of:
a. blood dyscrasias.
b. diabetes mellitus or cardiac disease.
c. hypertension or respiratory disorders.
d. liver disease.

Copyright © 2004 Mosby Inc. All rights reserved.

Drugs Affecting Neoplasms

Syllabus

CHAPTER CONTENT

Cancer and the Use of Antineoplastic Agents
   (p. 609)
Drug Therapy for Cancer (p. 610)
   Drug Class: Alkylating Agents (p. 614)
   Drug Class: Antimetabolites (p. 614)
   Drug Class: Natural Products (p. 614)
   Drug Class: Antineoplastic Antibiotics (p. 614)
   Drug Class: Hormones (p. 621)

CHAPTER OBJECTIVES

1. Cite the goals of chemotherapy.
2. Explain the normal cycle for cell replication and describe the effects of cell cycle-specific and cell cycle-nonspecific drugs within this process.
3. Cite the rationale for giving chemotherapeutic drugs on a precise time schedule.
4. State which types of chemotherapeutic agents are cell cycle-specific and those that are cell cycle-nonspecific.
5. Describe the role of immunomodulators and chemoprotective agents in treating cancer.
6. Study the nursing assessments and interventions needed for persons experiencing adverse effects from chemotherapy.
7. Develop patient education objectives for a patient receiving chemotherapy.

KEY TERMS

cancer
metastases
cell cycle-specific
cell cycle-nonspecific

palliation
combination therapy
immunomodulators
chemoprotective agents

ASSIGNMENTS

Read textbook, pp. 609-624.
Study Key Terms associated with chapter content.
Complete Collaborative Activities as assigned.
Study Review Sheet for Chapter 43.
Complete Chapter 43 Practice Quiz.
Complete End-of-Chapter Math Review and Critical Thinking Questions.
Complete Chapter 43 Exam.

WEB RESEARCH ACTIVITY

Access: www.cancer.org
Select: Clinical Trials
Review questions that should be asked by the patient when considering participation in a clinical trial protocol.

Register on the professional site.
Review upcoming events in your local area on cancer topics and identify local resources available.

COLLABORATIVE ACTIVITIES

Complete the following as preparation for in-class discussion and group work that may be assigned by the instructor.
Many times, a cancer patient will have an order for administration of a biologic response modifier. Research the following drugs:
1. Epoetin (Epogen, Procrit):
   What is the action of epoetin on blood cells?
   Why is epoetin also used in end-stage renal disease?
   What premedication assessments should be made prior to epoetin administration? What side effects may occur after the drug is administered?

Copyright © 2004 Mosby Inc. All rights reserved.

2. Filgrastim (Neupogen)
   What is the action of filgrastim on blood cells? What storage parameters are suggested for this drug?

3. Leucovorin calcium (Wellcovorin)
   What is a "leucovorin rescue"? What is the purpose of a leucovorin rescue and what nursing responsibilities are associated with its administration?

4. Mesna (Mesnex)
   What is the action of this drug? Why is it administered to patients receiving ifosfamide?

Copyright © 2004 Mosby Inc. All rights reserved.

Drugs Affecting Neoplasms

Review Sheet

The QUESTION column and the ANSWER column have been offset so that you can cover the answers while reading the questions, allowing you to assess your knowledge.

Question	Answer
1. What are the phases of the cell cycle?	
2. What is combination therapy?	1. See textbook, p. 609.
3. What are immunomodulators and chemoprotective agents?	2. Using both a cell cycle-specific and cell cycle-nonspecific agent at the same time for treatment of the cancer
4. State baseline assessments needed during the initiation of cancer therapy.	3. Immunomodulator drugs boost or strengthen the person's own immune system as a defense for the cancer; chemoprotective agents help reduce the toxicity of the chemotherapeutic agents.
5. Cite the goals of chemotherapy and specific factors affecting the patient dosage, drug identification, drug preparation, and drug administration.	4. The type of cancer being treated; the emotional status of the patient; the understanding the patient has of the diagnosis; the patient's usual methods of coping; the patient's degree of pain, usual eating pattern, and elimination pattern.
6. State the nursing interventions needed for persons experiencing adverse effects from chemotherapy.	5. Control of growth of the cancer cells is the primary goal of treatment. See other goals, textbook, p. 610. Since many of the cancer drugs have similar spellings, it is imperative to check the drug name closely. Cancer drugs are given in a variety of forms: orally, intravenously, by bolus, and so forth. Therefore, the physician's order must be checked carefully. Many cancer drugs require reconstitution—follow directions precisely. When drugs are given IV, check the IV site carefully for extravasation. During oral administration, maintain an accurate record of the medication on the flow sheet and record any side effects experienced.
7. State the five classes of antineoplastic agents.	6. See textbook for adverse effects associated with chemotherapy. Monitor for nausea and vomiting, hydration, positioning, changes in bowel patterns, stomatitis, alopecia, neurotoxicity, musculoskeletal complaints, bone marrow depression, infection, thrombocytopenia, and activity intolerance.

Copyright © 2004 Mosby Inc. All rights reserved.

8. Define *cell cycle-specific* and *cell cycle-nonspecific* antineoplastic agents.
9. When is chemotherapy most effective?

10. Why is it difficult to kill tumor cells in the G_O phase?
11. What criteria are used to choose the type of chemotherapy to be administered?

12. Examine Table 43-2, Immunomodulators, and study the action of agents listed. Which agent stimulates production of RBCs?
Which agent is known as a *human granulocyte stimulating factor*? Which agent is known as a *granulocyte macrophage colony stimulating factor* (GM-CSF)?
13. What is/are the action(s) of trastuzumab (Herceptin)?

14. Discuss the three chemoprotective agents amifostine, dexrazoxane, and mesna. What are they primarily used for?
15. List questions that may be asked when taking a health history of the risk factors the individual has for development of cancer.
16. What are the common side effects to expect/report associated with chemotherapy?
17. Why is it sometimes advisable to discuss birth control and reproductive counseling prior to initiation of chemotherapy?

18. What type of oral hygiene measures should be instituted when chemotherapy is administered?

19. What are common signs and symptoms of bleeding the nurse should assess for, especially when platelet counts are decreased?
20. What is meant by "neutropenic precautions"?

7. Alkylating agents, antibiotics, antimetabolites, natural products, and hormones
8. The action of cell cycle-specific antineoplastic agents occurs in a specific phase of the cell's growth. Cell cycle-nonspecific antineoplastics are active throughout the cell cycle.
9. When cells of the tumor are small in number and rapidly dividing
10. Many chemotherapeutic agents kill cells when in the replication phase. Cells in the resting phase (G_O) of the cell cycle are not dividing and therefore are not susceptible to destruction by chemotherapeutic agents.
11. Type of tumor cells, the rate of growth, and size of the tumor.

12. Examine Table 43-2, Immunomodulators, p. 620.
Epoetin alpha (Procrit), filgrastim (Neupogen), sargramostim (Leukine)
13. Used in treatment of breast cancer with HER_2 positive tumors. See Table 43-2 for more details.

14. Examine Table 43-3 for detailed discussion.

15. See textbook, p. 610.

16. It depends on the type of chemotherapy drug administered. Generally, myelosuppression, anemia, bleeding, stomatitis, diarrhea or constipation, alopecia, anorexia, nausea, and vomiting are common symptoms. See a medical-surgical textbook for specific interventions for each of these side effects. Also read implementation and health promotion, pp. 611-614.
17. Reproductive abilities may be affected and agents may pass through the placental barrier; thus being potentially harmful to a fetus.
18. See textbook, pp. 454-456. (See also Chapter 31.)

19. Epistaxis, hematuria, bruises, petechiae, dark, tarry stools, "coffee ground emesis," blurred vision, excessive menstrual flow, hemoglobin, hematocrit

Copyright © 2004 Mosby Inc. All rights reserved.

21. When several courses of intravenously administered chemotherapy are planned, the antineoplastic agents are frequently administered via _____.

22. What three types of emesis are associated with antineoplastic therapy?
23. Identify whether the following agents are cell cycle-specific or cell cycle-nonspecific: alkylating agents, antimetabolites, natural products, and antineoplastic antibiotics. What is the action of hormones?

20. Neutropenic precautions are designed to minimize the individual's exposure to microorganisms. Handwashing, avoiding exposure to individuals with infection, no fresh flowers or fruits and vegetables, no freestanding water (e.g., plants, flowers, humidifiers, denture cups). Avoid pets and persons receiving immunizations.
21. Implantable vascular access devices

22. Acute, delayed, and anticipatory emesis (see also Chapter 33)

23. Alkylating agents: cell cycle-nonspecific
Antimetabolites: many are cell cycle-specific S phase
Natural products: cell cycle-specific
Antineoplastic antibiotics: act through various mechanisms to prevent replication as well as RNA synthesis. See drug class for discussion of specific antibiotic agents that are cell cycle-specific and cell cycle-nonspecific.
Hormones: alter the hormone environment of the cell

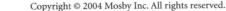

Copyright © 2004 Mosby Inc. All rights reserved.

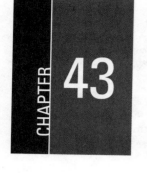

CHAPTER 43

Drugs Affecting Neoplasms

Practice Quiz

COMPLETION

Complete the following statements.

1. A patient with breast cancer is receiving chemotherapy with cyclophosphamide, Adriamycin, and fluorouracil. Her latest laboratory report shows:

Patient Report	Normal Range
WBC: 3,000	5,000 to 10,000/mm³
Hgb: 9.5	12–16 g/dl
Platelets: 100,000	150,000/mm³ to 400,000/mm³
RBC: 4.5	4.0–5.0 million/mm³

Use available resources to identify significance of this data and then develop nursing diagnoses to support your conclusions.

2. List nursing interventions appropriate for neutropenia.
3. Alkylating agents are cell cycle-_____.
4. Antimetabolites are cell cycle-_____.
5. Natural products are cell cycle-_____.
6. The primary therapeutic outcome desired of chemotherapy is _____.
7. Describe antiemetics administered in relation to the administration of IV chemotherapy.
8. What data should be collected to assess an individual's hydration status?
9. Describe nursing interventions needed for a neutropenic patient.
10. The patient has 1000 ml lactated Ringer's running at 80 ml/hr. Using a microdrip administration set, at what drip rate per minute should the IV be infused?

A patient weighing 135 lbs is to receive 5 mcg/kg/day, SC, of filgrastim. The drug is available for injection 300 mcg/ml.

11. How many kg does the patient weigh? _____ (Carry conversions to hundredths, round to tenths.)

12. Based on the data given, how many mcg of filgrastim would be administered?
    Give: _____ mcg.
13. Give _____ ml of filgrastim.
14. Mesna is used to prevent the toxic effects of what drugs on what organ?
15. Oprelvekin (Neumega) stimulates production of _____.
16. Trastuzumab (Herceptin) is used in the treatment of _____.
17. A _____ type of chemotherapeutic agent is dose-dependent.

END-OF-CHAPTER MATH REVIEW

1. Ordered: cefazolin 1 g, IV, q 8 h
   On hand: cefazolin 1 g, diluted in 50 ml D_5W
   To administer this medication over a 30-minute period on a pump that is calibrated in ml/hr, at what rate should the pump be set? _____
2. Ordered: PCA morphine sulfate 1 mg/dose, with 6-minute lockout/maximum 30 mg/q 4 h
   Discuss how to initiate the PCA setup on this patient and how to set up the initial settings on the PCA pump. Describe when and how to record the amount of morphine sulfate used each shift.

CRITICAL THINKING QUESTIONS

T.K., age 65, has small-cell cancer of the lung with brain and liver metastases. He has had several grand mal seizures in the past month. His orders read:

1. Daily weight
2. Assist with ambulation as tolerated
3. Routine vitals
4. Seizure precautions
5. Intake and output

Copyright © 2004 Mosby Inc. All rights reserved.

Student Name _____

6. Heparin lock the IV
7. Physical therapy consult to assist with plan for self-care at home
8. IV site dressing change q 72 h
9. Medications:
   Folic acid 1 mg, PO, q d
   Multivitamin 1 PO, q d
   Ensure 1 can, tid
   KCl 20 mEq, PO, bid
   Normal saline flush 2.5 ml, heparin lock after meds
   Ranitidine 300 mg, PO, q hs
   Ondansetron 32 mg, IV, 30 minutes before chemotherapy
   Dexamethasone 4 mg, IV, q 12 h
   Phenytoin 200 mg, PO, qd
   Lorazepam 1 mg, PO, q 12 h

Develop a Kardex for this patient and a Medication Administration Record that includes the scheduling of each medication.

For each medication prescribed, state the drug action and side effects to expect and report.

For IV medications prescribed, state the drug action, rate of administration, dilution for administration, monitoring required, and what type of IV setup would be required to initiate the intravenous delivery of the medications.

A 68-year-old patient has gastric cancer with liver metastasis. She has the following medication orders:

5% Dextrose/0.45% normal saline at 100 ml/hr
Ondansetron 32 mg, IV, in 50 ml D$_5$W to run for 15 minutes
Cisplatin 35 mg in 250 ml normal saline to run for 30 minutes
Add mannitol 12.5 g to cisplatin
Leucovorin 20 mg, IV push

1. To carry out these orders, what type of an intravenous setup would be required?
2. Because you are not "chemo certified" and could not start the chemotherapy drugs as a student nurse, what nursing responsibilities would you have during the execution of these drug orders?
3. What is the action of each medication, side effects to expect, and side effects to report?
4. How would you set a pump to deliver the ondansetron in 15 minutes? (The pump is calibrated in ml/hr.)

REVIEW QUESTIONS

_____ 1. When the drug monograph says that a particular chemotherapeutic agent may cause thrombocytopenia, it is important that the nurse teach the patient to:
   a. avoid having fresh flowers, vegetables, or fruit in the room.
   b. rise slowly from a sitting or lying position to avoid hypotension.
   c. report "coffee-ground" emesis, hematuria, or epistaxis.
   d. obtain adequate daily exercise.

_____ 2. The purpose of administering epoetin alfa (Procrit) to a patient receiving chemotherapy is to:
   a. stimulate WBC (white blood cell) production.
   b. stimulate RBC (red blood cell) production.
   c. prevent thrombocytopenia.
   d. protect the kidneys from toxic chemotherapy.

_____ 3. The drug mesna (Mesnex) is given to:
   a. stimulate WBC (white blood cell) production.
   b. stimulate RBC (red blood cell) production.
   c. prevent thrombocytopenia.
   d. protect the bladder from toxic chemotherapy.

_____ 4. The purpose of androgens in the treatment of cancer is to:
   a. alter the female hormone environment to prevent cancer cell growth.
   b. facilitate the development of testosterone to prevent cancer cell growth.
   c. inhibit RNA synthesis.
   d. provide a cell cycle-specific chemotherapeutic agent.

Copyright © 2004 Mosby Inc. All rights reserved.

44 Drugs Used to Treat the Muscular System

Syllabus

CHAPTER CONTENT

Muscle Relaxants and Neuromuscular Blocking
  Agents (p. 625)
Drug Therapy for Muscle Disorders (p. 628)
  Drug Class: Centrally Acting Skeletal Muscle
    Relaxants (p. 628)
  Drug Class: Direct-Acting Skeletal Muscle
    Relaxants (p. 630)
  Drug Class: Neuromuscular Blocking Agents
    (p. 631)

CHAPTER OBJECTIVES

1. Prepare a list of assessment data needed to evaluate a patient with a skeletal muscle disorder.
2. State the nursing assessments needed to monitor therapeutic response and development of
   side effects to expect and report from skeletal
   muscle relaxant therapy.
3. Develop a health teaching plan for patients receiving skeletal muscle relaxant therapy.
4. Describe the effect of centrally acting skeletal
   muscle relaxants on the central nervous system
   and the safety precautions required during their
   use.
5. Describe essential components of patient assessment used for patients receiving neuromuscular
   blocking agents.
6. State where information on the use of neuromuscular blocking agents in the patient's chart.
7. List the equipment that should be available in
   the immediate patient care area when neuromuscular blocking agents are to be administered.
8. Describe the physiologic effects of neuromuscular blocking agents.
9. Cite four uses of neuromuscular blocking
   agents.

10. Identify the effect of neuromuscular blocking
    agents on consciousness, memory, and the pain
    threshold.
11. Describe disease conditions that may affect the
    patient's ability to tolerate the use of neuromus-
    cular blocking agents.
12. List steps required to treat respiratory depres-
    sion.

KEY TERMS

cerebral palsy
multiple sclerosis
hypercapnia
muscle spasticity
hyperreflexia

clonus
stroke syndrome
neuromuscular
  blocking agents

ASSIGNMENTS

Read textbook, pp. 625-633.
Study Key Terms associated with chapter content.
Study Review Sheet for Chapter 44.
Complete Chapter 44 Practice Quiz.
Complete End-of-Chapter Math Review and Critical
  Thinking Questions.
Complete Chapter 44 Exam.

WEB RESEARCH ACTIVITY

Access: www.mdausa.org/
View the video on stem cell therapy.
What advances are being made in the field of stem
cell use to treat muscular diseases?

Copyright © 2004 Mosby Inc. All rights reserved.

CHAPTER 44

Drugs Used to Treat the Muscular System

Review Sheet

The QUESTION column and the ANSWER column have been offset so that you can cover the answers while reading the questions, allowing you to assess your knowledge.

Question	Answer
1. Describe the nursing assessments needed to evaluate a patient with a skeletal muscle disorder.	
2. What adjustments are usually required during the initial phase when treating an individual with muscle spasms and pain?	1. See textbook, pp. 625-628.
3. What nursing measures can be implemented to alleviate lower back pain?	2. Immobilize and elevate the affected part; range-of-motion exercises may be prescribed to prevent muscle atrophy and contractures.
4. Immediately following a muscle injury _____ packs will reduce the swelling.	3. Maintain proper body alignment; elevate the head of the bed 15–20 degrees and flex the knees slightly. Give prescribed analgesics and muscle relaxants.
5. To decrease swelling following an injury, how should the affected part be treated?	4. Ice
6. What two classes of drugs are used to relieve pain and inflammation associated with musculoskeletal disorders?	5. Elevated and immobilized
7. Compare the site of action of centrally acting and direct-acting muscle relaxants.	6. Analgesic agents are used for pain and anti-inflammatory agents are used to reduce the inflammatory response.
8. Both centrally acting and direct-acting skeletal muscle relaxants can produce hepatotoxicity. What are the signs and symptoms of this toxicity?	7. Centrally acting muscle relaxants depress the central nervous system. Their major benefit may be their sedative effects. Direct-acting skeletal muscle relaxants act directly on the skeletal muscle producing generalized, mild weakness of skeletal muscles.
9. What premedication assessments should be made before administering centrally acting skeletal muscle relaxants?	8. Anorexia, nausea, vomiting, jaundice, hepatomegaly, splenomegaly, and abnormal liver function tests (e.g., AST, ALT, LDH)
10. Which class of muscle relaxants can cause photosensitivity?	9. Baseline vital signs, mental status assessment, laboratory studies as ordered (e.g., liver function, complete blood count)
11. What are the primary uses of baclofen?	10. Direct-acting skeletal muscle relaxants
12. Describe the signs of respiratory depression.	11. Baclofen is used to manage muscle spasticity resulting from multiple sclerosis, spinal cord injuries, and other spinal cord diseases.

Copyright © 2004 Mosby Inc. All rights reserved.

13. What laboratory values would be used to confirm hypoxia and hypercapnia?

14. Why are centrally acting muscle relaxants not given to persons with long-term muscle spasticity?

15. What are the uses of dantrolene (Dantrium)?

16. Explain when and why neuromuscular blocking agents are administered.

17. What effect do neuromuscular blocking agents have on consciousness?

18. What nursing assessments should be made when a neuromuscular blocking agent has been administered?

19. Review the drug interactions that enhance therapeutic and toxic effects of neuromuscular blocking agents and identify the three classes of drugs commonly administered that may interact with neuromuscular blocking agents.

20. Where in the patient's chart is administration of a neuromuscular blocking agent recorded?

21. Name common neuromuscular blocking agents by their generic and brand names.

22. What premedication assessments should be done prior to the administration of a neuromuscular blocking agent?

23. Explain the treatment of overdose of neuromuscular blocking agents.

12. Early signs: restlessness; anxiety; decreased mental alertness; headache; increase in heart rate, blood pressure, and respiratory rate. Later signs: heart rate increases; blood pressure decreases; cyanosis; use of accessory chest, abdominal, and neck muscles in respiratory effort; flaring nostrils. Changes in mental status: confusion progressing to coma

13. Hypercapnia (elevated pCO_2), hypoxemia (decreased pO_2), and decreased oxygen saturation (SaO_2)

14. They would further reduce the functioning of the individual by reducing the overall strength of the remaining active muscle fibers.

15. Control spasticity of chronic disorders (e.g., cerebral palsy, multiple sclerosis, spinal cord injury, stroke syndrome). Dantrolene is also used to treat neuroleptic malignant syndrome.

16. To provide muscle relaxation during anesthesia, facilitate endotracheal intubation and prevent laryngospasm, decrease muscular activity in electroshock therapy, and aid in reducing muscle spasms associated with tetanus.

17. No effects. Unless anesthetized, the patient is fully conscious but unable to respond due to neuromuscular blockade.

18. Patent, adequate airway, check lung sounds bilaterally. Residual effects may be apparent for up to 72 hours especially in neonates and infants—watch for respiratory depression. Check cough reflex and ability to swallow. Question any antibiotic orders that prescribe aminoglycosides or tetracycline when neuromuscular blockers have been used.

19. Aminoglycoside antibiotics, beta-adrenergic blocking agents, and diuretics that cause potassium depletion.

20. Anesthesiologist's record

21. See Table 44-2, textbook p. 631.

22. See textbook, p. 631.

23. See textbook, p. 631.

Copyright © 2004 Mosby Inc. All rights reserved.

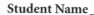

CHAPTER 44

Drugs Used to Treat the Muscular System

Practice Quiz

MULTIPLE CHOICE

Place the answer selected in the space that corresponds with the question being answered.

_____ 1. A 5-year-old patient is in the postanesthesia recovery area after having abdominal surgery. She received a neuromuscular blocking agent as part of her anesthetic and is now complaining of pain. What additional data are essential to collect before giving the prescribed analgesic?
    a. laboratory results for CBC and electrolytes
    b. vital signs
    c. family history
    d. estimated time of discharge

_____ 2. A drug used to treat neuroleptic malignant syndrome is:
    a. meperidine (Demerol).
    b. carisoprodol (Soma).
    c. dantrolene (Dantrium).
    d. baclofen (Lioresal).

_____ 3. Immediate treatment of a musculoskeletal injury would include:
    a. application of heat.
    b. TED (thromboembolic deterrent hose).
    c. application of ice.
    d. exercise of the affected part.

_____ 4. The primary use of centrally acting skeletal muscle relaxants is to:
    a. treat muscle spasticity.
    b. strengthen remaining active muscles.
    c. provide analgesia.
    d. relieve muscle spasms.

_____ 5. Centrally acting skeletal muscle relaxants may cause:
    a. blood dyscrasias and hepatotoxicity.
    b. blood dyscrasias and electrolyte imbalance.
    c. hepatotoxicity and nephrotoxicity.
    d. cardiac complications.

END-OF-CHAPTER MATH REVIEW

1. Ordered: methocarbamol (Robaxin) 1.5 g qid. Convert 1.5 g to _____ mg.

CRITICAL THINKING QUESTIONS

1. A patient was working in his garden and "pulled a muscle" in his back. The doctor prescribed cyclobenzaprine 10 mg tid, for 1 week. What health teaching should you provide the patient about the medication and temporary lifestyle changes?

2. Following an extensive major surgical procedure, the patient is transferred to the postanesthesia recovery unit with an endotracheal tube in place. The anesthesia record notes the administration of tubocurarine chloride during the surgical procedure. What criteria should be used to determine when to remove the endotracheal tube? What monitoring of the patient should be done to check for residual effects of the neuromuscular blocking agent?

Copyright © 2004 Mosby Inc. All rights reserved.

REVIEW QUESTIONS

_____ 1. Centrally acting skeletal muscle relaxant
drugs should NOT be given to patients
having:
   a.   muscle spasms.
   b.   cerebral or spinal cord disease.
   c.   a sprained ankle.
   d.   pulled back muscles.

_____ 2. Neuromuscular blocking agents require
the availability of _____ to treat an overdose.
   a.   dantrolene (Dantrium)
   b.   baclofen (Lioresal)
   c.   neostigmine methylsulfate
        (Prostigmin)
   d.   carisoprodol (SOMA)

Copyright © 2004 Mosby Inc. All rights reserved.

CHAPTER

45 Antimicrobial Agents

Syllabus

CHAPTER CONTENT

Antimicrobial Agents (p. 634)
Drug Therapy for Infectious Disease (p. 638)
    Drug Class: Aminoglycosides (p. 638)
    Drug Class: Carbapenems (p. 641)
    Drug Class: Cephalosporins (p. 642)
    Drug Class: Macrolides (p. 644)
    Drug Class: Penicillins (p. 645)
    Drug Class: Quinolones (p. 646)
    Drug Class: Streptogramins (649)
    Drug Class: Sulfonamides (p. 650)
    Drug Class: Tetracyclines (p. 651)
    Drug Class: Antitubercular Agents (p. 652)
    Drug Class: Miscellaneous Antibiotics (p. 655)
    Drug Class: Topical Antifungal Agents (p. 659)
    Drug Class: Systemic Antifungal Agents (p. 662)
    Drug Class: Antiviral Agents (p. 667)
Drug Therapy for Urinary Tract Infections (p. 676)

CHAPTER OBJECTIVES

1. Identify significant data in a patient history that could alert the medical team that a patient is more likely to experience an allergic reaction.
2. Identify baseline data the nurse should collect on a continual basis for comparison and evaluation of antimicrobial drug effectiveness.
3. Describe basic principles of patient care that can be implemented to enhance an individual's therapeutic response during an infection.
4. Identify criteria used to select an effective antimicrobial agent.
5. Differentiate between gram-negative and gram-positive microorganisms and between anaerobic and aerobic properties of microorganisms.
6. Explain the major actions and effects of drugs used to treat infectious diseases.
7. Describe the nursing assessments and interventions for the common side effects associated with antimicrobial agents: allergic reaction; direct tissue damage from nephrotoxicity, ototoxicity, or hepatotoxicity; secondary infection; and other considerations such as photosensitivity, peripheral neuropathy, and neuromuscular blockage.
8. Review parenteral administration techniques and the procedure for vaginal insertion of drugs.
9. Develop an education plan for patients receiving aminoglycosides; carbapenems, cephalosporins; penicillins; quinolones; streptogramins; sulfonamides; tetracyclines; and antitubercular, antifungal, and antiviral agents.

KEY TERMS

pathogenic
antibiotics
nephrotoxicity
ototoxicity
gram-negative
    microorganisms

gram-positive
    microorganisms
hypoprothrombinemia
thrombophlebitis
penicillinase-resistant
    penicillins

ASSIGNMENTS

Read textbook, pp. 634-378.
Study Key Terms associated with chapter content.
Complete Collaborative Activities as assigned.
Study Review Sheet for Chapter 45.
Complete Chapter 45 Practice Quiz.
Complete End-of-Chapter Math Review and Critical
    Thinking Questions.
Complete Chapter 45 Exam.

Copyright © 2004 Mosby Inc. All rights reserved.

WEB RESEARCH ACTIVITIES

Access: www.cdc.gov/health/diseases.htm
Select Health Topics A to Z
1. HIV–AIDS
2. Treatment HIV–AIDS
What kinds of problems are associated with antiretroviral drugs?
What new drugs are currently being studied as anti-HIV drugs?

COLLABORATIVE ACTIVITIES

Intravenous Antibiotic Therapy
Vancomycin hydrochloride 1 g added to 200 ml D_5W to be infused over 60 minutes using an infusion pump calibrated in ml/hr.
1. At what rate should the IV pump be set?
   Run at _____ ml/hr.
2. What premedication assessments should be made prior to the administration of vancomycin hydrochloride?
3. What is "red man syndrome"? What nursing actions should be taken when this occurs?
4. Research the correct procedure for planning or scheduling blood draws for vancomycin serum levels.

Oral Antibiotic Therapy
Zidovudine (AZT) 200 mg, PO, q 4 h is ordered for a patient with acquired immune deficiency syndrome (AIDS) and *Pneumocystis carinii* infection.
1. Explain the desired therapeutic outcome of this drug. Does taking it prevent the transmission of the disease to others?
2. What side effects may occur with the drug's administration and what health teaching should be completed in relation to the administration of this medication?
3. Examine the drug monographs for the antiviral agents used for the treatment of HIV-1.
   a. Do any of the drug monographs state that the use of the drug(s) prevents the spread of HIV through sexual contact or exposure to blood or body secretions?
   b. Which antiviral agents can produce anemia or granulocytopenia?
   c. Which agents can produce confusion?

Copyright © 2004 Mosby Inc. All rights reserved.

Antimicrobial Agents

Review Sheet

The QUESTION column and the ANSWER column have been offset so that you can cover the answers while reading the questions, allowing you to assess your knowledge.

Question	**Answer**
1. What criteria are used to select an antimicrobial agent?	
2. Describe the signs and symptoms of the common side effects seen with antimicrobial therapy.	1. The HCP must choose an antimicrobial agent that will be effective against the type of organism present and one that will not be too toxic to the patient.
3. Differentiate between gram-negative (Gm−) and gram-positive (Gm+) microorganisms, and anaerobic and aerobic properties of microorganisms.	2. Allergy: rash or skin reaction (e.g., hives with or without dyspnea, laryngeal edema, shock, stridor, and sternal retractions). Direct tissue damage: hepatotoxicity (liver damage) as noted by an elevation of AST, ALT, GGT, and alkaline phosphatase. Ototoxicity: dizziness, tinnitus, and progressive hearing loss. Nephrotoxicity [renal damage: as noted by an increase in serum creatinine, BUN, and by alterations in the urine (e.g., decrease in specific gravity, casts, or protein in the urine, and an excess of RBCs over 0–3)]. Secondary infection: stomatitis, glossitis, itching, vulvovaginitis, cold sores, or canker sores. See textbook, p. 637, Blood Dyscrasias, and p. 637, Nausea, Vomiting, and Diarrhea.
4. Describe basic principles of patient care that can be implemented to enhance an individual's therapeutic response during an infection.	3. Classification of microorganisms as gram-positive or gram-negative refers to the type of staining properties of a bacterium. Cells with a cell wall retain stain and are referred to as *gram-positive* cells. Cells without a cell wall do not retain the gram stain, and are referred to as *gram-negative* cells. Broad-spectrum antibiotics are effective against many gram-positive and gram-negative organisms. Anaerobic bacteria grow in the absence of oxygen; aerobic bacteria require oxygen to reproduce.
5. Review components of a baseline assessment to evaluate a patient's hydration status and assessments needed to detect renal or hepatic toxicity.	4. Adequate rest, hydration, and nutrients. Teach personal hygiene measures (e.g., handwashing, proper techniques for changing dressings).

Copyright © 2004 Mosby Inc. All rights reserved.

6. Identify significant data in a patient's history that could alert the medical team that the patient is more likely to experience an allergic reaction.

7. Describe the usual management of nausea, vomiting, and diarrhea when they occur in conjunction with antimicrobial therapy.

8. State the signs and symptoms of a secondary infection and actions that can be taken to minimize these effects.

9. Review techniques and procedures for parenteral administration and vaginal insertion of drugs.

10. Identify significant information relating to patient education when caring for a person receiving an antibiotic.

11. Cite the primary uses of aminoglycosides and the serious side effects that require close monitoring of the patient.

12. Identify precautions needed to prevent incompatibilities between aminoglycosides and other medications.

5. Hydration: skin turgor, intake and output, inspect mucous membranes for moisture or dryness, check firmness of eyeballs, check specific gravity of urine (see Table 39-1). Renal toxicity: decreasing urine output, increasing BUN and/or serum creatinine; check for presence of protein, blood, or casts in the urine. Hepatic toxicity: anorexia, nausea, vomiting, jaundice, hepatomegaly, splenomegaly, and abnormal (elevated) liver function tests (AST, ALT, LDH, GGT, alkaline phosphatase).

6. Before administering any antibiotic, check for any prior allergies to medications or foods or the presence of asthma. If the patient is allergic to anything, get details regarding the symptoms and previous treatment of the allergy.

7. Gather data relative to the patient's usual pattern of elimination (e.g., number of stools per day, consistency) and compare this information with the current data. Read individual drug monographs to identify antimicrobials that may cause diarrhea, nausea, or vomiting. Report these to the physician.

8. Be particularly alert for secondary infection in patients receiving broad-spectrum antibiotics and those patients who are immunosuppressed. Assess for white patches in the mouth, cold sores, canker sores, vaginal itching, diarrhea, and recurrent fever.

9. See Chapter 8: Percutaneous Administration; Chapter 10: Parenteral Administration: Safe Preparation of Parenteral Medications; Chapter 11: Parenteral Administration: Intradermal, Subcutaneous, and Intramuscular Administration; and Chapter 12: Parenteral Administration: Intravenous Therapy.

10. With the instructor's assistance, identify significant points relating to the prescribed drug therapy that should be taught to the patient for each class of antimicrobials ordered.

11. Aminoglycosides are used to treat gram-negative bacteria causing meningitis, wound infections, chronic urinary tract infections, and life-threatening septicemia. Monitor the patient closely for ototoxicity and nephrotoxicity. If the patient has had anesthesia within 48–72 hours that included the administration of a skeletal muscle relaxant, withhold aminoglycoside and ask health care provider for further instructions.

Copyright © 2004 Mosby Inc. All rights reserved.

13. State the mechanism of action of aminoglycosides on the bacterial cell.

14. What premedication assessments should be made before aminoglycoside therapy?
15. What is the mechanism of action of carbapenems?

16. Prior to administration of a carbapenem, what premedication assessments should be performed?
17. Why is it essential to report the occurrence of severe diarrhea with antibiotic therapy?

18. Explain the admixture compatibility of carbapenems.
19. Cite the effectiveness of cephalosporins, according to generation, against gram-positive and gram-negative microorganisms.
20. What premedication assessments should be performed before therapy with cephalosporins?

12. Do not mix aminoglycosides in the same syringe or infuse these drugs simultaneously with other medications. Tag the chart of any patient going to surgery who is receiving an aminoglycoside. Respiratory depression may occur when these agents are combined with skeletal muscle relaxants.

13. Aminoglycosides inhibit protein synthesis of bacteria.

14. Baseline assessment of allergies, presenting symptoms, T, P, R, BP, and hydration status. Check for any hearing disorders or deficits or renal disease. If present, hold drug and notify physician. Check for patient having received any skeletal muscle relaxants within the past 72 hours. If taking aminoglycosides, check serum level. Check for laboratory results ordered by the health care provider (e.g., CBC with differential).

15. Carbapenems inhibit bacterial cell wall synthesis.

16. Check T, P, R, BP, and hydration status for pre-existing gastric symptoms and any allergies (specifically to penicillin and cephalosporins), obtain laboratory studies, check for history of seizures and assess basic mental status and symptoms present.

17. Severe diarrhea with any antibiotic may indicate drug-induced pseudomembranous colitis.

18. See textbook, p. 642.

19. The first-generation cephalosporins have good activity against gram-positive bacteria and mild activity against gram-negative bacteria. The second-generation cephalosporins have somewhat increased activity against gram-negative bacteria but are much less active than the third-generation agents. The-third generation agents are less active than first-generation agents against gram-positive cocci. Some of the third-generation agents are also active against *Pseudomonas aeruginosa*, a very potent gram-negative microorganism. The third-generation cephalosporins have greater activity against gram-positive penicillinase-producing bacteria than first-generation cephalosporins. Fourth-generation cephalosporins are considered broad-spectrum, with both gram-negative and gram-positive coverage.

Copyright © 2004 Mosby Inc. All rights reserved.

21. State the mechanism of action of cephalosporins on the cell wall.

22. What types of infections can be treated effectively using cephalosporins?
23. What side effects from cephalosporins should be reported?

24. Why may hypoprothrombinemia occur with cephalosporin therapy?
25. What are the signs and symptoms of thrombophlebitis, which may occur with cephalosporin therapy?

26. What precautions should be instituted when cephalosporins are combined with probenecid or alcohol?
27. What is the difference between bacteriostatic and bactericidal?

28. Identify the uses of macrolides.

29. State the actions of penicillins on the bacterial cell.

30. Identify the clinical uses of penicillins.

31. For what types of adverse effects should a patient taking penicillin be monitored?

32. Cite questions that should be asked to screen a patient for a penicillin allergy before administration of the agent.

20. Baseline assessment of allergies, presenting symptoms, T, P, R, BP, and hydration status, symptoms of renal disease or bleeding disorder (hold drug and notify physician if present), and laboratory studies as ordered by physician (e.g., CBC with differential).

21. Interferes with synthesis of bacterial cell wall.

22. Respiratory, urinary, gastrointestinal, skin, and soft tissue infections, septicemia, meningitis, osteomyelitis, and certain sexually transmitted diseases

23. Diarrhea, secondary infections, abnormal liver and renal function tests

24. Although rare, hypoprothrombinemia may develop in the older adult, debilitated, or otherwise compromised patient with borderline vitamin K deficiency. Treatment with broad-spectrum antibiotics eliminates enough gastrointestinal flora to cause a further reduction in vitamin K synthesis.

25. Report redness, warmth, tenderness to touch, or edema in the affected part. Homans' sign in lower extremities.

26. Probenecid with cephalosporins may increase likelihood of toxicity. When combined with alcohol, cephalosporins may produce flushing, dyspnea, tachycardia, and hypotension. Do not ingest alcohol within 72 hours of taking cephalosporins.

27. Bactericidal agents kill the microorganism; bacteriostatic agents weaken the microorganism. Whether an agent is bacteriostatic or bactericidal depends on the organism and concentration of medication present.

28. Macrolides are used for respiratory, gastrointestinal tract, skin and soft tissue infections, and STDs, especially when penicillins, cephalosporins, and tetracyclines cannot be used.

29. Penicillins act by interfering with the synthesis of the bacterial cell wall. They are most effective against bacteria that are multiplying.

30. Treatment of middle ear infection, pneumonia, meningitis, urinary tract infections, syphilis, and gonorrhea; and as a prophylactic antibiotic before surgery or dental procedures for patients with a history of rheumatic fever.

31. Watch for diarrhea, abnormal liver and renal function tests, thrombophlebitis, and electrolyte imbalances from sodium or potassium types of

Copyright © 2004 Mosby Inc. All rights reserved.

33. Identify precautions necessary to prevent an incompatibility between penicillin and other medications given intramuscularly or intravenously.

34. Briefly describe the mechanisms of action of the quinolones and fluoroquinolones.

35. Review the multiple uses of quinolones and fluoroquinolones.

36. Why are the quinolones not used in children under the age of 12 years?
37. What premedication assessments should be made prior to beginning quinolone therapy?
38. Describe the effects of antacids, iron, and sucralfate on quinolones and the adaptations in scheduling required if both agents are prescribed concurrently.

39. Identify the drug interactions that may occur when quinolones are combined with concurrent use of NSAIDs, morphine sulfate, or sparfloxacin.

40. What is the mechanism of action of the new class of antibiotics known as *streptogramins*?
41. What are the uses of streptogramins?

42. What precautions need to be used when reconstituting streptogramins or administering them IV?
43. Cite the mechanism of action of sulfonamides and the importance of monitoring following administration.
44. State the effect of sulfonamides on persons taking sulfonylurea oral hypoglycemic agents.

penicillin. Elderly or debilitated patients with impaired renal function are more likely to develop adverse effects.
32. "Have you ever taken an antibiotic before?" "Do you have any known allergies to foods or medications?" If so, obtain further details, such as: "When you got sick while taking the medication, what symptoms did you have?" "What did the doctor tell you to do when this occurred?" "Do you have hay fever or asthma?"
33. Do not mix penicillin with other drugs in the same syringe or infuse together with other drugs.
34. Quinolones act by interfering with replication of bacterial DNA. Quinolones are effective against gram-negative and gram-positive bacteria, including anaerobes. Fluoroquinolones act by inhibiting activity of DNA gyrase, an enzyme essential for the replication of bacterial DNA.
35. See textbook, pp. 646-647.

36. Quinolones may cause permanent damage to cartilage in a pediatric patient.
37. Baseline assessment of allergies, presenting symptoms, T, P, R, BP, and hydration status, gastric symptoms present, baseline laboratory studies as ordered, check for pregnancy. Warn about possible photosensitivity with lomefloxacin.
38. Antacids, iron-containing products, and sucralfate may decrease the absorption of quinolones. The antibiotic should be scheduled 4 hours before or 4 hours after taking any of these medications.
39. See textbook, pp. 648-649.

40. Streptogramins (quinupristin, dalfopristin) act by inhibiting protein synthesis in bacterial cell wall.
41. These agents should be reserved for treatment of serious or life-threatening infections associated with vancomycin resistance.
42. See textbook, p. 650.

43. Sulfonamides inhibit bacterial biosynthesis of folic acid, leading to inadequate metabolism and cell death. Persons taking sulfonamides for 14 days or more need periodic monitoring of RBC and WBC (with differential) counts. All patients receiving sulfonamides need adequate hydration

Copyright © 2004 Mosby Inc. All rights reserved.

and should be encouraged to drink eight 12-oz glasses of water daily.

45. State the mechanism of action of tetracyclines.

44. Sulfonamides may displace sulfonylurea oral hypoglycemic agents from their protein binding sites, potentially resulting in hypoglycemia. Have patients taking these two agents concurrently test their blood glucose or urine 1/2 hour ac and hs to detect the development of a problem.

46. List a minimum of two types of antibiotics that may cause photosensitivity.
47. Identify the effects of administering tetracyclines during pregnancy and at the age of tooth development.

45. Tetracyclines inhibit protein synthesis by bacterial cells.
46. Quinolones, tetracyclines, sulfonamides, and griseofulvin may cause photosensitivity. Patients taking these antibiotics should be cautioned to avoid exposure to sunlight and ultraviolet lights. Discourage the use of artificial tanning lights and instruct patients to wear clothing that provides adequate coverage of the body when in the sunlight.

48. Describe the dosage and administration considerations when tetracycline is prescribed.

47. Do not administer tetracycline during the last half of pregnancy or to children through 8 years of age because it may cause enamel hypoplasia and permanent staining of the teeth. Do not administer to nursing mothers because it is secreted in breast milk.

49. Identify the causative organism and mode of transfer of tuberculosis.

48. Take medication 1 hour before or 2 hours after ingesting antacids; milk; dairy products; or products containing calcium, aluminum, magnesium (antacids), or iron (vitamins).
Exception: doxycycline is not affected by food or milk.
49. *Mycobacterium tuberculosis* is spread by airborne droplets from the cough or sneeze of a person infected with the organism.

50. Describe factors that need consideration to enhance a patient's response to antitubercular therapy.
51. Develop a teaching plan for persons receiving antitubercular agents.

50. Personal hygiene, nutritional status, and stress reduction are factors that must be considered during the treatment of tuberculosis.
51. Review your teaching plan with the course instructor.

52. Compare the mechanisms of action of ethambutol, isoniazid, and rifampin.
53. Identify the effects of rifampin on body secretions (e.g., urine, feces, saliva, and sputum).

52. Ethambutol inhibits TB bacterial growth by altering cellular RNA synthesis and phosphate metabolism. The mechanism of action of isoniazid is unknown. It appears to disrupt the *M. tuberculosis* cell wall and inhibit replication. Rifampin acts against enzymes in the bacterial cell required to produce DNA.
53. Rifampin may tinge urine, feces, saliva, sweat, and tears a reddish-orange color.

54. What drug interaction does rifampin have with oral contraceptives?

Copyright © 2004 Mosby Inc. All rights reserved.

55. What is the mechanism of action of monobactams?

56. What is the mechanism of action of chloramphenicol?

57. State specific limitations for the use of chloramphenicol.
58. Identify specific nursing assessments needed to detect possible serious hematologic effects from chloramphenicol.
59. What is the mechanism of action of clindamycin?

60. Describe effective treatment for diarrhea associated with clindamycin therapy.
61. State the primary clinical uses for metronidazole.

62. What premedication assessments should be done whenever metronidazole (Flagyl) is to be administered?
63. What is the mechanism of action of spectinomycin?
64. Identify the effectiveness of spectinomycin against gonorrhea and syphilis.
65. Cite specific recommendations for intramuscular administration of spectinomycin.

66. Why should serology testing for syphilis be done prior to initiating therapy using spectinomycin?

67. What is the mechanism of action of vancomycin?
68. Describe nursing assessments that may be used to detect ototoxicity.
69. Describe "red man syndrome" and identify the drug is associated with its occurrence.

54. Rifampin interferes with the contraceptive activity of birth control pills. Alternate methods of birth control should be used during rifampin therapy.
55. Monobactams are a new class of synthetic, bactericidal antibiotics that act by inhibiting cell wall synthesis.
56. Chloramphenicol acts by inhibiting bacterial protein synthesis.
57. Use only for serious infections; it is particularly effective in treating rickettsial infections, meningitis, and typhoid fever.
58. Check for sore throat, feelings of fatigue, elevated temperature, small petechial hemorrhages, and bruises of the skin. Report any of these symptoms immediately to the physician. Routine laboratory studies including RBC, WBC, and differential counts are scheduled for patients taking chloramphenicol 14 days or longer.
59. Clindamycin acts by inhibiting protein synthesis.
60. Do not self-treat diarrhea. (Kaopectate for persistent diarrhea from clindamycin therapy is used since it absorbs clindamycin. Do not use diphenoxylate, loperamide, or paregoric.) Patients should be instructed to contact the physician for specific directions and not to self-treat the diarrhea.
61. Metronidazole is used to treat trichomoniasis, giardiasis, amebic dysentery, amebic liver abscess, and anaerobic bacterial infections.
62. See textbook, p. 657.

63. Spectinomycin acts by inhibiting protein synthesis.
64. Spectinomycin is used to treat gonorrhea in both males and females. It is not effective in treatment of syphilis.
65. Use a 20-gauge needle, and inject into upper outer quadrant of gluteal muscle. Causes pain at injection site.
66. This drug masks symptoms of syphilis.

67. Vancomycin acts by preventing synthesis of bacterial cell wall.
68. Dizziness, tinnitus, and progressive hearing loss (e.g., turns the TV on louder, has to have conversation repeated).

Copyright © 2004 Mosby Inc. All rights reserved.

70. What type of dressings should be avoided with topical antifungal medications and what type of precautions should be taken to prevent accidental pregnancy when these drugs are administered intravaginally?
71. What is the mechanism of action of amphotericin B?

72. Cite the primary uses of amphotericin B.

73. Describe the systemic side effects seen with intravenous administration of amphotericin B.

74. Identify the monitoring parameters used to detect nephrotoxicity.

75. Cite specific dosage and administration characteristics associated with the use of amphotericin B.

76. Describe the effects of light on amphotericin B.
77. List medications that may occasionally be added to amphotericin B suspensions to minimize venous irritation.
78. Review procedures used to administer topical medications to the skin.

79. Describe the uses of fluconazole (Diflucan) and flucytosine (Ancobon, Ancotil).
80. Compare the premedication assessments needed for flucytosine (Ancobon, Ancotil), griseofulvin (Fulvicin, Grifulvin) , itraconazole (Sporanox), ketoconazole (Nizoral), and terbinafine (Lamisil).

81. What action prohibits the administration of itraconazole to a patient with heart failure?
82. What are the therapeutic outcomes from administration of abacavir (Ziagen)?

83. Describe the mechanisms of action and uses of griseofulvin (Fulvicin, Grifulvin).

69. "Red man syndrome" or "redneck syndrome" is caused by rapid IV infusion of vancomycin; symptoms include sudden hypotension with or without maculopapular rash over face, neck, upper chest, and extremities.
70. Avoid occlusive dressings. Alternative forms of birth control should also be used when antifungal ointments are instilled intravaginally. Diaphragms and condoms may deteriorate with prolonged contact with petroleum-based ointment.
71. Amphotericin B disrupts the cell membrane of fungal cells resulting in loss of cellular content and death of the cell.
72. Amphotericin B is used to treat systemic fungal infections and meningitis. Topically, it can be used for candidal infections.
73. Nephrotoxicity, electrolyte imbalances, chills, fever, malaise, headache, nausea and vomiting, and thrombophlebitis
74. Nephrotoxicity is indicated by increased excretion of uric acid, magnesium, oliguria, granular casts in urine, proteinuria, increased BUN, and serum creatinine. Report decrease in daily urine volume or changes in visual appearance of the urine.
75. See textbook, p. 662.
76. Amphotericin B deteriorates in the presence of light. Cover the solution to protect it from light during administration.
77. Heparin, hydrocortisone, or methylprednisolone may be added to infusion solution to diminish venous irritation.
78. See Chapter 8, Percutaneous Administration.

79. Fluconazole is used for cryptococcal meningitis and oropharyngeal, esophageal, vulvovaginal, or systemic candidiasis. Flucytosine is effective against susceptible candidal septicemia, endocarditis, urinary tract infections, cryptococcal meningitis, and pulmonary infections.
80. See textbook, pp. 664-667.

81. Itraconazole has the action of being a negative inotropic agent and may seriously aggravate a patient with heart failure.
82. Abacavir slows clinical progression of HIV-1 infection and reduces the frequency of opportunistic secondary infections.

Copyright © 2004 Mosby Inc. All rights reserved.

84. State laboratory tests needed periodically to monitor renal, hepatic, and hematopoietic function when griseofulvin is administered.
85. State the mechanisms of action and types of fungal infections for which itraconazole, ketoconazole, miconazole, and terbinafine are used.

86. What are the therapeutic outcomes of abacavir (Ziagen), efavirenz (Sustiva), and lamivudine (Epivir)?

87. Identify the mechanism of action of acyclovir (Zovirax), didanosine (Videx), famciclovir (Famvir), and valacyclovir (Valtrex).

88. Cite the potential effects of acyclovir on renal function.
89. Identify the first antiviral agent that is effective against respiratory viruses.

90. What is the drug lamivudine (Epivir) used to treat?
91. What is oseltamivir (Tamiflu) used to treat?

92. Explain the administration aerosol ribavirin powder using a small-particle aerosol generator (SPAG-2).
93. What is valacyclovir (Valtrex) used to treat?
94. Does zanamivir (Relenza) reduce the transmission of influenza to others?
95. Cite the clinical limitations of zidovudine in the treatment of human immunodeficiency virus (HIV).

83. Griseofulvin acts by stopping cell division and new cell growth and is used to treat ringworm of scalp, body, nails, and feet.
84. Hepatotoxicity (liver damage) is noted by an elevation in AST, ALT, GGT, and alkaline phosphatase. Nephrotoxicity (renal damage) is indicated by an increase in serum creatinine, BUN, and by alterations in the urine (e.g., decrease in specific gravity, casts or protein in the urine, and an excess of RBCs over 0–3). Hematologic: monitor for the development of sore throat, fever, purpura, jaundice, or excessive progressive weakness.
85. Ketoconazole, itraconazole, and miconazole act by interfering with cell wall synthesis, causing leakage of cellular contents. (Itraconazole, see textbook, p. 665.) Ketoconazole is used orally to treat candidiasis, chronic mucocutaneous candidiasis, oral thrush, coccidioidomycosis, histoplasmosis, chromomycosis, and paracoccidioidomycosis. Miconazole is used parenterally to treat similar fungal infections. Terbinafine is used to treat onychomycosis of the toenail or fingernail due to dermatophytes. (Terbinafine, see textbook, pp. 666-667.)
86. Abacavir (Ziagen), efavirenz (Sustiva), and lamivudine (Epivir) slow the progression of HIV-1 infection and reduce the frequency of opportunistic secondary infections.
87. These antiviral agents act by inhibiting the viral cell wall replication.
88. Transient elevation of serum creatinine. Patients who are poorly hydrated, have low renal function, or who receive acyclovir by a bolus are susceptible to renal tubular damage.
89. Ribavirin (Virazole)

90. Lamivudine (Epivir) is combined with zidovudine in treating HIV-1 infection.
91. See textbook, p. 673.

92. See textbook, pp. 673-674.
93. Acute herpes simplex virus (shingles)

94. No

Copyright © 2004 Mosby Inc. All rights reserved.

96. Identify the hematologic tests that should be completed periodically during the use of zidovudine.

97. Describe the effect of zidovudine on transmission of HIV to others through sexual contact or blood contamination.

98. Describe the proper schedule for administering zidovudine and essential health teaching needed.

99. Review current Centers for Disease Control recommendations for handling body secretions and blood for all patients.

100. Which of the antiviral agents may reduce pulmonary function?

101. Which antiviral agent may reduce the effectiveness of oral contraceptives?

102. Which antiviral agents may produce peripheral neuropathy?

103. Study the antibiotic tables throughout the chapter and identify common endings in the generic names of the antimicrobial agents.

95. It prolongs the lives of AIDS and AIDS-related complex (ARC) patients, reduces the risk and severity of opportunistic infections, and improves immune status. Zidovudine does not cure acquired immunodeficiency.

96. Monitor CBC with differential, platelets, hemoglobin, hematocrit, amylase, and liver function tests.

97. This drug does not reduce the risk of transmitting HIV to others through sexual contact or blood contamination.

98. Oral medication is taken every 4 hours around the clock even though it interrupts normal sleep. Do not share with other persons.

99. Check with your instructor to obtain the latest recommendations or research the information on the CDC website.

100. Both ribavirin and zanamivir may affect pulmonary function.

101. Amprenavir

102. Didanosine, lamivudine, zidovudine

103. See textbook Tables 45-1 through 45-9. Note: Because of the number of drugs included in these tables, ask the instructor to identify the more common drugs that will be encountered in the clinical site(s) where you are assigned.

Copyright © 2004 Mosby Inc. All rights reserved.

Antimicrobial Agents

Practice Quiz

CHAPTER 45

MATCHING

Match the definition with the term that it best describes.

_____ 1. A microorganism that is able to grow and function without oxygen.
_____ 2. Causing destruction or death of bacteria.
_____ 3. A microorganism that lives and grows with oxygen present.
_____ 4. Restrains or reduces the development or reproduction of bacteria.
    a. Bacteriostatic
    b. Anaerobic
    c. Bactericidal
    d. Aerobic
    e. Bacteremia

Match the definition with the term that it best describes.

_____ 5. Overgrowth of organisms resistant to current antibiotic therapy
_____ 6. Causes elevation in AST, ALT, LDH, and alkaline phosphatase
_____ 7. Causes increase in serum creatinine and BUN
_____ 8. Causes dizziness, tinnitus, and progressive hearing loss
    a. Ototoxicity
    b. Nephrotoxicity
    c. Secondary infection
    d. Pathogenic
    e. Hepatotoxicity

Match the definition with the term that it best describes.

_____ 9. An inflammation of a vein
_____ 10. Reduction in formation and excretion of urine
_____ 11. Characterized by poor blood clotting
_____ 12. Increased albumin in urine
    a. Thrombus
    b. Phlebitis
    c. Oliguria
    d. Proteinuria
    e. Hypoprothrombinemia

Match the drug with the corresponding drug classification. (Drug classifications can be used more than once.)

_____ 13. Ampicillin
_____ 14. Kanamycin
_____ 15. Dicloxacillin
_____ 16. Cephalexin
_____ 17. Gentamicin
_____ 18. Cefaclor
_____ 19. Sulfamethoxazole
_____ 20. Demeclocycline
_____ 21. Ciprofloxacin
_____ 22. Ketoconazole
    a. Cephalosporin
    b. Penicillin
    c. Sulfonamide
    d. Aminoglycoside
    e. Tetracycline
    ab. Quinolone
    ac. Topical antifungal

Copyright © 2004 Mosby Inc. All rights reserved.

TRUE OR FALSE

Mark "T" for true and "F" for false for each of the following statements. <u>Correct all false statements</u>.

_____ 23. Cephalosporins may be used as an alternative to penicillins for persons allergic to penicillin.

_____ 24. Aminoglycosides cause hepatotoxicity.

_____ 25. Tetracyclines (except doxycycline) should not be taken concurrently with iron- or calcium-containing foods.

_____ 26. Patients receiving aminoglycosides should have a warning sign placed on the front of the chart before a procedure requiring a general anesthetic.

_____ 27. Diarrhea may be a symptom of secondary infection.

_____ 28. Chloramphenicol may cause fatal bone marrow depression.

_____ 29. Patient education for persons taking antibiotics should stress taking all the prescribed medication.

_____ 30. Only drugs ending in "-mycin" are classified as macrolides.

_____ 31. Sulfonamides, when given to a patient taking sulfonylurea oral hypoglycemic agents, may cause hypoglycemia.

COMPLETION

Complete the following statements.

32. Two or more antitubercular drugs are often combined to _____.

33. _____ is an antitubercular drug that may interfere with the clinical efficacy of oral contraceptives. Other forms of contraception are recommended when this drug is prescribed.

34. When antibiotics are described as "broad spectrum" in their clinical activity, it means that the antibiotic is generally effective against both _____ and _____ bacteria.

35. Aminoglycoside antibiotics act by
_____.

36. The _____ class of antibiotics should not be administered during the last half of pregnancy or while breastfeeding; do not administer to children until permanent teeth are in place (usually by age 8 years).

37. The _____ class is not considered a true antibiotic; its action is to inhibit biosynthesis of folic acid, which results in bacterial cell death.

38. _____, an antitubercular drug, may tinge the urine, feces, saliva, sweat, and tears reddish-orange.

39. The _____ class of antimicrobials is reserved for serious life-threatening infections that are vancomycin-resistant.

40. _____ is required for aerobic bacteria growth.

41. Two major side effects associated with aminoglycoside antibiotics are _____ and _____.

42. In general, a person who is allergic to sulfonamides should not take _____ oral hypoglycemic agents.

43. _____ agents kill bacterial pathogens.

44. The administration schedule for zidovudine should be established so the medication is taken _____.

END-OF-CHAPTER MATH REVIEW

1. Order: chloramphenicol 50 mg/kg/24 hours, IV, in 4 equally divided doses for an infant 12 weeks old weighing 13 lbs.
   The infant's weight in kg is _____.
   The amount of chloramphenicol to be administered in a 24-hour period is _____mg.
   Each of the four divided doses is _____mg.
   On hand: chloramphenicol sodium succinate 100 mg/ml
   Give: _____ ml for each single dose.

2. Order: amoxicillin 150 mg, q 8 h, PO. After establishing this is a safe dose for the infant's weight, you prepare:
   On hand: amoxicillin oral suspension 125 mg/5 ml
   Give: _____ ml.

3. Order: cefazolin (Kefzol) 400 mg, IM, q 6 h
   On hand: cefazolin 330 mg/ml
   Give: _____ ml.

4. Order: An IV antibiotic for administration in 30 minutes. The administration set delivers 15 gtt/ml. Volume to be given is 50 ml.
   Set the drip rate at: _____ gtt/min.

Copyright © 2004 Mosby Inc. All rights reserved.

5. Order: vancomycin 1 g, in 150 ml D₅W over 1.5 hours.
   Using an infusion pump to deliver this IVPB, set the pump at: _____ ml/hr.

CRITICAL THINKING QUESTIONS

1. In math problem 1 above, the infant is 12 weeks old. After calculating the drug dose, what type of syringe and size needle would you use to administer the prescribed chloramphenicol? What site of administration would be best in an infant of this age? Give your rationale. Explain correct technique for administration, including landmark identification.

2. While providing care to a patient diagnosed 3 months ago with tuberculosis, you suspect nonadherence with the prescribed regimen. How would you proceed to verify this and what interventions would you attempt?

REVIEW QUESTIONS

_____ 1. Probenecid, when given with antibiotics that are excreted in the urine, causes:
   a. photosensitivity.
   b. increased serum levels by blocking urinary excretion of the prescribed anti-infective agent.
   c. increased incidence of nephrotoxicity.
   d. increased incidence of ototoxicity.

_____ 2. Ototoxicity is seen with:
   a. systemic antifungals.
   b. quinolones.
   c. carbapenems.
   d. aminoglycosides.

_____ 3. Cephalosporins, carbapenems, and _____ have the potential for cross-sensitivity.
   a. penicillins
   b. tetracyclines
   c. chloramphenicol
   d. quinolones

_____ 4. Photosensitivity may be seen with the administration of quinolones, sulfonamides, and _____.
   a. tetracyclines
   b. aminoglycosides
   c. choramphenicol
   d. cephalosporins

_____ 5. Many drugs are known to interact with antimicrobial agents by decreasing the absorption of the prescribed medication. When antacids are prescribed, it is safest to schedule antimicrobial drugs _____ hours before or after the antacid.
   a. 1–2
   b. 2–3
   c. 3–4
   d. 4–5

_____ 6. When looking at drugs within each classification in the various antimicrobial tables throughout the chapter, note that the quinolones all end in "-oxacin" except for:
   a. cephalexin.
   b. netilmicin.
   c. nalidixic acid.
   d. piperacillin.

Copyright © 2004 Mosby Inc. All rights reserved.

CHAPTER CONTENT

Principles of Nutrition (p. 679)
Dietary Reference Intakes (p. 681)
Physical Activity (p. 690)
Malnutrition (p. 691)

CHAPTER OBJECTIVES

1. Differentiate between information found in the dietary reference intake tables and the Recommended Dietary Allowances tables.
2. Identify the function of macronutrients in the body.
3. Research good dietary sources of fiber.
4. Identify the exercise guidelines currently recommended for people with different daily patterns of physical activity (sedentary, low active, and very active).
5. State the formula used to estimate basal energy expenditures for males and females.
6. Differentiate between fat-soluble and water-soluble vitamins.
7. List five functions of minerals in the body.
8. Describe nutritional assessments essential prior to administration of tube feedings and parenteral nutrition.
9. Describe physical changes associated with a malnourished state.
10. Cite common laboratory and diagnostic tests used to monitor a patient's nutritional status.
11. Discuss nursing assessments and interventions required during the administration of enteral nutrition.
12. Discuss home care needs of a patient being discharged on any form of enteral or parenteral nutrition.

KEY TERMS

dietary reference
   intakes (DRI)
recommended dietary
   allowances (RDA)
adequate intake (AI)
estimated average
   requirement (EAR)
tolerable upper intake
   level (UL)
kilocalories
carbohydrates
monosaccharides
disaccharides
polysaccharides
fiber
fats
lipids
essential fatty acids

proteins
gluconeogenesis
vitamins
minerals
water
physical exercise
marasmus
kwashiorkor
mixed kwashiorkor-
   marasmus
enteral nutrition
tube feedings
parenteral nutrition
total parenteral
   nutrition (TPN)
peripheral parenteral
   nutrition (PPN)

ASSIGNMENTS

Read textbook, pp. 679-700.
Study Key Terms associated with chapter content.
Complete Collaborative Activities as assigned.
Study Review Sheet for Chapter 46.
Complete Chapter 46 Practice Quiz.
Complete End-of-Chapter Math Review and Critical Thinking Questions.
Complete Chapter 46 Exam.

Copyright © 2004 Mosby Inc. All rights reserved.

WEB RESEARCH ACTIVITIES

Access: www.nutrition.gov
Quick Search: fiber in the diet
1. How much fiber per day does the typical American eat?
2. What foods are high in fiber?
3. What benefits does added fiber in the diet have on disease such as cancer, heart disease, and digestive disorders?

COLLABORATIVE ACTIVITIES

Answer the following questions. Be prepared to share your answers during in-class discussion and group work that may be assigned by the instructor.
1. Use a laboratory reference book to research the normal findings for the following lab tests used to assess lean body mass: albumin, prealbumin, retinol-binding protein, and transferrin.
2. Research the policy used at the clinical site where you are assigned for checking feeding tube placement and residual volumes.
3. Review the procedure manual at your clinical site to determine the procedure for monitoring total parenteral nutrition (TPN) (hyperalimentation).
4. Review the drug interactions listed for enteral and parenteral nutrition products.

Copyright © 2004 Mosby Inc. All rights reserved.

CHAPTER 46

Nutrition

Review Sheet

The QUESTION column and the ANSWER column have been offset so that you can cover the answers while reading the questions, allowing you to assess your knowledge.

Question	**Answer**
1. What factors affect one's nutritional requirements?	
2. What information can be found in the Dietary Reference Intake (DRI) table and Recommended Dietary Allowance (RDA) table?	1. See textbook, pp. 679-680.
3. What is the unit of measurement of energy requirements?	2. See Table 46-1 and 46-2, textbook pp. 682-686.
4. What does the Harris-Benedict equation calculate?	3. Kilocalories (kcal)
5. What are other names for simple carbohydrates?	4. The Harris-Benedict equation is one approach to calculating the total calories needed.
6. Fats, according to the Academy of Science report should be limited to _____ of total daily intake.	5. Simple carbohydrates are known as *monosaccharides* and *disaccharides*.
7. State the daily caloric needs from carbohydrates required.	6. 20–35%
8. Carbohydrates supply _____ kilocalories of energy per gram, fats supply _____ kilocalories of energy per gram, and proteins supply _____ kilocalories of energy per gram.	7. Range is from 3–5.5 grams/kg/day, depending on energy requirements for daily living, stress, and wound healing.
9. What are the end products of protein metabolism?	8. Carbohydrates supply 4 kilocalories, fats supply 9 kilocalories, and proteins supply 4 kilocalories.
10. How many water-soluble and fat-soluble vitamins are there to date?	9. Nitrogenous products such as urea, uric acid, ammonia, carbon dioxide, and water
11. Why are minerals essential to life?	10. Thirteen total vitamins; 9 water-soluble; 4 fat-soluble
12. Name three forms of malnutrition.	11. See textbook, p. 690.
13. What laboratory studies can be used to assess lean body mass?	12. Marasmus, kwashiorkor, and mixed kwashiorkor-marasmus
14. Differentiate between enteral and parenteral nutrition.	13. Albumin, prealbumin, retinol-binding protein, transferrin
15. Explain components of a nutritional assessment.	14. Enteral nutrition is administered orally; parenteral nutrition is given via venous access and implantable vascular access devices.
16. What physical changes are related to a malnourished state?	15. See textbook, pp. 691-692.

17. What are the general routines used for checking tube placement and residuals?

18. When is the use of enteral nutrition contraindicated?

19. What premedication assessments should be performed prior to administering enteral nutrition?

20. Differentiate among bolus, intermittent, and continuous feedings.

21. How should prescribed medications be administered via a feeding tube?

22. List side effects of enteral feedings that should be reported to the physician.

23. Review the drug monograph for enteral nutrition and note drugs that interact with grapefruit juice.

24. What is the difference between peripheral parenteral nutrition solutions (PPN), and total parenteral nutrition (TPN) solutions?

25. List premedication assessments that should be performed before administering TPN or PPN.

26. List side effects of parenteral feedings that should be reported to the physician.

27. List key signs and symptoms of fat-soluble and water-soluble vitamin deficiencies.

16. Height, weight, muscle circumference, skin fold thickness, skin integrity, cardiovascular, respiratory, neurological alteration, thyroid function, gastrointestinal symptoms

17. See textbook, pp. 694-695.

18. Enteral nutrition is contraindicated when the individual has intractable vomiting, a paralyzed ileum, or certain types of fistulas.

19. See textbook, pp. 694-695.

20. See textbook, p. 696.

21. See textbook, p. 696.

22. Pulmonary complications (aspiration), diarrhea, constipation, nausea, vomiting, increased residual volume, rash, chills, fever, and respiratory difficulty

23. See textbook, p. 697.

24. PPN solutions consist of 2–5% crystalline amino acid preparations and 5–10% dextrose with electrolytes and vitamins. TPN consists of 15–25% glucose, amino acids (3.5–15%), fat emulsion (10–20%), electrolytes, vitamins, and minerals. Due to high osmolality (see Chapter 12), TPN solutions must be administered through a central venous access line.

25. See textbook, p. 698.

26. Hypoglycemia, hyperglycemia, fluid imbalance, rash, chills, fever, respiratory difficulty, electrolyte imbalances, and hepatotoxicity

27. See textbook, p. 688.

Copyright © 2004 Mosby Inc. All rights reserved.

Nutrition

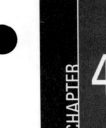

Practice Quiz

COMPLETION

Complete the following statements.

1. The new Harvard Food Pyramid has _____ as the foundation of the pyramid.
2. The _____ is used to calculate basal energy expenditure in kilocalories per day.
3. The daily carbohydrate needs are _____ grams/kg/day.
4. Carbohydrates and proteins supply approximately _____ kilocalories of energy per gram.
5. The fat-soluble vitamins are _____, _____, _____, and _____.
6. Kwashiorkor is caused by a diet deficient in _____.
7. From research on assigned laboratory studies, it is apparent that a decreased albumin level is related to the maintenance of _____ in the vascular system.
8. _____ is an indicator of recent catabolism in the body.
9. Osmolite is an example of a _____ formula.
10. Edema of the abdomen and subcutaneous tissue is a possible sign of _____ deficiency.
11. A _____ deficiency can increase the heart rate and heart size.
12. Stomach-content residuals from tube feedings are generally checked prior to each bolus feeding and once every _____ hours for continuous enteral feedings.
13. During _____ (type of feeding), the client is often placed on insulin by sliding scale.
14. Prior to hanging a _____ solution, two qualified nurses should check the contents of the container against the specific doctor's order.

15. The enteral feeding tube should be clamped _____ minutes before administering a prescribed medication that should be taken on an empty stomach.
16. Persons receiving continuous tube feedings should have the head of the bed elevated _____ degrees on a continuous basis.
17. _____ consists of a parenteral nutrition solution that is 2–5% crystalline amino acids, and 5–10% dextrose with added electrolytes and vitamins.
18. TPN solutions can be given directly via a(n) _____.
19. A pyridoxine deficiency can result in _____.
20. _____ (vitamin) deficiency can result in anemia, depression, and delayed wound healing.

END-OF-CHAPTER MATH REVIEW

1. M.B. has an order to receive Osmolite, full strength, at 80 ml per hour around the clock. The feeding is shut off for an hour 3 times per day when medications are administered that interact with the nutritional product. What adjustments in the rate of administration should be made to administer the full amount of prescribed formula during the hours it is running?
2. A client is receiving intermittent bolus feedings of Ensure 250 cc every 4 hours, followed by a water bolus of 150 ml per feeding. What is the individual's total fluid intake over a 24-hour period?

CRITICAL THINKING QUESTIONS

1. A client's TPN solution has gotten behind in the rate of administration. As the nurse, you realize the client needs the nutrients. What interven-

Copyright © 2004 Mosby Inc. All rights reserved.

tions could be initiated and what actions would be contraindicated? Give your rationale.

2. In a nursing home, the client on a continuous tube feeding could have the tube feeding scheduled to run at night, allowing greater mobility during the daytime. If the client needs an intake of 80 ml per hour over a 24-hour time span, how would the hourly intake be adjusted to administer the enteral product between 8 PM and 8 AM?

3. Explain teaching you would institute for an adult being discharged on bolus enteral feedings. How would you teach the person to administer the enteral product and what monitoring for complications should be done prior to discharge?

4. It is time to hang the next bag of TPN and it has not arrived from the pharmacy. What would be appropriate actions for the nurse to take?

5. While caring for an elderly client receiving continuous tube feedings using a kangaroo feeding pump, you suspect the patient has aspirated some of the formula. What symptoms would you assess for and what immediate nursing actions should you take?

REVIEW QUESTIONS

_____ 1. Select good food sources of dietary fiber from the following list.
   a. lettuce salad with dressing
   b. potatoes, pasta, and white bread
   c. cereal brans, sweet potatoes, vegetables, and fruits
   d. beef, chicken, fish, and tofu

_____ 2. Sources of the type of dietary fats that are cardioprotective include:
   a. corn oil, soybean oil, and safflower oil.
   b. coconut oil, olive oil, and peanut oil.
   c. olive oil, canola oil, and peanut oil.
   d. stick margarine, peanut oil, and corn oil.

_____ 3. The Harvard Health Eating Pyramid base is composed of:
   a. breads, cereal, rice, and pasta.
   b. dairy products.
   c. whole grains, fruits, and vegetables.
   d. activity and weight control.

_____ 4. Medications known to interact with grapefruit juice include:
   a. calcium channel blockers and barbiturates.
   b. cyclosporine, sulfonamides, and angiotensin-converting enzyme (ACE) inhibitors.
   c. triazolam and calcium channel blockers.
   d. prokinetic agents and calcium channel blockers.

_____ 5. New recommendations for daily nutritional distribution of CHO (carbohydrates), fats, and proteins to minimize chronic disease include:
   a. CHO 40–63%, fats 25–50%, proteins 12–20%.
   b. CHO 35–45%, fats 10–15%, proteins 30–50%.
   c. CHO 50–60%, fats 30%, proteins 10–20%.
   d. CHO 45–60%, fats 10–35%, proteins 20–30%.

Copyright © 2004 Mosby Inc. All rights reserved.

Herbal and Dietary Supplement Therapy

Syllabus

CHAPTER CONTENT

CHAPTER OBJECTIVES

1. Summarize the primary actions, uses, and interactions of the herbal and dietary supplement products listed.
2. Describe the possible impact of the use of herbal and dietary supplement products on cultural or ethnic beliefs.

KEY TERMS

dietary supplements   phytomedicine
herbal medicines   phytotherapy
botanicals

ASSIGNMENTS

Read textbook, pp. 701-713.
Study Key Terms associated with chapter content.
Complete Collaborative Activities as assigned.
Study Review Sheet for Chapter 47.
Complete Chapter 47 Practice Quiz.
Complete Critical Thinking Questions.
Complete Chapter 47 Exam.

WEB RESEARCH ACTIVITIES

Access: www.herbmed.org
1. Research black cohosh:
   What adverse effects have been reported with the use of this herb during pregnancy?
2. Research ginkgo:
   What interactions are there between ginkgo and prescribed cardiovascular medications?

COLLABORATIVE ACTIVITIES

Complete the following as preparation for in-class discussion and group work that may be assigned by the instructor.
1. Go to a health food store that sells herbal products and have the salesperson recommend some products for the treatment of depression, lack of energy, and general malaise. Ask the salesperson about his or her background or qualifications to make these recommendations.
2. Research the herbal products available at a pharmacy and their cost (e.g., St. John's wort).
3. Research cultural beliefs regarding herbal products.
4. Check for the resources available on herbal products at the clinical unit where you are assigned.

Copyright © 2004 Mosby Inc. All rights reserved.

47 Herbal and Dietary Supplement Therapy

Review Sheet

The QUESTION column and the ANSWER column have been offset so that you can cover the answers while reading the questions, allowing you to assess your knowledge.

Question	Answer
1. Define the key terms associated with this chapter.	
2. Describe the role of the Food and Drug Administration (FDA) in the regulation of herbal products.	1. See textbook, pp. 701 and 703.
3. What factors should be considered when recommending herbal products?	2. The FDA has no direct role in regulation of herbal products. The Dietary Supplement Health and Education Act (DSHEA) of 1994 governs the use of herbal medicines, vitamins, minerals, and amino acids. Under this Act, almost all herbal medicines, vitamins, minerals, amino acids, and other supplemental chemicals used for health were reclassified legally as dietary supplements, a food category. The labels and advertisements from the manufacturer must contain a statement that the product has not yet been evaluated by the FDA for treating, curing, or preventing any disease. The law does not prevent other persons from making claims (founded or unfounded) about the therapeutic effects of supplement ingredients. The end result of the new law is that dietary supplements are not required to be safe and effective and unfounded claims of therapeutic benefit abound. There are now hundreds of herbal medicines and other dietary supplements being marketed in the United States as single- and multiple-ingredient products for an extremely wide variety of uses, all implying that they will improve one's health. The vast majority of the popular claims made for herbal medicines and dietary supplements are unproven. There are also no standardized manufacturing practices that control the manufacture of most of these products as there are with medicines approved by the FDA.

Copyright © 2004 Mosby Inc. All rights reserved.

4. Prepare a list of herbal products listed in the chapter and insert the corresponding popular uses by lay persons of these herbal products.

5. What questions as part of a medication history should elicit information regarding the use of herbal products and other alternative medicines?

6. What potential drug interactions may occur with each herbal product listed?

3. See Box 47-1, p. 704.

4. *Herbal Product:*   *Use(s):*
   Aloe   See p. 703.
   Black cohosh   See p. 704.
   Chamomile   See p. 704.
   Echinacea   See p. 704.
   Ephedra   See p. 705.
   Feverfew   See p. 705.
   Garlic   See p. 706.
   Ginger   See p. 706.
   Ginkgo   See p. 707.
   Ginseng   See p. 707.
   Goldenseal   See p. 708.
   Green tea   See p. 708.
   Saw palmetto   See p. 709.
   St. John's wort   See p. 709.
   Valerian   See p. 710.
   Other Dietary Supplements:
   Co-Enzyme Q_{10} See p. 710.
   Creatine   See p. 710.
   Gamma-hydroxybutyrate (GHB)   See p. 711.
   Lycopene   See p. 712.
   Melatonin   See p. 712.
   S-adenosylmethionine (SAM-e)   See p. 713.

5. Consult with your instructor for assistance.

6. Review individual monographs throughout chapter.

Copyright © 2004 Mosby Inc. All rights reserved.

CHAPTER 47

Herbal and Dietary Supplement Therapy

Practice Quiz

TRUE OR FALSE

Mark "T" for true and "F" for false. <u>Correct all false</u> <u>statements</u>.

_____ 1. Alternate forms of medicine, including the use of herbal products, are increasingly popular in the United States.

_____ 2. The nurse should check the hospital policy regarding the methodology to be used in recording herbal products being taken or administered on the clinical unit.

_____ 3. Chamomile has been shown to be an effective antidepressant.

_____ 4. Black cohosh is sometimes used for reduction of symptoms of premenstrual syndrome, dysmenorrhea, and menopause.

_____ 5. Black cohosh may interact with hormone replacement therapy products and antihypertensive agents prescribed by the physician.

_____ 6. Echinacea is a bacteriostatic and bactericidal agent.

_____ 7. There are essentially no drug interactions with ephedra.

_____ 8. Feverfew is used as an antiplatelet and antihypertensive agent.

_____ 9. Garlic affects platelet aggregation and therefore should be used with caution for clients taking antiplatelet medications.

_____ 10. Ginseng may cause hyperglycemia.

_____ 11. Saw palmetto is used to treat symptoms of benign prostatic hyperplasia.

_____ 12. St. John's wort has an action similar to SSRIs.

_____ 13. Persons taking St. John's wort should be aware that exposure to sunlight may result in excessive sunburn.

_____ 14. Valerian is used as a sleep aid and as a mild tranquilizer.

CRITICAL THINKING QUESTIONS

1. Discuss the pros and cons of allowing a patient to use herbal products for self-treatment of such things as premenstrual syndrome (black cohosh), especially if the woman is using an estrogen/progestin replacement therapy hormone as well. What if the individual also has hypertension?

2. What recommendations should a nurse make to an immunocompromised patient who asks about taking echinacea as an anti-inflammatory agent for "arthritis"?

3. What is the law in the state where you reside with regard to the use of ephedrine?

4. What health teaching should be completed for a patient taking nonsteroidal anti-inflammatory agents and feverfew concurrently?

5. What herbal products listed in this chapter interact with anticoagulants?

REVIEW QUESTIONS

_____ 1. Saw palmetto is used to treat:
   a. gastrointestinal symptoms.
   b. cholesterol.
   c. benign prostatic hyperplasia.
   d. rheumatoid arthritis.

_____ 2. Coenzyme Q10 is used primarily as adjunctive therapy for:
   a. chronic heart failure.
   b. insomnia.
   c. depression.
   d. antiviral treatment of human immunodeficiency virus (HIV).

Copyright © 2004 Mosby Inc. All rights reserved.

_____ 3. Melatonin has become best known for use for/as:
a. a euphoriant.
b. prostate cancer.
c. colds.
d. sleep alterations.

_____ 4. SAM-e should not be used in patients diagnosed with:
a. fibromyalgia.
b. manic depression.
c. osteoarthritis.
d. eating disorders.

Copyright © 2004 Mosby Inc. All rights reserved.

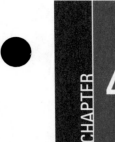

Substance Abuse

Syllabus

CHAPTER CONTENT

Definitions of Substance Abuse (p. 715)
Substances of Abuse (p. 715)
Theories on Why Substances Are Abused (p. 716)
Signs of Impairment (p. 716)
Screening for Alcohol and Substance Abuse (p. 717)
Health Professionals and Substance Abuse (p. 717)
Principles of Treatment of Substance Abuse (p. 721)

CHAPTER OBJECTIVES

1. Differentiate among key terms associated with substance abuse.
2. Explore biological, psychological, and sociocultural models that influence the assessment and treatment of substance abuse.
3. Describe the different types of screening tools used to assess alcohol and substance abuse.
4. Cite the responsibilities of professionals when suspecting substance abuse by a colleague.
5. Explain the primary long-term goals in the treatment of substance abuse.
6. Study the withdrawal symptoms and approaches to treatment and relapse prevention for major substances that are commonly abused.

KEY TERMS

substance abuse
impairment
dependence
addiction
illicit substance
intoxication

ASSIGNMENTS

Read textbook, pp. 715-730.
Study Key Terms associated with chapter content.
Complete Collaborative Activities as assigned.
Study Review Sheet for Chapter 48.
Complete Chapter 48 Practice Quiz.
Complete End-of-Chapter Math Review and Critical Thinking Questions.
Complete Chapter 48 Exam.

WEB RESEARCH ACTIVITIES

Access: www.alcoholics-anonymous.org
Select:
1. Alcohol and sexual assault
   Print the fact sheet on Binge Drinking: Alcohol and Sexual Assault and bring it to class for discussion.
2. Alcohol and violence
   What can be done to decrease the incidence of binge drinking and violence?

COLLABORATIVE ACTIVITIES

Answer the following questions. Be prepared to share your answers during in-class discussion and group work that may be assigned by the instructor.
1. Use a laboratory reference book to research the normal findings for the lab tests used to assess for substance abuse in the clinical site where you are assigned.
2. Research the protocol used for treating alcohol withdrawal at the clinical site where you are assigned.
3. Review the procedure manual at your clinical site to determine the documentation process used for persons suspected of substance abuse.

Copyright © 2004 Mosby Inc. All rights reserved.

4. Review the laws regulating nursing in your state that pertain to substance abuse. What are the responsibilities of a nurse who suspects a colleague of substance abuse? Is there an impairment program available for nurses?

5. Attend an Alcoholics Anonymous (AA) or Narcotics Anonymous (NA) meeting and identify strategies used by these groups to foster abstinence. Discuss findings in class.

Copyright © 2004 Mosby Inc. All rights reserved.

48 Substance Abuse

Review Sheet

The QUESTION column and the ANSWER column have been offset so that you can cover the answers while reading the questions, allowing you to assess your knowledge.

Question	**Answer**
1. Define *substance-related disorders, substance abuse, impairment, dependence, addiction,* and *illicit substances.*	
2. Differentiate among the biological model, psychological theories, and sociocultural factors that are associated with substance abuse.	1. See textbook, pp. 715-716.
3. List sociological signs of impairment associated with substance abuse.	2. Biologic model: caused by person's genetic profile. Psychologic theory: sees alcoholism as occurring in an individual who is fixated in the oral stage of development and is seeking oral gratification. This theory also recognizes a link to depression, anxiety, antisocial personality, and dependent personality. Sociocultural: the individual is influenced by such things as attitudes, norms, values, nationality, religion, gender, family background, and social environment.
4. List four tests used to screen for alcohol and substance abuse.	3. Substance abuse first affects the family life, then social life, and finally results in physical and mental changes.
5. What is the prevalence of substance abuse by health care professionals?	4. See Table 48-4.
6. Cite legal considerations associated with substance abuse and dependence in health care providers.	5. See textbook, p. 717.
7. List three long-term goals of treatment of substance abuse as defined by the American Psychiatric Association.	6. See textbook, pp. 720-721; research laws governing nursing in the state where you are practicing.
8. Cite examples of organizations that promote the goals of abstinence from substance abuse.	7. Reduction or abstinence in use and effects of substances; reduction in frequency and severity of relapse; and improvement in psychological and social functioning.
9. Compare the effects on the body of acute and chronic use of alcohol.	8. AA, NA, and others

Copyright © 2004 Mosby Inc. All rights reserved.

10. Define *alcohol intoxication* and *alcohol withdrawal*.
11. What drugs are used to treat alcohol withdrawal symptoms?
12. Describe components of an alcohol relapse prevention program.

13. Name two medications used to promote abstinence from alcohol use.
14. List commonly abused opiates.
15. List the signs and symptoms of opioid intoxication and opioid withdrawal.

16. What limitations does naltrexone (ReVia) have in the treatment of opioid addiction?
17. Name two new dosage forms of buprenorphine approved for opioid maintenance programs.

18. What effect does cocaine have on the CNS?

19. What is the difference between "freebase" and "crack" cocaine?

20. Describe the signs and symptoms of cocaine intoxication and withdrawal from cocaine.

21. List the nursing assessments that should be used when substance abuse is suspected or diagnosed.
22. What laboratory tests are routinely ordered for drug screening?
23. Study Table 48-3 to identify drugs, usage forms, possible side effects, signs of overdose, and long-term effects of drugs classified as stimulants, depressants, narcotics, cannabis, hallucinogens, and inhalants.

9. See textbook, pp. 722-723.

10. See textbook, p. 723.

11. Benzodiazepines are used for detoxification. Long-acting chlordiazepoxide, diazepam, and clorazepate most commonly used protocol for alcohol withdrawal.
12. See textbook, p. 723.

13. Disulfiram (Antabuse) and naltrexone (ReVia)
14. Heroin, morphine, hydromorphone, codeine, oxycodone, and hydrocodone; opiate-like substances (e.g., meperidine, fentanyl, others)
15. See textbook, pp. 723-724.

16. Naltrexone does not block the desire to get "high;" it only blocks the "high" when an opioid is used.
17. Buprenorphine (Subtex) and buprenorphine-naloxone (Suboxone)
18. Blocks metabolism of catecholamines in the brain, bringing on a sudden CNS stimulation with euphoria or a "rush"
19. "Freebase" is cocaine hydrochloride mixed with ammonia and dissolved in ether. As ether evaporates, it forms a powder residue that can be smoked for its "high." "Crack" cocaine is cocaine hydrochloride mixed with baking soda that is heated to form "rocks" which are then smoked.
20. See textbook, pp. 724-725.

21. See textbook, pp. 725-729.

22. See textbook, p. 727.

23. See Table 48-3.

Copyright © 2004 Mosby Inc. All rights reserved.

CHAPTER 48

Substance Abuse

Practice Quiz

COMPLETION

Complete the following statements.

1. THC, hashish, and marijuana are classified as _____.

2. LSD and PCP are classified as _____.

3. Nicotine, caffeine, amphetamines, and cocaine are classified as _____.

4. Loss of coordination, sluggishness, slurred speech, and disorientation are possible side effects of the use of drugs classified as _____.

5. The onset of major motor seizures during alcohol withdrawal usually occur _____ hours after alcohol is withdrawn.

6. Four possible consequences of severe cocaine intoxication are _____, _____, _____, _____, and _____.

7. _____ is a drug used for relapse prevention to block the pharmacologic effects of opioids and alcohol.

END-OF-CHAPTER MATH REVIEW

1. Order: chlordiazepoxide (Librium) 100 mg, IM
   On hand: chlordiazepoxide (Librium) 100 mg/ml
   Give: _____ ml.

2. Order: lorazepam (Ativan) 2 mg, IM, q 1 h until patient is moderately sedated.
   On hand: lorazepam (Ativan) 4 mg/ml
   Give: _____ ml.

3. Order: lorazepam (Ativan) 2 mg, PO, stat
   On hand: lorazepam (Ativan) 1 mg tab.
   Give: _____ tab.

CRITICAL THINKING QUESTIONS

1. Investigate the community resources available in your area for alcoholics, drug users, and families or significant others. Then attend a meeting to observe:
   a. How participants are guided to accept responsibility for their actions.
   b. How participants deal with the problem of relapse.
   c. What problems with sobriety participants discuss.
   d. The incidence of alcohol and drug use in teens, adults, and older adults.

2. Research the protocol used for treatment of alcohol withdrawal in the patient care units where you are assigned.

3. What medico-legal requirements are incorporated into emergency room procedures for persons admitted with suspected substance abuse?

REVIEW QUESTIONS

1. The _____ theory of substance abuse focuses on the patterns of relationships between family members through the generations.

2. The theory that attributes alcohol abuse to a person being fixed in the oral stage of development is an example of a _____ theory.

3. The alcohol withdrawal protocol lists the treatment for severe withdrawal as _____ _____ _____.

Copyright © 2004 Mosby Inc. All rights reserved.

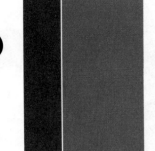

Answer Key

CHAPTER 1

Practice Quiz

1. pharmacology
2. drug
3. The chemical name describes the exact placement of atoms and molecular groupings of a chemical compound; it is of most value to the chemist. The brand name, also known as the trade name, is used by a particular manufacturer to market a drug. The brand name is capitalized and is followed by an ®, which is the symbol of a registered trademark. The generic name is given to a drug and is used as the official name for reference to the drug by any and all manufacturers and in all countries. It is not capitalized.
4. Brand names: Bayer®, Ecotrin®, Empirin® Generic name: aspirin
5. Brand names: Anacin-3®, Datril®, Tempra®, Tylenol® Generic name: acetaminophen
6. Brand name: Pepto-Bismol® Generic names: bismuth subsalicylate
7. Brand names: Maalox®, Gelusil II®, Aludrox® Generic name ingredients: magnesium hydroxide and aluminum hydroxide
8. Brand names: Motrin IB®, Advil®, Nuprin® Generic name: ibuprofen
9. Brand names: Tums®, Bio-Cal®, Cal-Sup® Generic name: calcium carbonate
10. *American Drug Index*: Index for all drugs available in U.S.
11. *American Hospital Formulary Service, Drug Information*: Contains drug monographs on every single-drug entity available in U.S.
12. *Facts and Comparisons*: Book is arranged by body systems. Each chapter is subdivided by therapeutic classes. The data in each monograph is the most current FDA-approved package insert information and includes publication from official groups; e.g., CDC and National Academy of Science.
13. *Martindale—The Complete Drug Reference*: Comprehensive text of drugs used throughout the world.
14. *Handbook of Nonprescription Drugs*: Most comprehensive book on medicines sold over-the-counter in the United States.
15. *Medical Letter*: A biweekly newsletter with comments on newly released drug products.
16. *Physicians' Desk Reference*: Reference on pharmacology

divided into seven sections. See p. 6 of textbook to further verify content of each section.
17. IV
18. IV
19. IV
20. II
21. II
22. II
23. III
24. III
25. III
26. II
27. II
28. The Controlled Substance Act of 1970 provides the legal basis for the drugs that are classified as controlled substances. This law establishes the degree of control, the conditions of record-keeping, the particular order forms required, and other regulations relating to these drugs depending on classification.
29. Nurses must administer controlled substances under the direction of a physician or dentist who has been licensed to prescribe these agents. Nurses may not have a controlled substance in their possession unless 1) they have been requested to administer it to a patient under a doctor's order, 2) the nurse is the patient for whom the controlled sub-

Copyright © 2004 Mosby Inc. All rights reserved.

prescribed, or 3) the nurse is the official custodian of a limited supply of controlled substances on a patient care unit of a hospital.

30. *Tyler's Honest Herbal* contains monographs on 120 individual herbal names with information on the herb's use and the author's judgment with regard to rational clinical uses of the herb.

31. Answers will be individual, based on the clinical setting.

32. preclinical phase
    clinical research and development
    new drug application review
    postmarketing surveillance

33. The cost of drug development for medicines used for rare diseases is so great that the companies cannot recover their expenses. Special benefits must be provided as an incentive for manufacturers to research and develop medicines for rare diseases.

CHAPTER 2

Practice Quiz

1. F, parenteral
2. T
3. T
4. T
5. F, percutaneous
6. T
7. F, do not stimulate a response.
8. T
9. F, inactivation of drug
10. T
11. T
12. F, metabolism
13. T
14. additive
15. synergistic
16. displacement
17. incompatibility

18. Drug tolerance occurs when increasingly larger doses are required to achieve the same effect that was achieved with a lesser dose previously.

19. Drug dependence means "addiction."

20. Adverse drug reactions are sometimes referred to as drug toxicity.

21. c
22. b
23. b
24. c
25. a
26. a

CHAPTER 3

Practice Quiz

1. T
2. F, not
3. F, does not have
4. T
5. F, does not
6. T
7. T
8. F, An elder has a lower percentage of body fluid than an infant.
9. T
10. T
11. T
12. F, Bound drug is unable to cause a drug action.
13. F, Infants are babies 1–24 months of age.
14. T
15. T
16. F, more rapid in women
17. T
18. T
19. F, do not
20. T

CHAPTER 4

Practice Quiz

1. subjective
2. assessment

3. medication history
4. defining characteristics, actual nursing diagnosis
5. action/intervention
6. measurable goal
7. the exact time the last dose of the medication was administered
8. before
9. risk
10. evaluation
11. nursing classification system

CHAPTER 5

Practice Quiz

1. F, cognitive
2. T
3. T
4. T
5. F, not
6. T
7. F, Referral may be necessary.
8. T
9. T
10. T

CHAPTER 6

Practice Quiz 1

1. 1
2. 3
3. 1
4. 2
5. 4
6. 1
7. 480
8. 60
9. 1
10. 1000
11. 1000
12. 1000
13. 15
14. multiply number of g by 15
15. divide number of gr by 15
16. divide by 1000; that is, move decimal point of milligrams three places to left
17. multiply the number of grains by 60 (60 mg/gr)

Copyright © 2004 Mosby Inc. All rights reserved.

Practice Quiz 2
1. v
2. viiss
3. iv
4. xv
5. xx
6. xxiv
7. 1
8. 2
9. 3
10. 2
11. 10
12. 2 as written or 12 as improper fraction
13. 10
14. 3
15. 1/8
16. 3/4
17. 1/100
18. 1/3
19. 7/8
20. 1/90
21. 1/4
22. 1/2
23. 1/2
24. 3/4
25. 1 2/3
26. 3 2/5
27. 1 3/4
28. 12 3/4
29. 2 1/2
30. 1/3
31. 0.875 = 0.88
32. 0.833= 0.83
33. 1.75
34. 0.666= 0.67
35. 0.9375 = 0.94
36. 0.333= 0.33
37. 0.625= 0.63
38. 0.777=0.78
39. 0.063= 0.06
40. 0.5
41. 1/12
42. 1/4
43. 7/16
44. 21/32
45. 2/7
46. 7/12
47. 1 1/8
48. 2 2/15
49. 0.76=0.8
50. 0.66=0.7
51. 2.22=2.2
52. 17.70=17.7
53. 61.46=61.5
54. 17.97=18
55. 1866.66= 1866.7
56. 3.81=3.8
57. 33.83=33.8
58. 0.56
59. 0.0066=0.66%
60. 66.6%
61. 0.75
62. 0.005
63. 75%
64. 87.5%
65. 1.23
66. 3/10
67. 3/1000
68. 3/100
69. 0.4
70. 0.04
71. 0.004
72. 3:4
73. 3:5
74. 1:200
75. 4
76. 16
77. 1
78. 30
79. 125
80. 360
81. 0.25
82. 4
83. 4 or 5
84. 2.73
85. 75

CHAPTER 7

Practice Quiz
1. d
2. a
3. e
4. c
5. ab
6. a
7. d
8. b
9. c
10. d
11. b
12. Check school policy, usually F
13. c
14. d
15. c
16. b
17. a
18. b
19. d
20. d
21. c
22. b
23. d
24. patient's full name, date, drug name, route of administration, dose, duration of the order, and signature of the order.
25. Response is clinical site-dependent.
26. Response is clinical site-dependent.

CHAPTER 8

Practice Quiz
1. See textbook, pp. 100-101.
2. See textbook, p. 101.
3. lotions
4. See textbook, p. 101; charting should be checked with course instructor.
5. See textbook, pp. 103-105.
6. See textbook, pp. 105-106.
7. Have A.H. turn on the call light whenever using the nitroglycerin. Obtain data regarding location, degree of pain being experienced, and relief obtained. As appropriate, take and record vital signs. Chart symptoms present, degree of relief, number of nitroglycerin tablets used for each attack, and vital signs. See also Chapter 10, p. 241.

Copyright © 2004 Mosby Inc. All rights reserved.

8. See charting—checked by instructor.

9. See textbook, pp. 108-110.

10. If inner canthus is not blocked, eye drops would drain immediately from the eye without coming in contact with the eye surface and being absorbed. There is also a greater likelihood that the patient may suffer systemic adverse effects of the drug if it is allowed to drain into the canal.

11. In a child under 3 years, the earlobe is pulled downward and back; in an adult, it is pulled upward and back.

12. Gently blowing the nose clears nasal passages and allows better contact and absorption of medication via mucous membranes.

13. Overuse of some nasal sprays causes "rebound" effect that will cause worsening of symptoms. If drug is not effective, call pharmacist or physician; do not increase the number of drugs or frequency of taking the medication.

14. See textbook, pp. 113-114.

15. See textbook, pp. 114-115.

CHAPTER 9

Practice Quiz

1. A capsule is a gelatin-type container holding dry or liquid drug.

2. Time-release tablets have layers of coating on the drug within the tablet so it dissolves at different rates.

3. oral; hold them in the mouth until they dissolve

4. water and alcohol

5. concentrated sugar with water

6. Emulsions are dispersed droplets throughout oil or water. Suspensions are liquid medications that require shaking before administration to disperse the insoluble drug throughout the solution.

7. 2

8. 5

9. F, Use accompanying dropper only; replace from pharmacy.

10. T

11. F, Clamp NG as fluid clears bottom of bulb syringe.

12. T

13. F, 24 hours

14. T

15. T

16. F, left

17. T

18. F, 1.0-6.0

19. F, yellow, bile-colored

20. F, Auscultation is not accurate.

CHAPTER 10

Practice Quiz

1. Figure 10-1, Parts of Syringe

2. 0.5 ml

3. 1.4 ml

4. 2.2 ml

5. 1.7 ml

6. 52 U

7. 64 U

8. 11 U

9. 0.05 ml

10. 0.65 ml

11. 0.71 ml

12. 0.13 ml

13. Figure 10-12, Parts of Needle

14. 0.01–0.1

15. 0.5–2.0

16. 0.5–2.0; 2 to 3 ml, see Note Table 10-1

17. 1000-2000 ml/24 hrs or as MD prescribes

18. Figure 10-20, p. 141.

19. Figure 10-21, p. 141.

20. Figure 10-22, p. 141.

21. See pp. 146-147.

CHAPTER 11

Practice Quiz

1. U-100 insulin syringe

2. tuberculin syringe

3. 3 ml syringe

4. 17 U

5. 1.7 ml

6. 0.07 ml

7. 2.6 ml

8. 0.86 ml

9. 36 U

10. 0.01–0.1 ml

11. 0.5–2 ml

12. 0.5–2 ml; divided 2–3 ml

13. 2 ml

14. 0.7 ml; TB or 3 ml syringe

15. 1.7 ml

16. a. Figure 11-1
    b. Figure 11-3
    c. Figure 11-5

17. label diagram

18. drawing, see Figure 11-6, p. 154

19. drawing, see Figure 11-18, p. 157

20. label

CHAPTER 12

Practice Quiz

1. macrodrip

2. syringe pump

3. over

4. midline access catheter

5. PICC

6. Groshong

7. arteries, veins, capillaries

8. 295–310

9. superior vena cava

10. CDC (Centers for Disease Control and Prevention)

11. no; promotes fungal infections and antimicrobial resistance

12. 2 ml saline

Copyright © 2004 Mosby Inc. All rights reserved.

13. Date and time tubing was opened; date and time tubing is to be changed; initials of person preparing the tubing.
14. q 24 hours
15. Fill volume chamber with specified amount of IV solution, clamp tubing between IV bottle or bag and the volume chamber, add medication via injection port, disperse medication throughout the solution in the volume chamber, adjust the flow rate.
16. 33 gtt/min
17. 31 gtt/min
18. 17 gtt/min
19. 31 gtt/min
20. microdrip chamber
21. over-the-needle catheter
22. Figure 12-11, p. 168.

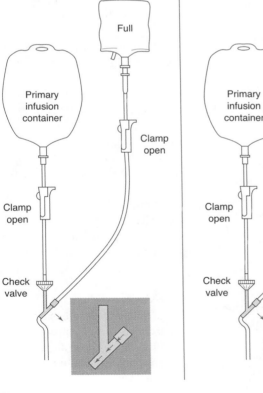

CHAPTER 13

Practice Quiz
1. norepinephrine, epinephrine, dopamine
2. kidneys, brain, and gastrointestinal tract
3. alpha, beta, and dopaminergic
4. parasympathetic
5. smooth muscle relaxation; bronchodilation
6. smooth muscle contraction; bronchoconstriction
7. vitals; blood pressure, check for use of bronchodilators and decongestants
8. tachycardia, orthostatic hypotension, dizziness, tremors, flushed skin
9. dryness of mucous membranes, urinary retention, constipation

10. "olol"
11. See textbook, p. 195.
12. See textbook, p. 193.
13. See textbook, p. 193.
14. See textbook, p. 193.

End-of-Chapter Math Review
1. 16 ml
2. 1 1/2 tablets
3. 0.4 mg; 1 ml

CHAPTER 14

Practice Quiz
1. initial insomnia
2. terminal insomnia
3. hypnotic
4. sedative
5. intermittent
6. hypnotic
7. nursing diagnosis: Sleep pattern disturbance r/t insufficient data m/b inability to sleep through the night
8. nursing diagnosis: Knowledge deficit related to hypnotic action/therapy m/b lack of understanding of long-term use of hypnotics for nightly sleep disturbance
9. barbiturates: hangover, sedation, lethargy; BZD: drowsiness, hangover, sedation, lethargy
10. Physical dependence to a drug is when the individual cannot function effectively without the drug.
11. See Review Sheet, Sedative-hypnotics, p. 85 of the Student Learning Guide. Benzodiazepines: see textbook pp. 204-205. Barbiturates: see textbook pp. 203-204.

End-of-Chapter Math Review
1. 2 tablets of 0.25 mg. General rule, when two dosages are available, give the least number of tablets to accurately fill the prescribed amount.

Copyright © 2004 Mosby Inc. All rights reserved.

2. 4 ml of 500 mg/5 ml syrup or 8 ml of 250 mg/5 ml chloral hydrate. Neither of capsules, 250 mg or 500 mg can be given to accurately prepare the ordered dose.
3. Safe dosage range is between 6 mg and 9 mg, therefore prescribed amount of 7.5 mg is reasonable.

CHAPTER 15

Practice Quiz
1. dopamine, acetylcholine
2. Regain dopaminergic activity as close to normal level of functioning; reduce symptoms of disease, thereby increasing the individual's quality of life.
3. See textbook, pp. 209-210.
4. Variable responses possible, check with instructor.
5. monitoring blood pressure q shift; provide for patient safety, etc.
6. Assess orientation to name, place, date, time, and basic functioning; e.g., confusion, alertness, etc.
7. Response time may vary and dosage will be individualized; response may not be immediate.
8. anticholinergic
9. See textbook, p. 217.
10. to reduce metabolism of levodopa
11. to cross into brain and be metabolized to dopamine to help restore deficient dopamine levels
12. is to reduce destruction of dopamine in peripheral tissue making more dopamine available in the brain
13. akinesia
14. livedo reticularis
15. sudden sleep events

End-of-Chapter Math Review
1. 1 tablet per dose of 25/100 strength
2. 1 tablet, 250 mg per dose of 250 mg strength
3. 1/2 tablet of 2.5 mg strength per dose

CHAPTER 16

Practice Quiz
1.-6. See textbook, pp. 225-226.
7. See textbook, pp. 226-229.
8. Provide for patient safety while intervening to reduce panic level.
9. benzodiazepines
Action: Stimulate neurotransmitter GABA that will reduce anxiety level.
Side effects: CNS depression (e.g. drowsiness, sedation, lethargy).
10. azapirones
Action: Midbrain modulator whose action is not fully understood; it is a partial serotonin agonist.
Side effects: CNS depression (e.g. drowsiness, sedation, lethargy).
11. hydroxyzine
Action: Antihistamine with several actions on CNS.
Side effects: CNS depression (e.g. drowsiness, sedation, lethargy) and anticholinergic activity (e.g. dry mucosa, blurred vision, constipation, urinary retention).
12. meprobamate
Action: Unknown mechanism of action
Side effects: CNS depression (e.g. drowsiness, sedation, lethargy)
Note: All of these drugs act on the CNS to produce some degree of depression.

13. level of anxiety present, vital signs including blood pressure in sitting and lying positions; check for history of blood dyscrasias or hepatic disease; determine if the patient is in the first trimester of pregnancy or is breast feeding

End-of-Chapter Math Review
1. 0.8 ml
2. 400 mg/dose
3. 0.75 ml

CHAPTER 17

Practice Quiz
1. euphoria or elation
2. depression
3. MAOIs
4. SSRIs
5. tricyclic antidepressants
6. miscellaneous agents (e.g., bupropion hydrochloride)
7. blood pressure and pulse
8. baseline blood sugar (diabetics)
9. meals with tyramine content
10. medical history (e.g., levodopa)
11. extrapyramidal symptoms
12. to check for therapeutic response
13. blocking reuptake or destruction of neurotransmitters (norepinephrine, dopamine, serotonin)
14. tyramine
15. SSRIs
16. the drug's anticholinergic effects (e.g., blurred vision, constipation, urinary retention, dry mucosa)
17. sedation
18. orthostatic hypotension
19. lab tests (e.g., electrolytes, FBS, BUN, creatinine clearance, urinalysis, thyroid function)
20. blood pressure

Copyright © 2004 Mosby Inc. All rights reserved.

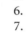

21. baseline weight and hydration status
22. signs of sodium depletion
23. 0.4–1.5 mEq/L
24. norepinephrine, dopamine, serotonin
25. mania
26. answers vary (e.g., blaming others, making excuses)
27. meperidine

End-of-Chapter Math Review
1. 2 tablets
2. Dosage available: 25, 50, and 75 mg tablets. Most likely 50 mg dispensed for this order. The 100 mg dose prescribed would require 2 tablets (50 mg strength).

CHAPTER 18

Practice Quiz
1. d
2. f
3. a
4. c
5. e
6. Thorazine
7. perphenazine
8. thioridazine
9. Clozaril
10. haloperidol
11. prochlorperazine

End-of-Chapter Math Review
1. 6.25 ml
2. 2 tabs
3. 0.6ml of 20 mg/ml or 1.2 ml of 10 mg/ml
   Use either available concentration.

CHAPTER 19

Practice Quiz
1. barbiturate, benzodiazepines, hydantoins, succinimides, miscellaneous agents
2. increases seizure threshold and regulates neuronal firing in the brain

3. tonic phase—loss of consciousness, body rigidity, intense muscle contractions
   clonic phase—alternate jerking and relaxation of extremities
4. benzodiazepines
5. hyperglycemia
6. Phenytoin, Tegretol, Primidone
7. antacid
8. See textbook, p. 268.
9. hypotension, dyspnea, edema, hepatotoxicity, blood dyscrasias, dermatologic reactions
10. carbamazepine (Tegretol)
11. zonisamide (Zonegran)
12. neuropathic pain; mania and depression

End-of-Chapter Math Review
1. Orders need clarification. What is the route of administration? What form of drug is to be used? Available in 50 mg tablets; 30 and 100 mg capsules; suspension 30 and 125 mg/5 ml and in 50 mg/ml injectable forms. Give 100 mg Dilantin capsules three times per day and at hs if PO route is used. Schedule: 8:00 AM, 1:00 PM, 6:00 PM, 10:00 PM (hs).
2. Using an oral syringe, measure 2.5 ml of Tegretol suspension to administer 50 mg. Give PO approximately every 6 hours.
3. Yes, this is a reasonable order. Valproic acid (Depakene) is only available in oral forms. At 15 mg/kg/24 hr, and 110 lb (50 kg), this means a total daily dose of 750 mg/24 hour or 250 mg tid. Depakene syrup is available 250 mg/5 ml. Give 5 ml, three times per day at 7:00 AM, 2:00 PM and 10:00 PM.

(The later dose would maintain more consistent blood level.)

CHAPTER 20

Practice Quiz
1. awareness of the sensation of pain
2. level at which pain is first felt
3. drugs that relieve pain without producing loss of consciousness
4. See textbook, pp. 287-288.
5. baseline neurologic assessment: vital signs, voiding and bowel pattern, prior use of analgesics, pain assessment
6. no
7. sedation, light-headedness, nausea, vomiting, sweating, orthostatic hypotension, constipation
8. for reversal of CNS depression effects of opiate agonists, opiate partial agonists and propoxyphene
9. gastric irritation
10. No, it is not an anti-inflammatory agent.
11. 21
12. 83
13. when the patient has abnormal liver function, or the drug causes these effects
14. salicylism: tinnitus, impaired hearing, decreased vision, sweating, fever, lethargy, dizziness, mental confusion
15. Nalmefene, naloxone, naltrexone
16. See drug monograph, textbook, pp. 304.

End-of-Chapter Math Review
1. 2 tablets
2. 3.8 ml
3. Give 1 ml, 15 mg/ml morphine

Copyright © 2004 Mosby Inc. All rights reserved.

4. Does not say PO; clarify order. Also, is this drug required qid or is it better on a q 4 h prn basis?

CHAPTER 21

Practice Quiz

1. atorvastatin, fluvastatin, lovastatin, pravastatin, simvastatin
2. decreased LDL, decreased total cholesterol, decreased triglycerides, increased HDLs
3. may cause hyperglycemia
4. baseline cholesterol, triglycerides, FBS (gemfibrozil), any GI symptoms, and liver function studies
5. fat-soluble vitamins, DEAK
6. thyroxine: early signs of hypothyroidism: fatigue, weight gain
    warfarin: anticoagulant properties would decline and patient would be prone to signs and symptoms of clot formation
7. T
8. F, increases HDL
9. T
10. T
11. F, decreases drug effectiveness
12. T
13. F, hyperglycemia
14. F, DEAK
15. 2 capsules

End-of-Chapter Math Review

1. 1 tablet/dose (500 mg tablet) total 1500 mg daily
2. 4 tablets

CHAPTER 22

Practice Quiz

1. e
2. a
3. c
4. b
5. b
6. a
7. ab
8. ac
9. c
10. T
11. F, Etiology is unknown.
12. T
13. F, Lifestyle changes are the first approach followed by the use of thiazide or thiazide-like diuretics.
14. T
15. F, vasoconstriction resulting in increased blood pressure
16. F, Take blood pressure in lying, sitting, and standing positions (usually done initially once a shift).
17. T
18. T
19. F, Start with thiazide or thiazide-like diuretics commonly.
20. F, Should also have baseline weight, hydration status, and laboratory studies deemed appropriate by the health care provider.
21. pulse
22. peripheral resistance
23. vasoconstriction; increased peripheral resistance
24. 60 gtt/min

End-of-Chapter Math Review

1. Call pharmacy and ask that 0.3 mg tablets be provided. Would only need 2 tabs of 0.3 mg administered twice daily. Otherwise, 1 tablet of 0.2 mg strength and 1 tablet of 0.1 mg strength or 3 tablets of 0.1 mg tablets could be administered twice daily.
2. 2 tabs per dose
    9:00 AM, 4:00 PM, and 10:00 PM or 0900, 1600, and 2200

CHAPTER 23

Practice Quiz

1. negative chronotropy
2. inotropic
3. digitalization
4. apical; one full
5. after meals; gastric irritation
6. reduce fluid and sodium overload
7. tachycardia resulting in increased cardiac output
8. reduce afterload by blocking angiotensin II-mediated peripheral vasoconstriction and help reduce circulating blood volume by inhibiting secretion of aldosterone
9. to increase renal output, thereby decreasing overall blood volume
10. intravenously
11. improves circulation and cardiac output by slowing the heart rate and strengthening force of each contraction

End-of-Chapter Math Review

1. 75 kg
    450 mcg or 0.45 mg
    Digoxin may be administered undiluted; or each 1 ml may be diluted in 4 ml sterile water. IV dose should be given slowly over at least 5 minutes. Give with caution with hypertension because IV administration may elevate blood pressure. It is compatible with normal saline, D_5W, or lactated Ringer's solution.
2. Give 0.5 ml of 0.25 mg/ml
3. Two alternatives:
    Give 1 tablet of 0.25 mg and 1 tablet of 0.125 mg or
    Give 3 tablets of 0.125 mg digoxin
    Which method would be most accurate? Discuss with the clinical instructor.

Copyright © 2004 Mosby Inc. All rights reserved.

CHAPTER 24

Practice Quiz

1. restore normal sinus rhythm
2. restore normal cardiac function
3. prevent life-threatening arrhythmias
4. poor tissue perfusion to brain cells
5. myocardial depression by preventing sodium ion movement
6. prolongs duration of electrical stimulation on cells and refractory time between electrical impulses
7. decreases heart rate
8. decreases systolic blood pressure
9. decreases cardiac output
10. Local anesthetic lidocaine contains a preservative and may have epinephrine added; either of which may be harmful to a patient with an arrhythmia.
11. rash, chills, fever, tinnitus from quinidine
12. SA node to AV node to Bundle of His to Purkinje fibers to the heart tissue of the myocardium
13. electrocardiogram
14. dyspnea
15. fatigue
16. edema
17. chest pain
18. syncope
19. palpitations
20. T
21. F; hypoglycemic symptoms
22. T
23. F; Class 1c antiarrhythmics
24. T
25. F, difference between systolic and diastolic blood pressure readings
26. F, lidocaine

End-of-Chapter Math Review

1. 4 tablets/ dose
   2.4 g in 24 hours
2. 4 capsules/dose

CHAPTER 25

Practice Quiz

1. See textbook, pp. 368-369.
2. See textbook, pp. 369-370.
3. See textbook, p. 370.
4. Up to 3 tablets sublingually over 15 minute period (5 minutes apart). If no relief is obtained, seek additional treatment from health care provider or emergency department.
5. q 8–12 h
6. Transmucosal tablets are placed under the upper lip or buccal pouch. One tablet tid, one on arising, pc lunch, and pc evening meal.
7. See textbook, pp. 372-373
8. See answer to Review Sheet, answer 6.
9. See Tables 25-2, 13-3, 22-5
10. See individual drug monographs.

End-of-Chapter Math Review

1. 2 tablets
2. 1 capsule
   Sublingual administration; puncture capsule with needle and squeeze medication under the tongue.
3. 2 ml

CHAPTER 26

Practice Quiz

1. T
2. F, seek medical treatment from health care provider
3. F, tolerance of exercise should increase
4. T
5. T

6. See textbook, p. 378.
7. See textbook, pp. 378-380.
8. See textbook, p. 379.
9. improvement in tissue perfusion, decreased pain, increase in exercise tolerance, and improvement in peripheral pulses
10. See textbook, p. 380

End-of-Chapter Math Review

1. 400 mg dose x 4 days requires 4 tablets; the next 5 days require 10 tablets
2. 2 capsules per dose

CHAPTER 27

Practice Quiz

1. heart failure
2. hypertension
3. hematocrit
4. hemoglobin
5. BUN
6. electrolytes (also skin turgor, I/O, breath sounds, others)
7. 135–145 mEq/L
8. 3.5–4.7 mEq/L
9. furosemide
10. ototoxicity
11. hyperglycemia
12. hyperuricemia
13. orthostatic hypotension or dehydration
14.–16. Bumetanide (Bumex), ethacrynic acid (Edecrin), furosemide (Lasix) or torsemide (Demadex)
17.–19. See Table 27-1, 27-2
20. amiloride (Midamor), spironolactone (Aldactone), or triamterene (Dyrenium)
21. Data are used as a baseline for comparison with subsequent data to evaluate response to diuretic therapy.
22. Decreased uric acid excretion may result in hyperuricemia; prevented by administering allopurinol especially in patients who

Copyright © 2004 Mosby Inc. All rights reserved.

have a history of previous gouty arthritis attacks.

23. Potassium and sodium; occasionally magnesium and chloride

24. Diuretics can cause excessive excretion of potassium resulting in hypokalemia while loss of fluid may cause increased concentrations of the digoxin leading to signs of digoxin toxicity.

25. aminoglycosides

26. furosemide and torsemide = loop diuretic
    hydrochlorothiazide = thiazide diuretic
    spironolactone = potassium-sparing diuretic

27. Combination diuretics contain both a thiazide and potassium-sparing diuretic in an attempt to prevent hypokalemia associated with the use of a thiazide diuretic alone.

28. Hyperkalemia (more likely in persons with diabetes mellitus or renal impairment)

End-of-Chapter Math Review

1. 100 ml/hr
2. 2 tablets

CHAPTER 28

Practice Quiz

1. embolus
2. thrombus
3. platelet inhibitors and anticoagulants
4. fibrinolytic agents
5. APTT
6. 1.5–2.5 times the control APTT value
7. daily platelet counts
8. periodic CBC
9. stools for occult blood
10. bleeding at any site

11. signs and symptoms of shock
12. blood in stools or urine
13. platelet count at or below 100,000 mm^3
14. vitamin K
15. b
16. c
17. 8 ml/hr
18. 80 gtts/min

End-of-Chapter Math Review

1. 0.2 ml
2. 2.7 ml/hr
   2400 U have already infused.
   4 ml/hr
3. 28 tablets

CHAPTER 29

Practice Quiz

1. vasoconstrict
2. following prescribed dosage and duration of therapy
3. antihistamines or H$_2$ receptor antagonists
4. on a regular schedule whether or not an allergen or symptoms are present
5. See textbook, p. 423.
6. See Chapter 8, pp. 111-112.

End-of-Chapter Math Review

1. 10 ml daily (using 5 ml/tsp equivalent)
2. Two 5 mg tablets or one 10 mg tablet
3. 10 ml

CHAPTER 30

Practice Quiz

1. See textbook, p. 427.
2. See textbook, p. 426.
3. See textbook, p. 432.
4. See textbook, p. 432.
5. liquefy mucus
6. suppress cough center in brain
7. acts directly on mucus plug(s) to reduce thick-

ness and/or dissolve mucus plug(s)
8. SaO$_2$
9. Asthma
10. spirometer
11. expectorant
12. potassium iodide
13. Acetylcysteine (Mucomyst)
14. palpitations and/or tachycardia
15. Corticosteroids
16. Antileukotriene

End-of-Chapter Math Review

1. 9.4 ml or 2.7 tsp using equivalent 4 ml/tsp or 1.8 tsp using equivalent 5 ml/tsp
2. 0.25 ml
3. Give 87.95 = 88 mg/*individual dose*
4. Give 8.8 ml/*individual dose*

CHAPTER 31

Practice Quiz

1. cold sores caused by herpes simplex type I virus
2. fungal infections caused by *Candida albicans*
3. foul odor from the mouth
4. partial or complete stoppage of saliva in the mouth
5.-9.   lidocaine
    Milk of Magnesia
    Kaopectate
    nystatin liquid or clotrimazole
    lozenges
    sucralfate suspension
    oral or parenteral analgesics

CHAPTER 32

Practice Quiz

1. F, ineffective
2. T
3. F, increases pH
4. T
5. T
6. T

Copyright © 2004 Mosby Inc. All rights reserved.

7. F, coats ulcer crater
8. F, increases peristalsis
9. T
10. Sucralfate
11. aluminum and magnesium ions
12. with
13. H_2 antagonists
14. acid rebound
15. See Table 32-4, textbook p. 470
16. See Table 32-2, textbook p. 464
17. 2.5 ml
18. 1 tab ac
2 tab at hs

End-of-Chapter Math Review
1. 300 ml/hr
2. 0.875 = 0.88 ml

CHAPTER 33

Practice Quiz
1. a pregnant woman with persistent vomiting that affects electrolyte, fluid and nutritional status
2. self-induced vomiting in response to an unpleasant stimulus
3. chemotherapy-induced emesis
4. suppression of vomiting center
5. interruption of impulses going to or from vomiting center
6. inhibiting dopamine receptors in pathway to vomiting center
7. CIE and postoperative nausea and vomiting
8. motion sickness
9. as soon as nausea is initially experienced
10. stimulation of labyrinth system of the ear with subsequent transmission of stimulus to vomiting center

11. 24–120 hours
12. dopamine antagonists, serotonin antagonists, anticholinergic agents, corticosteroids, benzodiazepines, and cannabinoids
13. See textbook, p. 475.
14. See textbook, p. 477, dopamine antagonists.
See textbook, p. 477, serotonin antagonists.
See textbook, p. 482, anticholinergic agents.
See textbook, p. 482, corticosteroids.
See textbook, p. 483, benzodiazepines.
See textbook, p. 483, cannabinoids.

End-of-Chapter Math Review
1. 61.36 kg; 9.2 mg of ondansetron; set infusion pump to 150 ml/hr
2. 1.5 ml

CHAPTER 34

Practice Quiz
1. a. retains H_2O in stool, stimulates peristalsis
   b. softens stool and lubricates intestinal mucosa, peristalsis not increased
   c. adsorbs excess H_2O to cause stool to be formed
   d. decreased peristalsis and GI motility
2. foods contaminated with bacteria or protozoa or contaminated drinking water
3. high-fiber diet with adequate fluids for hydration, especially water
4. magnesium
5. bulk-forming laxatives

CHAPTER 35

Practice Quiz
1. 2-4 oz fruit juice with 2 tsp sugar or honey, 1 c skim milk, 4 oz nondiet soft drink, or 1 piece of candy (not chocolate)
2. insulin
monitoring of blood glucose and ketones
hospitalization
identify underlying cause
if severe, usually requires rehydration and normalization of electrolytes
3. the brain
4. Regular
5. Ultralente
6. refrigerated except current bottle in use at room temperature
7. cannot; Regular insulin is only insulin approved for IV administration at this time
8. hyperglycemia and ketosis. The "fruity smell" is that of elevated ketones in the body, particularly acetone.
9. 10–15
10. between 3 PM and supper
11. Hyperglycemic
12. Lipodystrophy
13. 100 units
14. 126 mg/dl or greater
15. glycosylated hemoglobin or hemoglobin A_{1c}
16. hyperglycemia
17. gestational diabetes
18. 5–10
19. long-acting
20. 1; 2
21. less 100 or more than 250
22. paresthesia
23. beta cells; pancreas
24. 0.5–1 hour

End-of-Chapter Math Review
1. Volume of NPH:
0.22 ml. Can use TB syringe or measure 22 U NPH in an insulin syringe.

Copyright © 2004 Mosby Inc. All rights reserved.

2. a.   Volume of NPH:
0.27 ml. Use TB syringe
or 27 units NPH in an
insulin syringe
    b.   Volume of regular
insulin:
0.07 ml. Use TB syringe
or 7 U in an insulin
syringe
    c.   Total volume to inject:
0.27 ml NPH plus 0.07
ml regular= 0.34 ml or a
total of 34 U (27 U NPH
+7 U regular)

CHAPTER 36

Practice Quiz

1. T
2. F, Replaces T_3 and T_4 hormones that are deficient.
3. T
4. F, hypoactive
5. F, high
6. F, weight gain
7. antithyroid medications
8. See textbook, pp. 516-517;
517-519; 522.
9. See textbook, p. 524.
10. See textbook, pp. 522-523.

End-of-Chapter Math Review

1. 2 tablets
2. 0.2 mg

CHAPTER 37

Practice Quiz

1. F, adrenal cortex
2. T
3. T
4. T
5. F, does mask signs and
symptoms of infection
6. T
7. T
8. F, 2/3 before 9 AM; 1/3 late
afternoon
9. T

End-of-Chapter Math Review

1. 10 kg
2. 1 mg; 1.5 mg

CHAPTER 38

Practice Quiz

1. testes
2. ovaries
3. fostering implantation
4. fertilization of ovum and
maintaining pregnancy
5. preparing breast for lactation
6. pregnant or not
7. weight
8. vital signs, especially blood
pressure
9. thromboembolic disorders
or cancer of reproductive organs
10. maturation of ovarian follicle
11. inhibit ovulation
12. masculinization
13. progestin
14. androgen
15. estrogen

End-of-Chapter Math Review

1. 1.5 ml
2. 0.2 ml

CHAPTER 39

Practice Quiz

1. Glucocorticoids
2. negative
3. elevated
4. one; two
5. ophthalmic tetracycline;
ophthalmic erythromycin
6. bradycardia (below 120);
tachycardia (over 160)
7. late in third trimester
8. stimulant
9. Ergonovine malate; methylergonovine maleate
10. oxytocin
11. increase; increase

12. Terbutaline
13. 4–8
14. magnesium sulfate toxicity
15. Calcium gluconate 10%
16. Lateral aspect of thigh

End-of-Chapter Math Review

1. Available 0.2 mg/ml
Give 1 ml
2. 62.5 ml/hr

CHAPTER 40

Practice Quiz

1. estrogen; progestin
2. 21
3. every
4. minipill
5.-9.   nausea, headache, weight
gain, spotting, depression,
fatigue, chloasma, yeast
infections, vaginal itching
or discharge, alteration in
libido
10. Estrogen blocks folliclestimulating hormone (FSH),
thereby preventing an ovarian follicle from developing.
11. 3; During fourth week of
menstrual cycle, no patch is
worn.
12. NuvaRing contains an estrogen (ethinyl estradiol) and a
progestin (norelgestromin).

End-of-Chapter Math Review

1. 1000; 70
2. 12

CHAPTER 41

Practice Quiz

1. formaldehyde
2. False
3. rust-brown to yellow
4. nonobstructive urinary retention
5. fosfomycin (Monurol)
6. 5.5
7. vitamin C

Copyright © 2004 Mosby Inc. All rights reserved.

8. urinalysis, gram stain of bacteria present, culture and sensitivity of bacteria
9. fosfomycin (Monurol)
10. glucose-6-phosphate dehydrogenase deficiency
11. bladder spasms
12. 30 minutes
13. reduce the urgency and frequency of bladder contractions and delay initial desire to void in patients with overactive bladder

End-of-Chapter Math Review
1. 0.5
2. 7.5

CHAPTER 42

Practice Quiz
1. os
2. od
3. ou
4. block inner canthus
5. 1–2
6. acetylcholine
7. miosis
8. dilation (mydriasis)
9. reduce volume of intraocular fluid
10. decrease production of aqueous humor
11. hazy vision, lacrimation, redness and burning of eyes, and sensitivity to bright lights
12. allergic reaction of the eye and other acute, noninfectious inflammatory conditions
13. inhibition of the enzyme carbonic anhydrase, which results in a decrease of aqueous humor production, thereby lowering IOP
14. respiratory conditions (e.g., bronchitis, emphysema, asthma) because beta blockers may produce severe

bronchoconstriction. Use in patients with heart failure should be limited to those persons whose disease is under control because hypotension, bradycardia, and/or heart failure may develop with use of these agents.
15. pulse rate
16. sulfonamides

End-of-Chapter Math Review
1. 70.9
106 g

CHAPTER 43

Practice Quiz
1. See instructor.
2. Post sign on door: "neutropenic precautions," initiate nursing interventions, and update care plan. See textbook p. 613.
3. nonspecific
4. specific, S phase
5. specific, during mitosis
6. eradication of malignant cells
7. See textbook, Ch. 33.
8. skin turgor (not an accurate indicator in the elderly), mucous membrane moistness, softness versus firmness of eyeballs, electrolyte reports, fluid balance (I&O)
9. See textbook, p. 613.
10. 80 gtt/min
11. 61.5
12. 307
13. 1.02 = 1
14. ifosfamide and cyclophosphamide; bladder tissue
15. platelets
16. Breast cancer HER_2-positive tumors
17. nonspecific cell cycle

End-of-Chapter Math Review
1. 100 ml/hr

2. Check directions on type of PCA pump used in the clinical setting where you are assigned and discuss method of initiating PCA pump settings and recording amount of morphine sulfate used in the narcotic records.

CHAPTER 44

Practice Quiz
1. b
2. c
3. c
4. d
5. a

End-of-Chapter Math Review
1. 1500

CHAPTER 45

Practice Quiz
1. b
2. c
3. d
4. a
5. c
6. e
7. b
8. a
9. b
10. c
11. e
12. d
13. b
14. d
15. b
16. a
17. d
18. a
19. c
20. e
21. ab
22. ac
23. T
24. F, nephrotoxicity and ototoxicity
25. T

Copyright © 2004 Mosby Inc. All rights reserved.

26. T
27. F, may be side effect of anti-microbial agents
28. T
29. T
30. F, macrolides and aminogly-cosides
31. T
32. prevent development of re-sistant organisms
33. Rifampin (Rifadin)
34. Gm+; Gm–
35. inhibiting protein synthesis of bacterial cell wall
36. tetracyclines
37. sulfonamides
38. Rifampin
39. streptogramins
40. Oxygen
41. ototoxicity; nephrotoxicity
42. sulfonylurea
43. Bactericidal
44. q 4 h around the clock

End-of-Chapter Math Review

1. 5.9
   295
   Each dose is 73.7 mg = 74 mg
   Give 0.74 ml, using a tuber-culin syringe
2. 6
3. 1.2
4. 25
5. 100

CHAPTER 46

Practice Quiz

1. weight control and activity
2. Harris-Benedict equation

3. 3–5.5
4. 4
5. D, E, A, and K
6. protein
7. oncotic pressure
8. Prealbumin
9. tube feeding
10. protein
11. thiamine
12. 8, or by institutional policy
13. total parenteral nutrition
14. TPN
15. 30–60
16. 45
17. Peripheral parenteral nutri-tion
18. central intravenous line or port
19. neuropathy
20. Vitamin C

End-of-Chapter Math Review

1. Increase hourly rate by 11.4 ml/hr to a total of 91.4 or 91 ml/hr
2. 2400 ml

CHAPTER 47

Practice Quiz

1. T
2. T
3. F, anti-inflammatory and an-tibacterial properties
4. T
5. T
6. F, has neither of these prop-erties

7. F, interacts with beta-ad-renergic blockers and mon-amine oxidase inhibitors
8. F, used for migraine head-aches and as an anti-inflam-matory for rheumatoid ar-thritis
9. T
10. T
11. T
12. T
13. T
14. T

CHAPTER 48

Practice Quiz

1. cannabinoids
2. hallucinogens
3. stimulants
4. depressants
5. 8–24
6. hyperpyrexia, seizures, respi-ratory depression, coma, and death
7. Naltrexone (ReVia)

End-of-Chapter Math Review

1. 1
2. 0.5
3. 2

Copyright © 2004 Mosby Inc. All rights reserved.

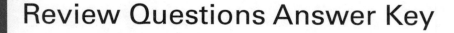

Chapter 1
1. a; 2. a

Chapter 2
1. d; 2. b; 3. c

Chapter 3
1. d; 2. b; 3. c

Chapter 4
1. b; 2. c

Chapter 5
1. b; 2. d

Chapter 6
Perform Questions throughout chapter.

Chapter 7
1. c; 2. d; 3. a

Chapter 8
1. c; 2. d; 3. c

Chapter 9
1. c; 2. c or d, depending on clinical site; 3. c

Chapter 10
1. b; 2. c

Chapter 11
1. b; 2. a; 3. a

Chapter 12
1. a; 2. a; 3. b; 4. d; 5. d

Chapter 13
1. d; 2. c

Chapter 14
1. a; 2. b; 3. b

Chapter 15
1. c; 2. c

Chapter 16
1. a; 2. d

Chapter 17
1. c; 2. c; 3. a

Chapter 18
1. d; 2. d

Chapter 19
1. a; 2. c

Chapter 20
1. d; 2. b; 3. a; 4. a; 5. b

Chapter 21
1. c; 2. a; 3. b; 4. d; 5. b

Chapter 22
1. c; 2. c; 3. b; 4. d; 5. c; 6. a; 7. b

Chapter 23
1. c; 2. c; 3. a; 4. b

Chapter 24
1. b; 2. b; 3. c; 4. d

Chapter 25
1. b; 2. a; 3. c; 4. c; 5. a

Chapter 26
1. a; 2. a; 3. b

Chapter 27
1. a; 2. c; 3. b; 4. c

Chapter 28
1. b; 2. a; 3. c; 4. d

Chapter 29
1. c; 2. a; 3. c

Chapter 30
1. c; 2. b; 3. b; 4. b; 5. c

Chapter 31
1. c; 2. c

Chapter 32
1. a; 2. c; 3. d; 4. a

Chapter 33
1. d; 2. d; 3. a; 4. c

Chapter 34
1. b; 2. c; 3. c; 4. d

Chapter 35
1. a; 2. c; 3. d; 4. d; 5. c

Chapter 36
1. c; 2. c; 3. b

Chapter 37
1. a; 2. d; 3. a

Chapter 38
1. d; 2. b; 3. c; 4. a

Chapter 39
1. c; 2. c; 3. b; 4. d

Chapter 40
1. c; 2. d; 3. c; 4. b

Chapter 41
1. b; 2. a; 3. b; 4. d

Chapter 42
1. a; 2. b; 3. c; 4. c

Chapter 43
1. c; 2. b; 3. d; 4. a

Chapter 44
1. b; 2. c

Chapter 45
1. b; 2. d; 3. a; 4. a; 5. c; 6. c

Chapter 46
1. c; 2. c; 3. d; 4. c; 5. d

Chapter 47
1. c; 2. a; 3. d; 4. b

Chapter 48
1. family systems; 2. psychoanalytical; 3. textbook p. 723

Copyright © 2004 Mosby Inc. All rights reserved.